The Artinian Intersystem Model

Barbara M. Artinian, PhD, RN, is professor emeritus in the School of Nursing, Azusa Pacific University. She has taught courses in community health nursing, family theory, nursing theory, and qualitative research methodology. She developed the Artinian Intersystem Model based on the work of Alfred Kuhn and Aaron Antonovsky. She published several articles about the model in the 1990s that culminated in the publication of the book entitled *The Intersystem Model: Integrating Theory and Practice* by Sage Publications (1997). The model has been used in a variety of practice settings and was used by David Taylor as a framework for his doctoral dissertation work done at the University of Wollongong, Wollongong, Australia. This book presents work done by students who were introduced to the model during their studies or from reading the publications about the model.

Dr. Artinian has served as advisor for grounded theory research for five doctoral and 24 master level students. The work of these students was reported in the book *Glaserian Grounded in Nursing Research: Trusting Emergence* by Springer Publishing Company (2009). This book has received excellent reviews.

Dr. Artinian grew up in Wisconsin and graduated from Wheaton College in Wheaton, Illinois. She attended Case Western Reserve University where she received a degree in nursing. She completed her graduate work at the University of California, Los Angeles, earning an MSN degree. At the University of Southern California, she earned a PhD in sociology with a major emphasis in family theory. She completed a postdoctoral research fellowship at the University of California, San Francisco, in the area of chronic illness and was introduced to the methodology of grounded theory at that time. Her knowledge of grounded theory research has enhanced her understanding of the process of the Artinian Intersystem Model.

Katharine S. West, MPH, MSN, RN, CNS, PHN, is a Nurse Clinical Systems Project Manager at Kaiser Permanente-Southern California Permanente Medical Group and a Professor for the Southern California campus of the University of Phoenix undergraduate and graduate nursing programs. She is on the forefront of innovative nursing practice through her position at Kaiser Permanente to develop solutions for clinical documentation in the electronic medical record.

A Phi Beta Kappa graduate of USC, West has master's degrees from UCLA (MPH) and Azusa Pacific University (MSN). Her expertise in nursing as a Maternal-Child Health Clinical Nurse Specialist and certified Public Health Nurse is based on broad clinical experiences ranging from in-patient care to insurance-based case management, maternal-child home health care, nursing and public health informatics, including implementation of a statewide public health program for newborn hearing screening in California.

West is a contributing author to books on qualitative research and rural nursing and has created online content for textbooks on maternal-newborn nursing and served as a reviewer for the leading nursing informatics text. Since 1992, she has taught nursing at all levels from vocational to graduate with an emphasis on Public Health nursing. Her extensive experience coupled with her scholarship and abilities to communicate make her an outstanding educator of computer technologies applied to health care. Her podium and paper presentations on using computer technologies in nursing are enthusiastically received at local, regional, national, and international conferences.

West has been recognized with several awards, including a Sigma Theta Tau research grant, Dale Carnegie Leadership awards, and service awards from employers. West's varied and dynamic experience is distinctive among nurses, as she discerns health care trends, translates them into pragmatic learning opportunities, and articulates the implications for clinical care.

Margaret M. Conger, EdD, MSN, RN, is professor emeritus in the School of Nursing, Northern Arizona University. Her fields of concentration include educational theory, nursing case management, and leadership/management. She holds a BSN and MSN from Azusa Pacific University. She also has an MS in Biology from California State University, Long Beach, an MS in Leadership from Webster University, and an Ed.D. in Adult Education from Nova University.

She is the coauthor of the book *The Intersystem Model* (1997) and author of *Managed Care: Practice Strategies for Nursing* (1999). She has published numerous journal articles in the areas of nursing education, case management, and international nursing. She has been a presenter at many conferences in the United States and keynote speaker at conferences in the Netherlands, Sweden, Lithuania, and the Czech Republic.

As an educator, Dr. Conger was instrumental in developing a rural clinical specialist program at Northern Arizona University. She has also taught extensively in the area of nursing case management and nursing leadership. She served as Associate Director of the School of Nursing at Northern Arizona University. She developed and coordinated an intercultural institute to bring nurses from the United States and Europe and Africa together to explore nursing care delivery to underserved populations. Her current interests lie in the area of working with nursing programs in Eastern Europe and Africa to assist them in developing professional nursing education.

The Artinian Intersystem Model

Integrating Theory and Practice for the Professional Nurse

Second Edition

Editors
Barbara M. Artinian, PhD, RN
Katharine S. West, MPH, MSN, RN, CNS, PHN
Margaret M. Conger, EdD, MSN, RN

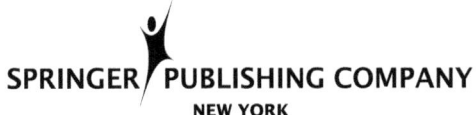

SPRINGER PUBLISHING COMPANY
NEW YORK

Copyright © 2011 Springer Publishing Company, LLC

All rights reserved.

No part of this publication may be reproduced, stored in a retrieval system, or transmitted in any form or by any means, electronic, mechanical, photocopying, recording, or otherwise, without the prior permission of Springer Publishing Company, LLC, or authorization through payment of the appropriate fees to the Copyright Clearance Center, Inc., 222 Rosewood Drive, Danvers, MA 01923, 978-750-8400, fax 978-646-8600, info@copyright.com or on the web at www.copyright.com.

Springer Publishing Company, LLC
11 West 42nd Street
New York, NY 10036
www.springerpub.com

Acquisitions Editor: Allan Graubard
Production Editor: Dana Bigelow
Cover Design: David Levy
Compositor: Newgen Data Services

ISBN: 978-0-8261-0752-7
E-book ISBN: 978-0-8261-0753-4

The author and the publisher of this Work have made every effort to use sources believed to be reliable to provide information that is accurate and compatible with the standards generally accepted at the time of publication. The author and publisher shall not be liable for any special, consequential, or exemplary damages resulting, in whole or in part, from the readers' use of, or reliance on, the information contained in this book. The publisher has no responsibility for the persistence or accuracy of URLs for external or third-party Internet Web sites referred to in this publication and does not guarantee that any content on such Web sites is, or will remain, accurate or appropriate.

Library of Congress Cataloging-in-Publication Data
The Artinian intersystem model : integrating theory and practice for the professional nurse. — 2nd ed. / editors, Barbara M. Artinian, Katharine S. West, Margaret M. Conger.
  p. ; cm.
  Rev. ed of: Intersystem model.
  Includes bibliographical references and index.
  ISBN 978-0-8261-0752-7 — ISBN 978-0-8261-0753-4 (E-book)
  1. Nurse and patient. 2. Nursing—Psychological aspects. 3. Nursing models. I. Artinian, Barbara M. II. West, Katharine S. III. Conger, Marge. IV. Intersystem model.
  [DNLM: 1. Nurse-Patient Relations. 2. Models, Nursing. 3. Nurses—psychology. WY 88]
  RT86.3.I585 2011
  610.73—dc22   2011000400

Special discounts on bulk quantities of our books are available to corporations, professional associations, pharmaceutical companies, health care organizations, and other qualifying groups.

If you are interested in a custom book, including chapters from more than one of our titles, we can provide that service as well.

For details, please contact:
Special Sales Department, Springer Publishing Company, LLC
11 West 42nd Street, 15th Floor, New York, NY 10036-8002
Phone: 877-687-7476 or 212-431-4370; Fax: 212-941-7842
Email: sales@springerpub.com

Printed in the United States of America by Gasch Printing.

We dedicate this book to

*Avo Artinian, Barbara's husband,
who has participated in discourse
about the model since its inception,*

Our mothers, who modeled scholarship and creativity, and

*All of our students who have used the model
to develop mutual plans of care with their patients and clients.*

Contents

Contributors		*xi*
Foreword Evelyn M. Wills, PhD, RN		*xv*
Preface		*xvii*
Acknowledgments		*xxi*

I.	**Theoretical Background of the Artinian Intersystem Model** Barbara M. Artinian	*1*
1.	Development of the Artinian Intersystem Model Barbara M. Artinian	3
2.	Situational Sense of Coherence: The Salutogenic Model Barbara M. Artinian	31
3.	Developing a Sense of Coherence: The Developmental Environment Katharine S. West and Barbara M. Artinian	49
4.	The Context of Involvement: The Situational Environment Barbara M. Artinian	59
II.	**Increasing Sense of Coherence in Aggregates** Barbara M. Artinian	67
5.	Family as Client: An Interactive Interpersonal System Barbara M. Artinian	69
6.	Institution As Client: Institutional Interaction Margaret M. Conger and Lourdes Casao Salandanan	81
7.	Community, State, or Nation as Client: Public Health Nursing Katharine S. West	103

III.	**The Artinian Intersystem Model in Educational Settings** *Barbara M. Artinian*	*133*
8.	Learning Theories to Enhance Clinical Practice *Margaret M. Conger and Rosalinda Haddon*	*135*
9.	The Artinian Intersystem Model in Nursing School Education *Pamela H. Cone, Barbara M. Artinian, and Katharine S. West*	*147*
10.	An Emerging Nursing Program In A Developing Country *Darlene E. McCown and Barbara M. Artinian*	*173*
11.	Fostering Mutuality in Clinical Practice *Margaret M. Conger*	*181*
IV.	**The Artinian Intersystem Model in Practice** *Barbara M. Artinian*	*199*
12.	Advanced Practice Nursing in an Ambulatory Setting *Christine Erdmann-Nell*	*201*
13.	Delegation Decision Making *Margaret M. Conger*	*207*
14.	Care Management of Heart Failure Patients in the Outpatient Setting *Laurie Carson and Louise Della Bella*	*219*
15.	Excellence in Practice: A Resident-Centered Care Program in a Long-Term Facility *Margo Y. Babikian, Barbara M. Artinian, and Victoria Winter*	*237*
16.	Integrating Theory and Practice Using the Artinian Intersystem Model *Barbara M. Artinian*	*257*
	Appendix A: AIM Block Care Plan Template for Undergraduate Students	*275*
	Appendix B: AIM Community Health Care Plan Template	*281*
	Appendix C: AIM Standard Care Plan Template	*287*
	Appendix D: AIM Narrative Care Plan Template for Graduate Students	*291*
	Index	*293*

Contributors

*Barbara M. Artinian, PhD, RN
Professor Emeritus
Azusa Pacific University
Azusa, California

Margo Y. Babikian, MS, RN
Executive Director
Ararat Nursing Facility
Mission Hills, California

*Mary Barkman, MSN, RN
Retired, Pulmonary Case Manager
Glendale Adventist Medical Center
Glendale, California

Margaret Bond, MSN, RN
Coordinator, Medical Information Services
Northern Arizona HealthCare
Flagstaff, Arizona

*Beverley Brownell, PhD, RN
Instructor
Department of Nursing
Golden West College
Huntington Beach, California

Laurie Kay Carson, MSN, FNP-BC
Heart Failure Outreach Care Coordinator
Department of Disease Management
Saddleback Memorial Medical Center
Laguna Hills, California

*Pamela H. Cone, PhD, RN, PHN, CNS
Associate Professor
School of Nursing
Azusa Pacific University
Azusa, California

*Margaret M. Conger, EdD, MSN, RN
Professor Emeritus
School of Nursing
Northern Arizona University
Flagstaff, Arizona

Louise Della Bella, RN, MN, ONE-C
Executive Director, Clinical Resource and
 Social Services
Saddleback Memorial Medical Center
Laguna Hills, California

*Christine Erdmann-Nell, MSN,
 RN, FNP
Dermatology Nurse Practitioner
Ava MD Dermatology
 and Aesthetics
Beverly Hills, California

Abigail Evangelista, BSN, RN
Night Relief—Assistant Department
 Administrator
Emergency Services
Kaiser Foundation Hospital
West Los Angeles, California

* Contributor to online adjunct manual.

*Maureen Friesen, MSN, RNC, CNS
Patient Flow Coordinator in
  Labor & Delivery
Huntington Memorial Medical Center
Pasadena, California
Adjunct Faculty
School of Nursing
Azusa Pacific University
Azusa, California

*Tove Giske, PhD, RN
Associate Professor
Haraldsplass Deaconess University College
  and Haraldsplass Deaconess Hospital
Bergen, Norway

Rosalinda Haddon, MA, RN
Associate Clinical Professor
Northern Arizona University
Flagstaff, Arizona

Antonius Hardianto, BSN, RN
Hospice Case Manager
Vitas Hospice Care
Covina, California

*Esther Hjälmhult, PhD, MAEd,
  RN, RPHN
Associate Professor
Faculty of Health and Social Sciences
Center of Evidence Based Practice
Department of Postgraduate Studies
Bergen University College
Bergen, Norway

Mary Hull, MSN, FNP-C
Certified Family Nurse Practitioner
Minute Clinic
Los Angeles, California

Elena Kirschner, BSN, RN
Staff Nurse
Northern Arizona HealthCare
Flagstaff, Arizona

Vince Martinez, BSN, RN
Paramedic Services
Guardian Medical Transport Service
Flagstaff, Arizona

Darlene E. McCown, PhD, RN,
  PNP, FNP
Director, School of Nursing
Hope Africa University
Bujumbura, Burundi

Katrina Perez, BSN, RN
Staff RN Mother-Baby Unit
Hoag Hospital
Newport Beach, California

*Darya Ratliff, BSN, RN
Staff RN—Telemetry Unit
Santa Monica-UCLA
  Medical Center
Santa Monica, California

Lourdes C. Salandanan, MSN,
  RN-BC, FNP
Corporate Director of Education
Citrus Valley Health Partners
Covina, California

Michelle Song-Howe, BSN, RN
Staff RN ICU
San Gabriel Valley Medical Center
San Gabriel, California

Amy M. Stilley, BSN, RN
Wound Care Specialist
Northern Arizona HealthCare
Flagstaff, Arizona

Sarah J. Templeton, MSN,
  RN, FNP-C
Nurse Practitioner
Student Health Center
Biola University
La Mirada, California

* Contributor to online adjunct manual.

*Katharine S. West, MPH, MSN, RN, CNS, PHN
Nurse Clinical Systems Analyst
 Project Manager
Kaiser Permanente–Southern
 California Permanente
 Medical Group
Pasadena, California
Faculty
Department of Nursing
University of Phoenix
Southern California Campus
Costa Mesa, California

Evelyn M. Wills, PhD, RN
Professor Emeritus
Department of Nursing
College of Nursing & Allied Health
 Professions
University of Louisiana at Lafayette
Lafayette, Louisiana

*Victoria Winter, MSN, RN, CNS, CCRN
Clinical Nurse IV
Childrens Hospital Los Angeles
Los Angeles, California
Adjunct Faculty
School of Nursing
Azusa Pacific University
Azusa, California

Foreword

Work on the Artinian Intersystem Model (AIM) began in the 1980s by Dr. Barbara Artinian. The model was refined over the next years with a focus on the interaction between the nurse and the client who could be a patient, a family, an institution, or a community. After a series of journal publications, the model was published as a much-awaited book in 1997. The model explains, as does no other, the process that takes place between the nurse and client in resolving a concern of either nurse or client.

Adopting the concept of sense of coherence (SOC) from Antonovsky's work, she refined and adapted the concept into the real world-nursing construct that she called situational sense of coherence (SSOC). SSOC corresponds more closely to the reality of professional nursing practice. Antonovsky saw SOC as a stable trait, resistant to change in adults whereas Artinian views its logical offspring, SSOC, as a process through which a patient or client in a state of disorganization can be helped to recover or increase the level of SOC during recovery.

Artinian's work is modern, logical, and it flows from a lifelong practice of observing how with appropriate nursing interventions, clients during health and illness can move from disorganization to reorganization leading to improved health. This is a model that is imminently useful to nurses in any area of nursing practice. It can be used as much by the bedside nurse as the community health nurse, the critical care nurse, the school nurse, the nurse providing elder care, or the nurse working with large institutions.

The research process inherent in this model is as important to the academic nurse as the nursing process she has provided is for the practice of nursing. In the grounded theory research process, the research is directed to understanding how a group of clients resolve their main concern. In the AIM, the effort is directed to assisting the client to resolve the individual main concern through use of the steps of the model. It provides a basis for the professional nurse to evaluate a client's state of health and plan cooperatively with the client for nursing interventions. The results of these interventions can be analyzed by measuring change in the client's SSOC.

This model is the result of Dr. Artinian's life work grounded in practical experience with clients and application of literature and research findings. It reflects her careful thought about what it means to be a nurse, an individual patient, or an aggregate in a state of needing nursing attention.

I am most pleased to be able to recommend this work to all nurses who want to have an organized, well researched, and thoroughly thought out structure for their nursing in any theater of nursing.

Evelyn M. Wills, PhD, RN
Professor Emeritus
College of Nursing & Allied Health Professions
University of Louisiana at Lafayette

Preface

This book came about because a graduate student asked "How do you develop a model?" This book answers that question and also the next logical question, "How do you use a model in daily professional nursing?" The Artinian Intersystem Model (AIM) is unique among nursing models because in addition to being used in daily professional nursing, it helps the nurse address both qualitative and quantitative aspects of patient care. It requires the nurse to ask the patient, "What is your Main Concern?" and then negotiate what the patient can do and is willing to do in the formation of a mutual plan of care. The model also provides for quantification of nursing care by establishing a baseline score on the patient's SSOC followed by a summation score that simply and easily identifies change that occurred in response to nursing care.

To answer the second question, this book gives recommendations for developing programs to promote health and provides examples of such programs. One of these is a program that encourages heart failure patients to participate in decision making to promote self care practices. Another is a resident-centered program in a nursing home that is designed to preserve the identity of the resident. Whereas most nursing theorists state that their models can be used at the individual level as well as the family level, the AIM provides examples of how the model is actually being used at individual, family, institutional, and community or national levels. The book also provides examples of how research can be used to inform nursing practice. Six of the studies presented in the companion book, *Glaserian Grounded Theory in Nursing Research: Trusting Emergence* (Artinian, Giske, & Cone, 2009), are given to show how nursing practice can be enhanced with the use of a grounded theory.

In essence, the AIM is a model of the nursing process that guides the nurse or provider to make it possible for the patient to participate in the planning of care on a more equal basis (shared decision making). This is done by reducing the inequality of power distribution by assessing the patient's own knowledge, by being attentive to values, and by assessing behaviors about the main concern before engaging in interaction to resolve the concern. The AIM is also based on the concept that each person or client is an intrasystem in his or her own right, made up of a biological self, a psychosocial self, and a spiritual self. Foundational to the model is the mutuality of the interaction between the patient/client and nurse/provider intrasystems that fosters mutual problem solving. Gone are the days of patronistic interactions where the "Doctor or Nurse knows best" and soliciting information from the patient was deemed inconsequential. The AIM fits well with today's healthcare paradigm where patients desire a central role in decisionmaking and in all aspects of their care.

An earlier iteration of the model had been presented in the 1990s in a series of journal articles and then presented in depth in the book *The Intersystem Model: Integrating Theory and Practice* (Artinian & Conger, 1997). Because few institutions used the model for planning care at that time, the focus of that book was on presenting theories associated with each aspect of the model accompanied by a care plan related to that aspect. This second edition contains many refinements of the model based on actual use in professional nursing. The most important of these is the refinement of Artinian's Situational Sense of Coherence Theory of Recovery that is incorporated into the model. This theory is based on the definition of SSOC as the meaning that patients bring to the events of their lives during times of stress or disorganization. Antonovsky described SOC as a relatively stable aspect of a person that changes only slightly after early adulthood. Many social scientists want to use the concept of SOC in their practice, where the goal is behavioral change, but are unable to because Antonovsky did not indicate how change can be brought about. The SSOC Theory of Recovery answers this dilemma and, by using the process of the AIM, a method has been developed that enables a health care professional to guide the client to actually improve the level of SSOC using the situation itself as the catalyst for change. This increased SSOC is reflected in the new level of SOC the person achieves following the period of disorganization.

The main benefits of using the AIM are summarized in the following. The Model:

- Makes it possible for the patient to participate in the planning of care on a more equal basis (shared decision making)
- Demonstrates a systematic way to assess the patient and provide care
- Places the spiritual subsystem at the core of the person
- Respects the dignity of patients by collaborating with them in the decision-making process

- Explores what the patient knows about the Main Concern, what the patient wants to do about it, and the resources the patient has to resolve the Main Concern
- Allows negotiation of values to develop a mutual plan of care
- Scores patient on SSOC using a simple descriptive scoring measurement of high, medium, or low on each aspect of SSOC
- Evaluates the effectiveness of the intervention by re-scoring on SSOC

This book is divided into four sections. Part I provides the theoretical background of the model and, with the core concept throughout of promoting the equalization of power, introduces the main concepts of the model: the developmental environment, the situational environment, the SSOC, and resolution of the main concern. Part II illustrates the way the model is used with aggregate populations to increase their SOC. Part III describes the use of the model in educational settings, and Part IV gives examples of actual use of the model in practice settings. The relationship between theory and practice is illustrated in care plans informed by qualitative research. An online adjunct manual contains many of the forms used in the practice settings and all of the care plans referred to in many of the chapters. It is available at www.springerpub.com/artinian.

Barbara M. Artinian, PhD, RN
Katharine S. West, MPH, MSN, RN, CNS, PHN
Margaret M. Conger, EdD, MSN, RN

Acknowledgments

We are most grateful to Allan Graubard, Executive Editor of Springer Publishing, for his vision and understanding the importance of this model for nursing practice and to Dana Bigelow for her excellent editorial assistance. We acknowledge the contribution of Ruth V. Matheney in the futuristic book of 1960, *Patient-Centered Approaches to Nursing* (New York: Macmillan Company), for introducing Dr. Artinian to the concept of patient-centered care. We thank all the authors who contributed to this book. Your innovative uses of the model have shown the creativity and varied applications of the model. We appreciate your scholarly work. We also thank your institutions and agencies where you use the model to direct practice. We thank Paulette Hardy for her availability and skills to assist with the manuscript preparation at many stages. Our gratitude for expert graphic design consultation for the current AIM diagram goes to Jane Schneider. We also thank Dr. Pamela Cone for her assistance in editing the final manuscript. We are grateful for the ongoing support of our families and friends who assisted us in bringing this book to completion. Finally, our prayer is that this book will glorify God.

PART

I

THEORETICAL BACKGROUND OF THE ARTINIAN INTERSYSTEM MODEL

Barbara M. Artinian

PART I PROVIDES the theoretical foundations of the Artinian Intersystem Model (AIM). Chapter 1 describes how the Model was developed to provide a framework for assessing the interaction between nurse and client in developing a joint plan of care. It presents the stages in the developmental process of integrating the theories of Robert Chin: *The Utility of System Models and Developmental Models for Practitioners* (1967), Alfred Kuhn: *The Logic of Social Systems* (1974), Aaron Antonovsky: *Unraveling the Mystery of Health* (1987), Herbert Blumer: *Symbolic Interactionism* (1969), Stallwood and Stoll: *Spiritual Dimensions of Nursing Practice* (1975), and Knickrehm: *The origins of inequality: A theoretical synthesis* (1994). The integration of these theories resulted in the AIM. All of these theories are described and the adaptation of each for describing the nursing metaparadigm concepts is discussed.

The AIM describes the interaction of nurse and client when the client has a main concern that cannot be resolved without nursing intervention. This is in contrast to the majority of nursing models in which the nurse initially determines the main concern of the client based on medical and nursing diagnoses, and then seeks to gather client data to support those assumptions. This is also in contrast to the work of a Glaserian grounded theorist who seeks to find out how the subjects by themselves resolve their main concern. Two care plans are presented one of which describes the process of resolving the main concern of the patient and the other shows how the main concern of the nurse was resolved in interaction with the patient by using the steps of the model. In each of these cases, the health providers were not familiar with the framework of the model, but they used the principles of the model in their interaction with patients.

Chapter 2 describes the use of the *situational sense of coherence* (SSOC) construct in clinical practice. The development of the SSOC theory of recovery is given to show how the theory is useful in understanding the process of recovering from a major stress. Recommendations for developing treatment programs based on salutogenic principles derived from the dissertation work of Taylor (1997) are presented.

The client is described in Chapter 3 as an individual composed of *biological, psychosocial,* and *spiritual subsystems.* The way in which these subsystems interact in a cultural environment to develop the *sense of coherence* of the person is described. An introduction to a care plan illustrating the interaction of the *biological, psychosocial,* and *spiritual subsystems* is provided.

In Chapter 4, the characteristics of client, change agent, setting, and the interpersonal behaviors of the client and change agent are described as they influence the development of a mutual definition of the situation within the context of inequality of power (Knickrehm, 1994). A discussion follows illustrating how these characteristics interact to form the interactional context in which a patient concern can be resolved.

REFERENCES

Antonovsky, A. (1987). *Unraveling the mysteries of health: How people manage stress and stay well.* San Francisco, CA: Jossey-Bass.

Blumer, H. (1969). *Symbolic interactionism.* Englewood Cliffs, NJ: Prentice Hall, Inc.

Chin, R. (1969). The utility of system models and developmental models for practitioners. In W. Bennis, K. Benne, & R. Chin, *The planning of change* (pp. 247–266). New York, NY: Holt, Rinehart and Winston, Inc.

Knickrehm, B. (1994, August). *The origins of inequality: A theoretical synthesis.* Paper presented at the 1994 American Sociological Association Meeting, Los Angeles, CA.

Kuhn, A. (1974). *The logic of social systems: A unified deductive, system-based approach to social science.* San Francisco, CA: Jossey-Bass.

Stallwood, J., & Stoll, R. (1975). Spiritual dimensions of nursing practice, Part C. In I. Beland & J. Passos (Eds.), *Clinical nursing* (3rd ed., pp. 1086–1098). New York, NY: Macmillan Publishing Company.

Taylor, D. (1997). *The implications of sense of coherence for the early treatment of people who have had a traumatic spinal cord injury.* Doctoral dissertation, University of Wollongong: Wollongong, Australia.

1

DEVELOPMENT OF THE ARTINIAN INTERSYSTEM MODEL

Barbara M. Artinian

THE ARTINIAN INTERSYSTEM Model describes the interactional process that takes place between the nurse/provider and patient/client when nursing assistance is needed. The assistance can be in the form of health promotion or resolution of a health concern. In the model, the client can be an individual, a family, an institution, a community, a state, or a nation each with its own network of significant others. Likewise, the nurse can be an individual or a health provider system in an institutional context each with its own network. In the interactional process, the two systems come together to form an intersystem characterized by the specific set of relations that connect them to each other. Intersystem interaction is mutually influencing and focuses on how information is communicated, how values are negotiated, and how behaviors are organized to implement a mutual plan of care that will increase the client's situational sense of coherence (SSOC).

DEVELOPMENT OF THE MODEL: EARLY PHASES

The first patient-centered model I used was the Clinical Analysis Record developed by Matheney (1960). I began teaching in a diploma school of nursing at the midpoint of a semester. At the end of the semester, much to my dismay, the care plans turned in by the students were very specific about the type of surgery a patient had had even to describing the size of the suture, but nothing was said about the patient's response to the surgery. During the Christmas recess, I found the book *Patient-centered Approaches to Nursing* by Abdellah, Beland, Martin, and Matheney (1960). In Matheney's chapter "Application of a Patient-centered Curriculum in an Associate Degree Program," I found a model for analyzing patient care. I modified the Clinical Analysis Record (Matheney, p. 82) to allow students to state a nursing problem in their own terms rather than using the "21 Problems" as described earlier in Matheney's chapter. The modified Clinical Analysis Record simply asked students to identify the following four areas: nursing care problem of the patient, scientific basis for problem, nursing care given, and scientific basis for care.

This helped students focus on the patient response to a problem and the reason for the problem as well as describe what the nurse did to alleviate the problem and why she had chosen that approach. I used the definition that Matheney used to describe the problem-solving process related to health, "A nursing problem is defined as a condition and/or situation faced by a patient, or his family, which the nurse can assist him to meet through the performance of her professional function" (1960, p. 80). By using this approach to analyze patient care, the curriculum at the diploma school was transformed and the students became adept at focusing on the problems presented by the patient.

While I was a graduate student at the University of California, Los Angeles (UCLA), I was introduced to the concepts developed by Peplau (1952) and Orlando (1961). Although these concepts provided a rationale for practice, they did not provide a structure for practice. It was when I found the work of Robert Chin (1969) that I realized that the essence of interpersonal relationships is an intersystem model. Chin writes that an intersystem model has the following characteristics (pp. 304–305):

- An intersystem model involves two open systems connected to each other. A visualization of this type of an intersystem model would be two systems side by side, with separately identified links (see Figure 1.1).
- Connectives represent the lines of relationships of the two systems. Connectives tie together parts.
- The intersystem model exaggerates the virtues of autonomy and the limited nature of interdependence of the interactions between the two connected systems.
- The external change-agent…does not completely become a part of the client-system. He must remain separate to some extent; he must create and maintain some distance between himself and the client, thus standing apart "in another system" from which he re-relates.
- Intersystem analysis of the change-agent's role leads to fruitful analysis of the connectives—their nature in the beginning, how they shift, and how they are cutoff.
- Intersystem analysis also poses squarely an unexplored issue, namely the internal system of the change-agent, whether a single person, consultant group, or a nation. Helpers of change are prone at times not to see that their own systems as change-agents have boundaries, tensions, stresses and strains, equilibria, and feedback mechanisms which may be just as much parts of the problem as are similar aspects of the client-systems.

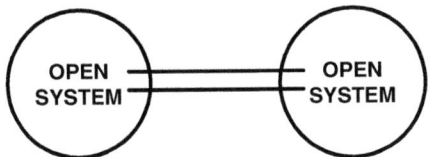

FIGURE 1.1 Representation of Chin's Intersystem Model (1969).
Source: Artinian (2011).

TABLE 1.1   A Therapist-Family Intersystem Model

1. Goal of action	Changing the processes of coping for each individual, thus altering the system to produce new ways of communication and increased productivity so that each system can identify and use its own resources.
2. Patiency [sic]	A family system that is dysfunctional because family rules for interacting do not fit needs for survival, growth, getting close to others, and productivity on the part of each member of the system.
3. Actor	*Place*: Outside target system bound to system by connectives such as social contract of mutual role expectation *Role*: Actively assists family system to accomplish change necessitated by inadequate interactional patterns
4. Source of difficulty	Family relationships that hamper growth and development
5. Intervention	*Focus*: Dysfunctional communication patterns which produce directly observable behavior *Mode*: A collaborative process to change communication patterns
6. Consequences	Reorganization in family members' ways of extending and maintaining self-esteem, use of feedback, and the use of words making it possible for members to give, receive, and check out communication meanings
7. Unintended consequences	If interaction has not been collaborative and therapist has not accurately assessed system needs, action may: ▪ not benefit subsystems or family system ▪ cause condition of system to become less organized ▪ be wasteful of material or of personnel time and effort

Source: Unpublished work from Artinian (1971).

An understanding of these characteristics has been the foundation for my work with intersystem models. Using these concepts from Chin (1969), I developed a Therapist-Family Intersystem Model (Artinian, 1971). Many of the units of this model have been carried over into the present Artinian Intersystem Model (see Table 1.1).

DEVELOPMENT OF THE INTERSYSTEM MODEL

When I was introduced to the book *The Logic of Social Systems* (Kuhn, 1974), I immediately recognized the value of this model in fostering interpersonal interaction and its use in nursing practice. The Kuhn model had many of the same principles developed by Chin, but it provided a more specific framework

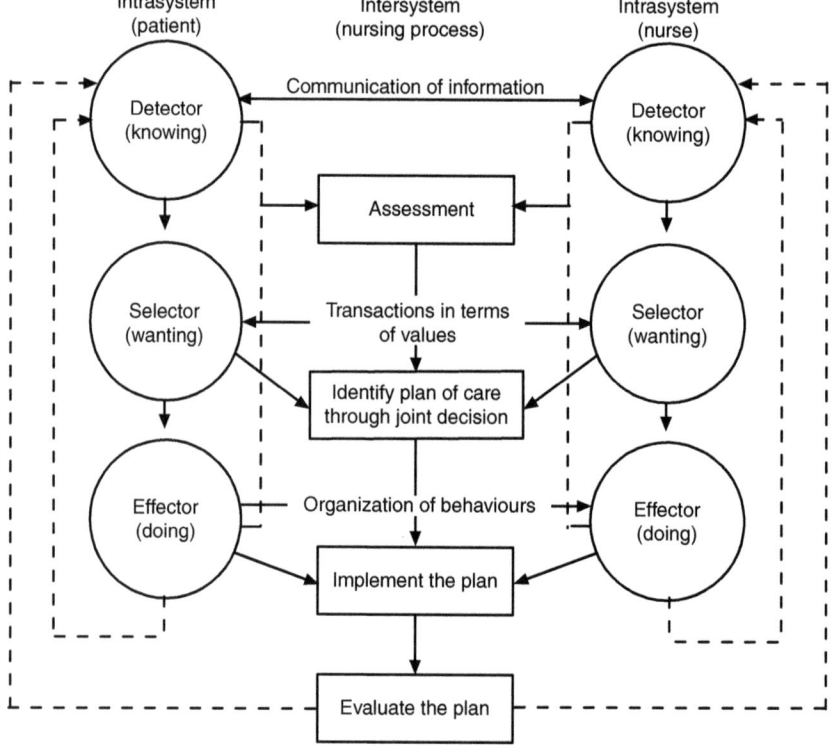

FIGURE 1.2 Early Intersystem Model diagram.
Source: Artinian (1975).

for using them. The Kuhn model is explicitly system-based and "system concepts form an integral part of the analytic structure in his model" (1974, p. xiii). Although Kuhn was an economist, he envisioned his model to be the central core of social science. When I began teaching pediatric nursing at UCLA, I introduced elements of the nursing process into the structure of the Kuhn model and used it in my teaching (see Figure 1.2). The use of this model assisted the students in including the patients in the planning of care. I discussed my adaptation of this intersystem model with Kuhn at a sociological conference in 1975, and he was pleased with the way I had adapted it for the nursing profession.

The first use of the model outside of the educational setting was in 1982 in a large public hospital when a nursing care plan study was carried out (Artinian, 1982). The same diagram of the model that I had used at UCLA was given to participants in the study and they used it in analyzing care plans. At that time, the nurses listed information they had about all of the patient problems and the plan for meeting each problem was placed next to each item. They did the same analysis for the values and the behaviors related to the identified problems (see Table 1.2). By identifying more than one problem, this approach was similar to the Clinical Analysis Record developed by Matheney (1960).

TABLE 1.2 Sample of Nursing Process Study Care Plan (1982)

Knowledge about patient	**Plan**
Patient is not eating because of nausea and vomiting	NG tube
Patient becomes nauseated during radiation therapy	Give medication before going
Patient has experienced side effects in previous chemotherapy	Watch for side effects
Patient has poor veins	Give hot packs before inserting needles
Family does not accept terminal diagnosis	Talk with family
Values or preferences of patient	**Plan**
Patient has poor appetite but likes milk	Offer milk with meal
Patient wants to know schedule of procedures	Keep patient informed
Patient dislikes _____ type of dressing	Use type of dressing
Behavior of patient	**Plan**
Patient is experiencing pain	Establish optimum drug schedule
Patient is confused	Give instructions clearly: observe
Patient is fatalistic about dying process	Understand and encourage patient
Patient is worried about dying	Initiate talk when he desires; provide respite

Source: Artinian (1982).

The next step in clarifying the model was to limit the focus of interaction to one specific problem and introduce a concept of person. The same diagram that had been used at UCLA and for the nursing care study was published in separate articles in 1983 and in 1984 (see Figure 1.2). These discussions of the model described the model in detail showing how the identified problem was the main focus of concern and how collaborative planning was carried out to meet that concern. These articles presented a clearer picture of the collaborative nature of intersystem interaction and how the nurse focused on only one problem until it was resolved. At that time, I depicted person as a person with social, psychosocial, and biological subsystems.

When I began teaching at Azusa Pacific University (APU), the faculty was using a model they called "The Nursing Process Systems Model based on the Developmental-Stress Model" developed by Chrisman at UCLA (1974). The model incorporated the concept of person as having three subsystems: spiritual, psychosocial, and biological as described by Stallwood and Stoll (1975; see Figure 1.3).

Stallwood and Stoll's concept of person was viewed to be the framework in which to perform the various components of the nursing process. In using the Nursing Process Systems Model, the nurse "looks at the patient's systems in terms of the stressor encountered and the degree of success of the stress

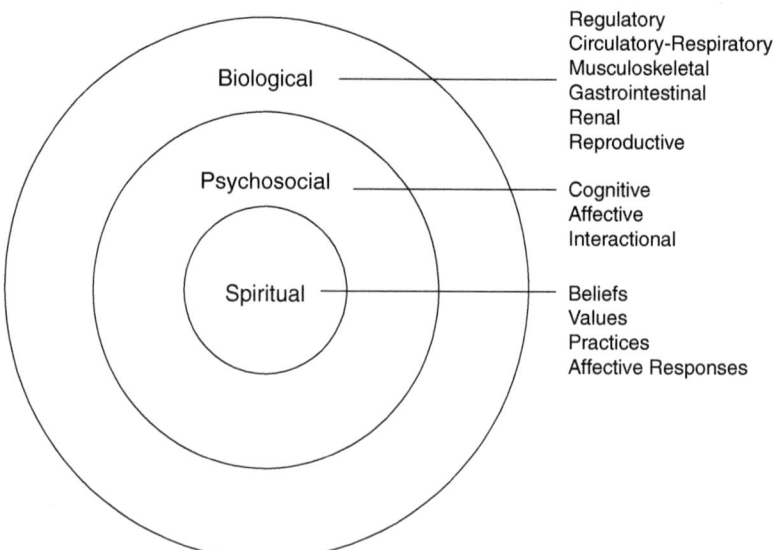

FIGURE 1.3 Description of person.
Source: Artinian (1991, 2011). Adapted from Stollwood & Stoll (1975).

response. This helps in identifying problem areas and in determining appropriate methods of intervention to assist in the attempt toward adaptation and equilibrium" (Brown, 1981, p. 39). The description of person developed by Stallwood and Stoll (1975) formed the structure of the Nursing Process Systems Model (see Figure 1.4).

Since the Nursing Process Systems Model did not provide an explicit framework for guiding practice and many of its concepts were in the already published Intersystem Model, the APU dean, Dr. Marilyn Wood, encouraged me to integrate the concepts from the Nursing Process Systems Model into the Intersystem Model framework. To gain acceptance of the Intersystem Model by the APU faculty, a document was used for several years, which placed all aspects of the Nursing Process Systems Model into the structure of the Intersystem Model. In

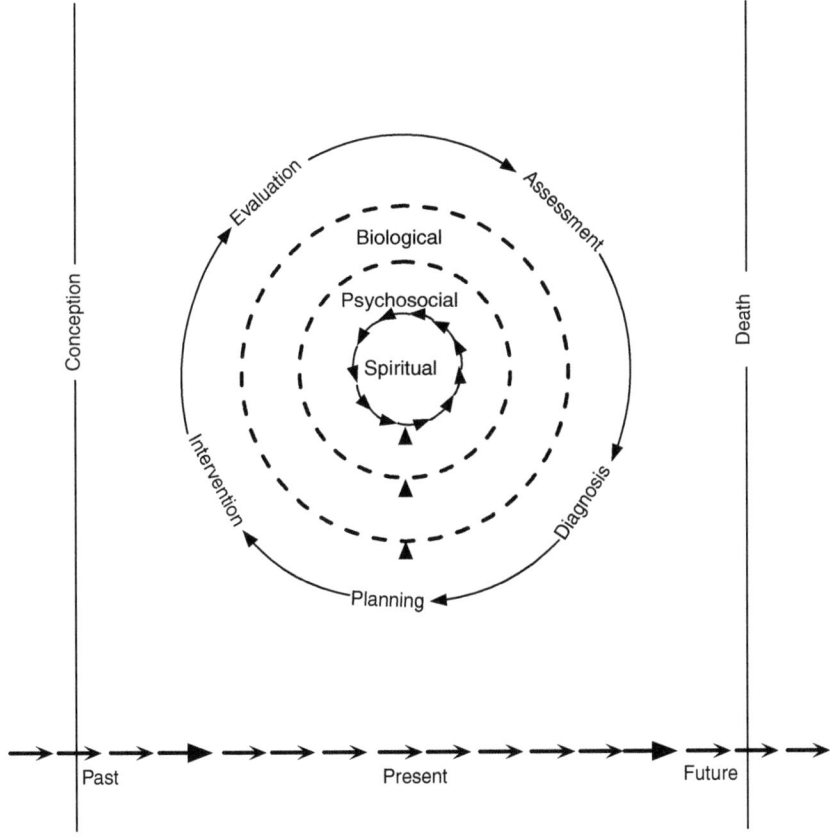

FIGURE 1.4 Nursing Process Systems Model.
Copyright © 1979 Azusa Pacific College.

this working document, I had initially identified all of the four nursing metaparadigm concepts except for the concept of health. I wanted a definition of health that would allow a person to be classified as healthy while dying. A new construct, *SSOC*, adapted from Antonovsky's (1987) *sense of coherence* concept (SOC), was incorporated into the model to equate the client's integrative potential in his or her response to an illness situation with health. This completed the model, and the Intersystem Model was adopted by the faculty at APU as the model for curriculum development. The name "Intersystem Model" reflects the interactional process that takes place between client and nurse in using the nursing process to develop a collaborative plan of care. The new diagram added the SSOC construct to the figure and replaced the action of "transactions in terms of values" with the action of "negotiating values" (see Figure 1.5).

In order to clarify the steps to follow in using the model, a flow chart was developed (see Figure 1.6). This flow chart and the revised version of the

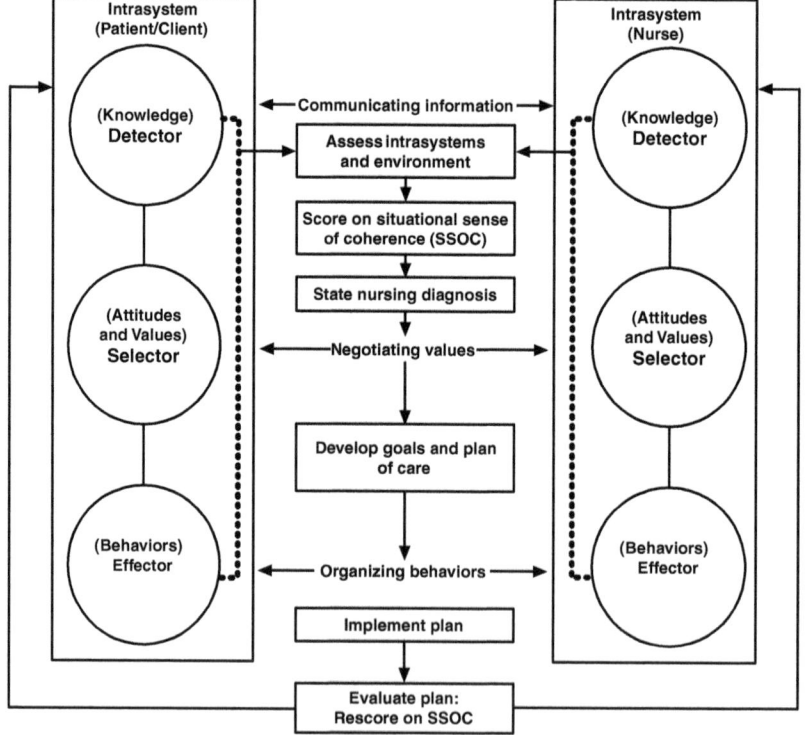

FIGURE 1.5 Early Intersystem Model.
Source: Artinian (1991, 1997).

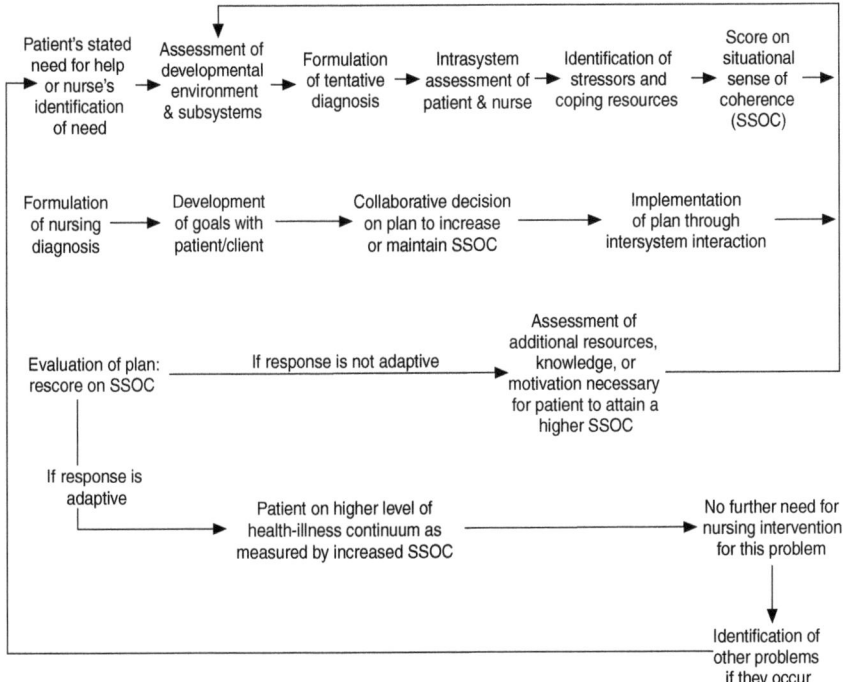

FIGURE 1.6 Flowchart of the nursing process in implementing the Intersystem Model (1991).
Copyright © 1991 B. Artinian.

model were reported in a journal article (1991) and in book form (1997). The flow chart was incorporated into the later versions of the model.

TRANSITION TO THE ARTINIAN INTERSYSTEM MODEL

The reconceptualization of the model that prompted the change of the name from the Intersystem Model to the Artinian Intersystem Model (AIM) introduced changes into the diagram of the model. An intermediate version of the model was prepared in 2009 using the flowchart format (see Figure 1.7).

Because the process depicted in the 2009 diagram was not clear to persons unfamiliar with the model, a new diagram of the model was developed. This latest revision of the Artinian Intersystem Model diagram made few changes in the concepts of the model, but the diagram depicting the concepts was changed to include all aspects of the model in one diagram (see Figure 1.8).

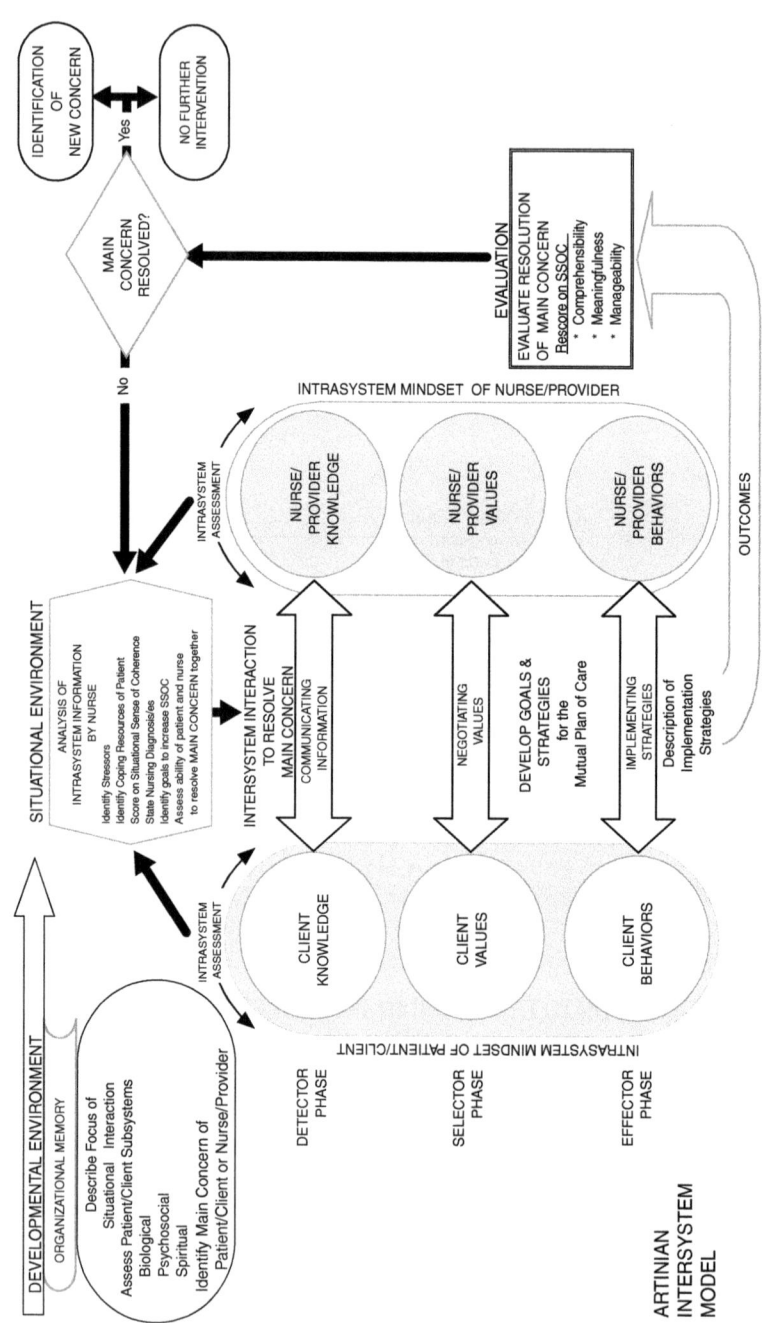

FIGURE 1.7 The Artinian Intersystem Model (2009).
Source: Adapted from A. Kuhn (1974). The Logic of Social Systems published by Jossey-Bass.

By integrating the theories of Chin (1969), Kuhn (1974), Antonovsky (1987), Blumer (1969), Stallwood and Stoll (1975), and Knickrehm (1994), the AIM provides a way of looking at person as a whole dynamic entity in a hierarchical relation of subsystems and suprasystems in mutual interaction. The model focuses on the main concern of the patient or of the nurse and how they work together to resolve the concern using the steps of the Artinian Intersystem Model. This model has been published in a series of articles and a book (1983, 1984, 1991, and 1997). The major concepts of the model are summarized within the metaparadigm concepts of nursing, which are person, environment, health, and nursing action.

Person

In the Artinian Intersystem Model, a person is viewed as a coherent being or aggregate that continually strives to make sense of the world. Person is seen as a system made up of various subsystems that can be viewed in terms of change over time. The subsystems that make up the whole person are the biological, psychosocial, and spiritual subsystems depicted as a series of concentric circles (Stallwood & Stoll, 1975) (see Figure 1.3). The biological subsystem is on the outside since it is through the body that the psychosocial and spiritual subsystems are manifested in the environment. The spiritual subsystem is in the center since the spirit is the core of the individual person or aggregate. Although person is viewed as having three subsystems, the "system must be understood as a whole and cannot be comprehended by examining its individual parts in isolation from each other" (Whitchurch & Constantine, 1993, p. 328).

When person is an individual, either the term "client" or "patient" can be used in the AIM. When person is an aggregate, the term "client" is used. The term client is derived from the Latin word meaning "to lean on" and implies that the person as client needs the professional advice or services of the nurse. The term patient is derived from the Latin word meaning "to suffer" and implies that the person as patient needs the caring the nurse can provide in a time of distress. Therefore, the choice of term will depend on the need of the patient/client in a particular interactional situation.

Environment

Developmental Environment

Merriam-Webster's School Dictionary (1999) defines *environment* as "the social and cultural conditions that influence the life of a person or human community" (p. 296). Therefore, the developmental environment can be defined as all the events, factors, and influences that affect the system experienced through its biological, psychosocial, and spiritual subsystems as it passes through its developmental stages. In systems theory, whatever is not the system is its environment. In this way, each suprasystem or subsystem is the environment for a particular system.

The developmental environment is the arena in which the system is developed and provides the context for the interaction at the time of a specific encounter in which nursing service is offered to assist with an illness or management problem that the system is unable to resolve independently. Symbolic interaction theory helps in understanding the interaction that takes place in the developmental environment. Symbolic interaction theory focuses on the nature of human social interaction by examining the connection between symbols (shared meanings) and interactions (verbal and nonverbal) with which individuals in relation to each other create symbolic worlds. Blumer (1969) says that people "act toward things on the basis of the meanings that the things have for them" and that "these meanings are socially derived" (p. 2). This provides the "integrative and interpretative framework" for judging life events and "the standard by which reality is managed and pursued" (Olthuis, 1989, p. 29). As such, it has a major impact on the health beliefs and practices held by individuals and aggregates. It also strongly influences the orientation the person has to life as being comprehensible, meaningful, and manageable—that is, the SOC as defined by Antonovsky (1987). A worldview is socially acquired within a cultural community and is shared by that community.

The set of environmental factors that bring the patient and nurse together form the focus of the interaction. During the interaction of the nurse/provider with the patient/client, the nurse is able to assess the effect of both the external and internal environments on the biological, psychosocial, and spiritual subsystems of the individual or aggregate. In addition, data are collected about the intrasystem functions of the person, which are the knowledge, values, and behaviors of the person (Kuhn, 1974). By analyzing all the factors in the developmental environment, the nurse can identify the main concern of the patient or nurse. When the nurse has previously interacted with the patient, knowledge of previous interactions with health professionals and the community at large facilitates the analysis since each interaction in a situational environment becomes part of the person's developmental environment when it is finished. This knowledge is stored as the organizational memory about the patient.

Situational Environment

It is in the situational environment that the nurse and client organize a plan of care and implement it. All the unique characteristics of the nurse and of the client as well as the characteristics of the setting interact to make the experience what it is. Different nurses with differing life experiences would make the encounter a different type of experience for a particular client, as would different characteristics of the setting. The situational environment includes all the details of the encounter such as the place, time, circumstance, motivational state, and receptivity of the care provider and recipient.

Following the identification of the main concern of the client or nurse in the developmental environment, intrasystem analysis and intersystem interaction take place in the situational environment to resolve the main concern of the client or nurse using the framework adapted from Kuhn (1974) and the SSOC scoring evaluation of the outcome adapted from Antonovsky (1987).

Nurses bear initial and ongoing responsibility for establishing relatedness with clients. The client approaches the interaction because of a need for assistance in matters of health and well-being. It is important for the nurse to assess how the client is interpreting the illness and what treatments are believed to be appropriate. Effective nursing requires that nurses become skilled in recognizing and responding to the client's need for help and become sufficiently involved to explore the client's interests.

Health

Health and disease are viewed on a multidimensional health/disease continuum. It would be difficult to find a person in perfect health, totally sound in body, mind, and spirit with full vigor and freedom from all signs of disease. On the other hand, as long as individuals live, they have some measure of health. Antonovsky (1987) suggests that people can manage stress and stay well by developing a strong SOC.

When individuals have a strong SOC, they can use a variety of coping strategies, which Antonovsky defines as generalized resistance resources in seeking a solution to a problem. If a person has a low SOC or the stressor generates more tension than can be managed, the person experiences a generalized resistance deficit and is in need of assistance to develop strategies to cope with the problem.

Antonovsky (1987) views the SOC as a "deeply rooted, stable dispositional orientation of a person" (p. 124) but states that there can be fluctuations around a mean, as in a time of crisis. Because the global SOC construct is conceived to be stable over the life span, a new construct, the SSOC has been developed (Artinian, 1991). This narrower construct describes the response that occurs in the period of disorganization in which a client is attempting to deal with a serious life event. When nursing assistance is provided, the SSOC theory of recovery describes how nursing action is given to assist the person to increase in SSOC when confronted with stressors that cannot be managed independently. These components are scored on a scale from 1 to 3 (high, medium, or low) with 3 being the highest. The SSOC contains the same three dimensions identified in the SOC, but they are defined by Artinian (1991) to reflect a present, specific orientation rather than a global orientation. When a successful stress response occurs, the response is adaptive and is reflected in a higher SSOC and a higher SOC.

By using the SSOC theory of recovery as implemented in the AIM, the nurse helps ensure that the client will be able to achieve the best possible state of health or outcome given the circumstances. Through strengthening a person's SSOC, health is achieved by successful adaptation to the stressors in the internal and external environments. Therefore, in the AIM, health is defined as a strong SOC. This means that the person has confidence that events are comprehensible, are worth investing in, and are manageable.

To assist the client to increase in SSOC, the goals of both the nurse/provider and patient/client must be met. The nurse as a professional person has knowledge, values, and behavioral skills that help to identify tentative goals for the person. This is done by assessing the client's knowledge about the main concern (*comprehensibility*), the resources available to make it manageable (*manageability*), and the client's motivation to accept the challenges created by the problems (*meaningfulness*).

Nursing Action

A systematic way has been developed to explore the definitions of the situation held by patient and nurse so that a plan of care that is acceptable to both can be made. This is done using the framework of the AIM adapted from Alfred Kuhn (1974). The Kuhn model consists of two interrelated models: the intrasystem model and the intersystem model. Kuhn states that any controlled adaptive system must use knowledge, preferences or values, and behavioral responses. Intrasystem analysis assesses the knowledge, values, and behaviors of both the nurse and the client in relation to the main concern. Based on these data, the nurse can assess the SSOC of the patient and develop a nursing diagnosis and tentative goals. If the nurse determines that he/she has the necessary knowledge and resources available to help, and that the nurse and client can work together to resolve the main concern, then intersystem interaction begins.

An intersystem model consists of two intrasystem models that are connected to each other through a specific set of relations. Intersystem interaction differs from the interaction of two open systems with each other because in the intersystem model the autonomy of each system is retained but the connectives which "represent the lines of relationships of the two systems" can be described (Chin, 1969, p. 304). In the Kuhn model, when two intrasystems interact, the focus is on how information is communicated between the two intrasystems, how values are negotiated to develop a joint plan of care, and how behaviors are organized to implement the plan that will resolve the main concern. For the nursing process to be effective, the priorities of both intrasystems must be taken into account. Through feedback loops, the intrasystems' knowledge, values, and behaviors are progressively clarified and modified to develop a joint plan of care.

The relationships between the developmental environment and the situational environment where the interaction occurs to resolve the main concern are diagrammed in Figure 1.8. This diagram traces the thought process of the nurse from understanding the situation that brings the nurse and patient together in interaction to collect intrasystem data in the Developmental Environment about the patient's biological, psychosocial, and spiritual subsystems. This leads to a tentative identification of the main concern of the patient or the nurse. The Main Concern is validated through assessment of the intrasystem functions of the patient and of the nurse in terms of their knowledge, values, and behaviors or resources in relation to the main concern.

The diagram specifies the link between the Developmental Environment and the Situational Environment through the Analysis of Intrasystem Data done by the nurse/provider. This includes identifying patient stressors and coping resources and scoring the patient on SSOC in order to make nursing diagnoses. The nurse then develops goals to increase the SSOC of the patient and assesses the ability of the nurse to resolve the main concern in interaction with the patient. If the nurse determines that patient and nurse can work together, Intersystem Interaction begins to resolve the main concern. This is done by communicating information, negotiating values, developing joint goals, and strategizing a mutual plan of care. The plan is implemented and evaluated by the nurse by re-scoring on SSOC. If the main concern is not resolved, the nurse must return to collecting and reanalyzing data from the intrasystems and begin

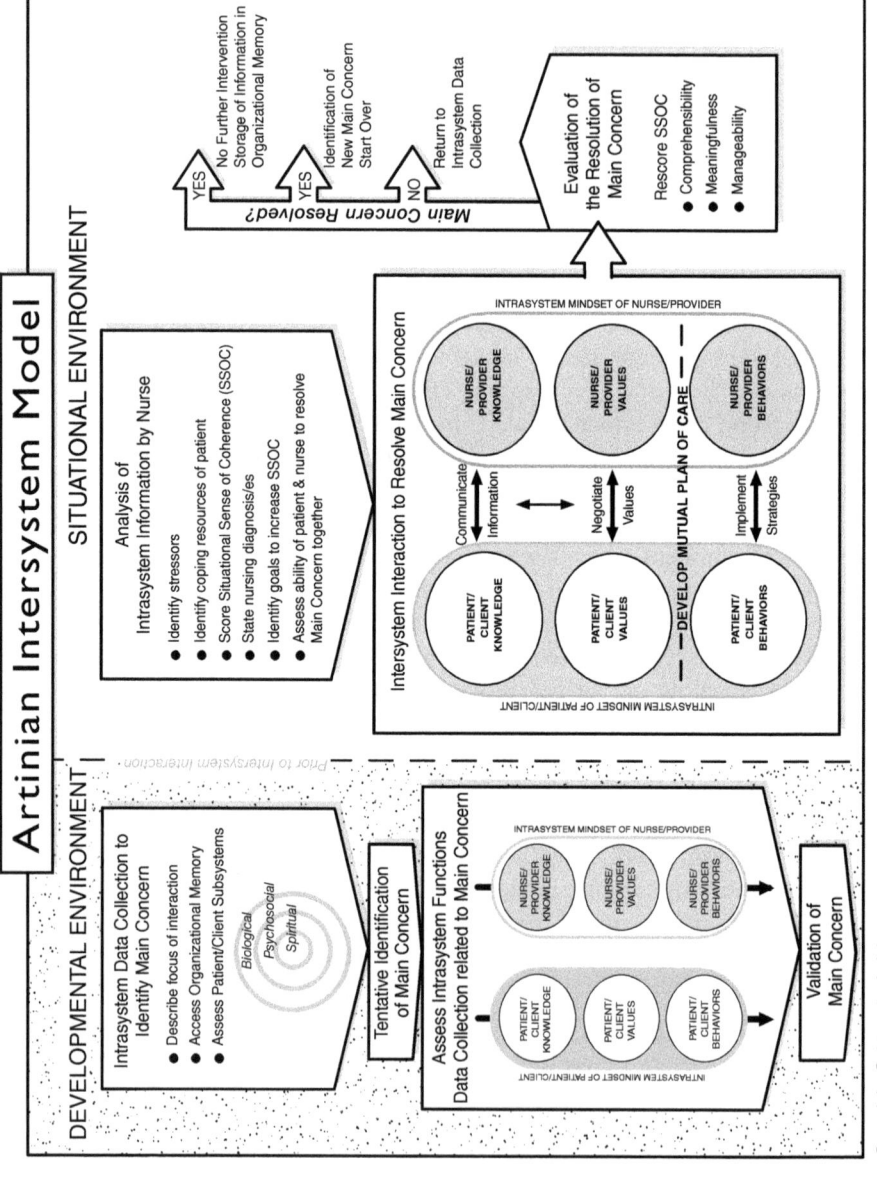

FIGURE 1.8 The Artinian Intersystem Model (2011)—opposite page.
This diagram of the current model also functions as a map guiding the nursing process using the Artinian Intersystem Model (AIM). Each section of this model corresponds to an equivalent section of the AIM Care Plan templates (see appendices). To use the model, start in the upper left corner, The Developmental Environment column, and perform the required tasks in sequence in each subsection, leading to the Validation of Main Concern at the bottom of the Developmental Environment. Next, proceed to the top of the Situational Environment section to begin the Analysis of Intrasystem Information by Nurse. Perform the required tasks in sequence in each subsection, through Develop Mutual Plan of Care and Implement Strategies (located in the Intrasystem Interaction to Resolve Main Concern section). Continue by following the arrow to the third column to the Evaluation of the Resolution of Main Concern section and complete the Rescore SSOC task in that box. Finally, answer the question "Was the Main Concern Resolved?" with one of the three options. Depending on the answer, conclude care or return to the appropriate section of the AIM and continue care.
Copyright © 2011 B. Artinian.

interaction again to resolve the main concern. If the interaction resolved the main concern, information about the interaction is stored in the organizational memory to be used if a new concern arises.

Because the Artinian Intersystem Model allows assessment of both the individual systems and the interaction between them, it provides a systematic way to assess the initial SSOC of the client about the main concern, provides a framework for increasing SSOC, and provides a means of evaluating the resolution of the main concern. If the concern is not resolved, a reassessment that focuses on the main concern is done. As client and nurse work together to develop successful coping strategies, both increase in their ability to resolve the main concern and to face new problems in the future. The same process occurs when the client is an aggregate. Just as input into the individual system is a life event that creates change, input into the aggregate is also a change event that is processed through the biological, psychosocial, and spiritual subsystems of the aggregate.

The most recent diagram of the AIM (2011) was developed to clarify the process of first completing intrasystem assessment followed by analysis of intrasystem information. This analysis is done prior to intersystem interaction.

If the client and the nurse are not able to agree on a plan of care, the nurse will need to begin another round of communication and negotiations in an effort to develop a plan of care that is mutually acceptable. When either the emotional or physical safety of the client is in question, the nurse must exercise professional power to protect the client while recognizing that this action constitutes a failure of the interactional process. This was illustrated in the research of Vuckovich (2003) who reported that when nurses were compelled to take legal action to force patients to take medications that they believed would be effective in helping the patients; they then justified their coercion so that they could see themselves as good nurses. Vuckovich (2009) published her study in *Glaserian Grounded Theory: Trusting Emergence* (Artinian, Giske, & Cone, 2009).

INTRODUCTION TO CARE PLANS

Although the AIM provides a specific framework to assist the nurse to make a collaborative plan of care with patient, the underlying principles of the model can be used by any health care provider who truly wants to include the patient in the planning of care. Two examples are given of mutual plans of care that were developed by professionals who were unfamiliar with the AIM. The first of these is a report of an interaction by an anesthesiologist who used the principles of the model to resolve the main concern of a patient having eyelid surgery and illustrates how the main concern of the patient was resolved (see Care Plan 1.1). The second example was developed from a first person account of pain management for a patient following surgery that was published in the American Journal of Nursing (Gordon & Ward, 1995). The patient feared becoming addicted to pain medication and the nurses knew that pain management was necessary for her recovery (see Care Plan 1.2). It illustrates how the main concern of the nurses was resolved. Both of the examples are concerned with pain management. In each case, the patient was reluctant to take the prescribed medication. In the first example, through negotiation, an alternative plan was strategized. In the second example, the patient was persuaded that she needed pain medication and a plan was set up to put her in control. The first care plan presents a truncated form of analysis that can be used by providers who can quickly assess the intrasystems of patient and self and make a diagnosis and determine their ability to resolve the main concern of the patient. The second example is one that can be used to teach students to critically analyze each aspect of the model.

The management of postoperative pain is just one aspect of providing care for the cancer patient. With the focus on helping the patient accept the need for setting a goal for pain management, many other issues are not addressed. The trust and confidence in the nurse and the institutional setting that were developed during this interactional sequence, however, will become part of the developmental environment of the patient and will influence future interactions. Issues such as further treatment for the cancer and the ambiguity of whether the cancer will become worse will need attention as they are introduced by the patient. This analysis of the interaction around the need for goal setting for pain relief illustrates that in using the AIM format it is permissible, based on the intrasystem assessment of the patient and self, for the nurse to introduce her concerns for the patient that the patient did not even know should be a concern.

CONCLUSION

The AIM can be used in brief nurse–client encounters or in long-term interactions. Each time the feedback loop is completed, the nurse and client will know more about each other, and the plan they organize can be more appropriate to resolve the main concern of either the client or the nurse. The information about the interaction is stored in the organizational memory. The AIM can be used by the novice practitioner as well as by the expert because the complexity of the model derives from the knowledge base of the user, not from the structure of the model.

In conclusion, the AIM has been developed from the work of many theorists. I am indebted to these theorists who understood the need for mutual interaction from a patient-centered perspective. This chapter illustrates how nursing knowledge advances based on the work of preceding theorists.

REFERENCES

Abdellah, F., Beland, I., Martin, A., & Matheney, R. (1960). *Patient-centered approaches to nursing*. New York, NY: The Macmillan Company.

Antonovsky, A. (1987). *Unraveling the mysteries of health: How people manage stress and stay well*. San Francisco, CA: Jossey-Bass.

Artinian, B. (1971). *A therapist-family intersystem model for conjoint family therapy*. Unpublished paper. Los Angeles, CA: University of Southern California.

Artinian, B. (1982). *Nursing care plans: An exploratory study*. Unpublished paper. Los Angeles, CA: LA County–USC Medical Center.

Artinian, B. (1983). Implementation of the intersystem patient-care model in clinical practice. *Journal of Advanced Nursing, 8*, 117–124.

Artinian, B. (1984). Collaborative planning of patient care in the prenatal, labor and delivery, and neonatal settings. *Journal of Obstetric, Gynecological and Neonatal Nursing, 13*, 105–110.

Artinian, B. (1991). The development of the intersystem model. *Journal of Advanced Nursing, 16*, 164–205.

Artinian, B., & Conger, M. (1997). *The intersystem model: Integrating theory and practice*. Thousand Oaks, CA: Sage.

Artinian, B., Giske, T., & Cone, P. (2009). *Glaserian grounded theory: Trusting emergence*. New York, NY: Springer Publishing.

Blumer, H. (1969). *Symbolic interactionism*. Englewood Cliffs, NJ: Prentice Hall.

Brown, S. J. (1981). The nursing process systems model. *Journal of Nursing Education, 20*, 36–40.

Chin, R. (1969). The utility of system models and developmental models for practitioners. In W. Bennis, K. Benne, & R. Chin, *The planning of change* (pp. 297–312). New York, NY: Holt, Rinehart and Winston, Inc.

Chrisman, M., & Riehl, J. (1974). The systems-developmental stress model. In J. Riehl & C. Roy (Eds.), *Conceptual models for nursing practice* (pp. 247–266). New York, NY: Appleton-Century-Crofts.

Environment. (1999). In *Merriam-Webster's school dictionary*. Springfield, MA: Merriam-Webster.

Gordon, D., & Ward, S. (1995). Correcting patient misconceptions about pain. *American Journal of Nursing, 95*, 43–45.

Kuhn, A. (1974). *The logic of social systems: A unified deductive, system-based approach to social science*. San Francisco, CA: Jossey-Bass.

Matheney, R. (1960). Application of a patient-centered curriculum in an associate degree program. In F. Abdellah, I. Beland, A. Martin, & R. Matheney. *Patient-centered approaches to nursing*. New York, NY: The Macmillan Company.

Olthuis, J. (1989). On worldviews. In P. Marshall, S. Griffioen, & R. Lieuw (Eds.), *Stained glass, worldviews, and social science*. New York, NY: University Press of America.

Orlando, I. J. (1961). *The dynamic nurse patient relationship*. New York, NY: G.P. Putnam.

Peplau, H. E. (1952). *Interpersonal relations in nursing*. New York, NY: G.P. Putnam.

Stallwood, J., & Stoll, R. (1975). Spiritual dimensions of nursing practice, Part C. In I. Beland & J. Passos (Eds.), *Clinical nursing* (3rd ed., pp. 1086–1098). New York, NY: The Macmillan Company.

Vuckovich, P. (2003). *Justifying coercion: Nurses' experiences medicating involuntary psychiatric patients*. PhD dissertation, University of San Diego, San Diego, CA.

Vuckovich, P. (2009). Justifying coercion. In B. Artinian, T. Giske, & P. Cone, *Glaserian grounded theory in nursing research: Trusting emergence* (pp. 197–209). New York, NY: Springer Publishing.

Whitchurch, G., & Constantine, H. (1993). Systems theory. In P. Boss, W. Doherty, R. La Rossa, W. Schumm, & S. Steinmetz (Eds.), *Sourcebook of family theories and methods* (pp. 325–352). New York, NY: Plenum Press.

1. Development of the Artinian Intersystem Model

CARE PLAN 1.1 Illustrating the Resolution of the Main Concern of Patient (Short Form to be used by an expert practitioner)

DEVELOPMENTAL ENVIRONMENT[1]	
COLLECTION OF INTRASYSTEM DATA TO IDENTIFY MAIN CONCERN	
Describe Focus of Interaction	When the patient first considered surgery for eyelid repair, she was told that she would be awake during the procedure. Later she was told that she would be given "twilight sleep." She almost cancelled the surgery because of reports of situations in which people had died during cosmetic surgery and the previous experiences she had had with anesthesia. This information was relayed to the surgeon and he called back to let her know that he could do the procedure with local anesthesia. He also said that he would discuss the preference of the patient with the anesthesiologist.
Access Organizational Memory	Clinic chart provided to anesthesiologist.
Assess Patient/Client Subsystems	
Biological Subsystem	Vital signs monitored.
Psychosocial Subsystem	Determined and articulate.
Spiritual Subsystem	Fear of dying under anesthesia.
Validation of Main Concern of Patient/Client or Nurse/Provider	Patient fears the use of analgesia to produce "twilight sleep."
SITUATIONAL ENVIRONMENT	
Assess Ability of Patient and Nurse to Work Together to Resolve Main Concern	Excellent. Values of both the same.
INTERSYSTEM INTERACTION TO RESOLVE MAIN CONCERN	
Communicate Information	The patient told anesthesiologist that since she rarely takes pain medication, she is very sensitive to medications and that she sometimes experiences sharp drops in blood pressure and pulse. The anesthesiologist told the patient that he has had much experience in providing anesthesia to patients with cardiac problems.

(Continued)

---

[1] See Figure 1.8

CARE PLAN 1.1 (Continued)

Negotiate Values	The anesthesiologist assured the patient that he wants to follow the patient's wishes unless they could lead to harm.
Develop Mutual Plan of Care	
Develop Joint Goals	1. Make patient comfortable about procedure. 2. Decrease anxiety about the use of anesthesia.
Develop Joint Objectives	To keep patient pain-free during procedure
Develop Implementation Strategies	Congruency of values made possible the development of joint plan of care. 1. A small amount of relaxant would be given initially to reduce anxiety. 2. The surgeon would inject local anesthesia. 3. At any time during the procedure if she experienced pain, the surgeon would signal the anesthesiologist to provide medication. 4. She was to use breathing techniques to promote relaxation. At this point the patient told the surgeon and anesthesiologist that they had practiced all the principles of the Intersystem Model. The anesthesiologist asked: "Doesn't everyone do this?"
Implement Strategies	Local anesthesia was injected into both eyelids. During the procedure while the second eye was being repaired, the local anesthesia had lost some effect and the patient signaled that she felt the procedure. The eyelid was again injected with anesthesia. The second time the patient indicated that she was having pain, the surgeon said that he was at a point where he couldn't stop and he instructed the anesthesiologist to provide medication. During the procedure her vital signs remained stable and she was relaxed. She was confident that the surgeon was able to complete the procedure successfully because during the time of the surgery, the anesthesiologist asked the surgeon how he had become so skillful. The surgeon replied that after his residency he had visited the major eye centers in the country and had observed the best surgeons performing the operation and had picked up some hints from them.

(Continued)

CARE PLAN 1.1 (Continued)

EVALUATION OF RESOLUTION OF MAIN CONCERN		
Score Patient on Situational Sense of Coherence (SSOC) (high = 3, medium = 2, or low = 1)		
Comprehensibility	3	The patient learned it is possible to have surgery while awake.
Meaningfulness	3	The patient acknowledged it was worthwhile to have had the procedure because the experience had not been stressful and she anticipated having better vision.
Manageability	3	The patient tolerated the procedure as planned according to the desired goal.
Reassess Need for Further Interaction		
Main Concern Is Resolved *No Further Intervention. Storage of Information in Organizational Memory.*	Procedure successful. Patient was satisfied with anesthesiologist's adaptation to patient's needs.	

CARE PLAN 1.2 Illustrating the Resolution of the Main Concern of the Nurse

DEVELOPMENTAL ENVIRONMENT[1]	
COLLECTION OF INTRASYSTEM DATA TO IDENTIFY MAIN CONCERN	
Describe Focus of Interaction	The nurse asks the patient a question that she has not thought about: "On the 0–10 scale, what's your goal? What level of pain relief do you want to achieve?" The interaction that takes place focuses on helping the patient understand what she could expect in terms of pain control and what goals are possible for her and on helping the nurse understand the patient's perspective on pain control. The purpose is to provide a target and sense of direction for the pain management plan.
Access Organizational Memory	First admission.

(Continued)

---

[1] See Figure 1.8

CARE PLAN 1.2 (Continued)

Assess Patient/Client Subsystems	
Biological Subsystem	J. S., age 42, had had a hysterectomy for uterine cancer 48 hours prior to this interaction. She is a patient on a surgical gynecology unit and has been asked frequently to describe the intensity and type of pain she is feeling. She reports a pain level of 4 to 7 depending on her activity.
Psychosocial Subsystem	She prides herself on her ability to "tough things out" and has rarely taken analgesics. She has teenage children and has worked hard to keep them off drugs. She believes that the misuse of drugs will cause her to get hooked on them and may lead to their ineffectiveness at a later time.
Spiritual Subsystem	Nothing is known about her spiritual orientation at this time. With further interaction, particularly if her cancer is not cured, she may discuss this with the nurse.
Tentative Identification of Main Concern of Patient or Provider	The patient did not have a goal for pain management.
ASSESSMENT OF INTRASYSTEM FUNCTIONS RELATED TO MAIN CONCERN	
Intrasystem Information About Nurse/Provider Related to Main Concern	
Knowledge	The patient believes that some pain is associated with cancer and surgery and is not aware of the negative consequences of pain on her recovery. She is not aware of breathing and splinting techniques to relieve pain. She has misconceptions about addiction and pain relief. She believes that the nurses are doing everything they can to control her pain.
Values	The patient would like to be free of pain but does not expect to be. She does not see herself as a complainer. She is more concerned about her future need for effective analgesics than for the pain she is currently experiencing.
Behaviors	The patient is using a patient-controlled analgesia (PCA) pump to give her own morphine but is reporting a pain level of 4 to 7 depending on her activity. Although she is experiencing pain, she is able to do some coughing and deep breathing exercises.

(Continued)

CARE PLAN 1.2 (Continued)

Intrasystem Information About Nurse/Provider Related to Main Concern	
Knowledge	The nurse understands the principles of pain control management and their benefit for comfort and recovery and the adverse effects of analgesic drugs. She understands that although the patient expresses satisfaction with the pain relief provided, it may be a result of not providing the patient with enough information to make a proper evaluation. She knows that she could be doing a better job. She understands the need for patients to define a goal for pain relief.
Values	The nurse values knowing patient expectations and preferences for pain control. She values patient teaching so that the patient can be a participant in planning care by knowing how to develop a goal that would assist her to make informed decisions about her care.
Behaviors	The nurse assessed patient's physiologic and behavioral responses to pain by monitoring pain level every 2 to 4 hours and noting drug usage and possible adverse effects of drugs. The behavior of the nurses displayed accurate perception, confidence, and the ability to provide anticipatory guidance.
Validation of Main Concern of Patient/Client or Nurse/Provider	The Main Concern of the Nurse is that the patient will benefit from active pain management, but patient does not believe it is possible.

SITUATIONAL ENVIRONMENT

ANALYSIS OF INTRASYSTEM INFORMATION BY NURSE

Identify Stressors of Patient	Diagnosis of cancer Pain from recent surgery
Identify Coping Resources of Patient	Previous experience with "toughing things out" Teenagers who are important to her Available analgesics Supportive nursing staff

Score Patient/Client on Situational Sense of Coherence (SSOC)
(high = 3, medium = 2, or low = 1)

Comprehensibility	1		Patient does not know the benefits of pain relief and the negative consequences of pain. She is concerned about getting hooked and fears she will develop tolerance to medications so that

(Continued)

CARE PLAN 1.2 (Continued)

		they will be ineffective in the future is her cancer is not cured.
Meaningfulness	1	The nurse believes that a goal for pain management is important, but the patient does not see the importance of having a goal.
Manageability	2	Since surgery, pain has not been kept within acceptable limits because of inadequate goals. The patient, however, is well educated and able to process the information effectively and can learn to develop adequate goals if she sees the importance of pain relief. The institution has the needed resources for pain management in terms of effective nursing staff, adequate equipment, and analgesics.
State Nursing Diagnosis/es		Inadequate management of pain related to knowledge deficit about adequate pain relief.
Identify Goals to Increase SSOC		1. Instruct patient about the benefit of pain management. 2. Negotiate a plan for pain management patient sees as beneficial for her.
Assess Ability of Patient and Nurse to Work Together to Resolve Main Concern		The nurse had the necessary knowledge and patient was willing to work with her.
INTERSYSTEM INTERACTION TO RESOLVE MAIN CONCERN		
Communicate Information		In response to the patient's misconceptions about the use of analgesics, information was given in a way that would not make her feel foolish. Authoritative literature was provided that would dispel her fears about addiction, tolerance, and side effects. Pillow splinting and breathing techniques to lessen pain while coughing and deep breathing were demonstrated. This information was accepted because the patient recognized its validity and perceived that the nurse was accurate in her assessment of her need for pain relief. The patient recognized that although this was a new and uncertain situation for her, the nurse had experienced it before and was competent to provide guidance for her.
Negotiate Values		Although the nurse and patient were far apart in their perception of the value of pain management at

(Continued)

CARE PLAN 1.2 (Continued)

	the beginning of the interaction, through the caring behaviors of the nurse, her value of needing to set a goal for pain relief was recognized by the patient as being appropriate for her and was accepted as her own. When she realized that the valued behavior of "toughing it out" was actually detrimental to her recovery process, she reinterpreted the situation so that both patient and nurse shared the same interpretation of the value of goal setting for pain management. At the beginning of the interaction, the patient was in a position of low power because of inadequate knowledge. Through appropriate teaching, the patient was brought to the place where she could make an informed decision about her care. She was no longer satisfied with a pain rating of 4 or more. This made it possible for a goal to be determined that would be both reasonable and realistic and acceptable to both patient and nurse.
Develop Mutual Plan of Care	
Develop Joint Goals	1. Patient will study information provided by nurse and test the effectiveness of new pain control techniques. 2. Patient will monitor her pain during times of rest and activity to identify a reasonable pain goal linked to activities necessary for her recovery. 3. Patient will evaluate the new program.
Develop Joint Objectives	Manage pain to stay within patient's stated acceptable pain range of 2–3.
Develop Implementation Strategies	Because the patient did not like to focus on pain, with the consent of the surgeon a continuous hourly basal infusion of analgesic was added to her PCA regimen while still allowing her to have personal control over additional medication during activity. The nurse continued to monitor her use of analgesics and asked, "Do you feel we need to adjust your dose?"
Implement Strategies	With reassessments of pain control during the next 12 hours, the patient's self report of pain was brought down to her desired goal of 2 or 3. She was able to switch to an oral analgesic. She continued to direct her pain management program and recommended that her dosing schedule be

(Continued)

CARE PLAN 1.2 (Continued)

	changed based on her activities so that she took the analgesic 1 hour before bathing, ambulating, and family visits.
EVALUATION OF THE RESOLUTION OF MAIN CONCERN	
Re-score Patient on SSOC (high = 3, medium = 2, or low = 1)	
Comprehensibility — 3	The patient has full understanding of the pain management program and was able to set a realistic goal for herself and meet it.
Meaningfulness — 3	The patient recognized the value of setting a goal for pain relief in terms of her overall recovery and actively developed her own program.
Manageability — 3	The patient had the resources to manage her pain and the needed assistance to use them Her pain was maintained at the desired goal.
Assess Effectiveness of Implementation Strategies	
Identify Strengths and Weaknesses of Implementation by Nurse	The negotiations that took place within the structural context of the surgical gynecology unit led to a mutual definition of the situation and a negotiated order that was exemplified in the plan for meeting the patient's goal for pain relief.
Reassess Need for Further Interaction (*select one of the following three options*)	
Main Concern Is Not Resolved *Return to Intrasystem Data Collection and Care Plan Process.*	
Main Concern Is Resolved *Identification of New Main Concern. Start Over.*	
Main Concern Is Resolved *No Further Intervention. Storage of Information in Organizational Memory.*	She was able to be more active and independent, and by the next day, she was able to switch to an oral analgesic.

Source: Gordon & Ward (1995).

2

SITUATIONAL SENSE OF COHERENCE: THE SALUTOGENIC MODEL

Barbara M. Artinian

SENSE OF COHERENCE

IN AN ATTEMPT to answer the question "What promotes health?" Antonovsky (1987) developed the *sense of coherence* (SOC) construct. It was designed to predict and explain movement toward the healthy end of the "health-ease/disease continuum" (p. 3). The SOC construct refers to "an integrated way of looking at the world in which one lives" (Antonovsky, 1993a, p. 117). It allows adaptability to whatever life has in store for the person. SOC describes a "salutogenic" orientation to life that makes possible successful coping by enabling individuals to learn to use their own resources to their best advantage when dealing with life's challenges. The focus is on health, psychological strength, and successful adaptation to the stressors of life. It is the opposite of a pathogenic orientation, which focuses on the disease process. It produces an inclination to have a particular set of behavioral responses during a time of stress. The construct SOC is incorporated within the framework of systems theory, which rejects linear causality and sees the development of SOC as being interactive with health in a recursive pattern. Antonovsky states that it "leads one to think in terms of factors promoting movement toward the healthy end of the continuum" (1987 p. 6). Antonovsky defines SOC as:

> ...a global orientation that expresses the extent to which one has a pervasive, enduring though dynamic feeling of confidence that 1) the stimuli deriving from one's internal and external environments in the course of living are structured, predictable, and explicable; 2) the resources are available to one to meet the demands posed by these stimuli; and 3) these demands are challenges, worthy of investment and engagement. (1987, p. 19)

An important factor in determining the level of SOC that is achieved by a person is the degree to which that person has had participation in making decisions about the tasks to be done so that the person has performance responsibility. This makes the person believe that performance has an effect on the outcome of the experience.

Components of SOC

The three components of SOC are comprehensibility, meaningfulness, and manageability. These are described in the following definitions:

Comprehensibility—the extent to which one perceives the stimuli that confront deriving from the internal and external environments, as making cognitive sense, as information that is ordered, consistent, structured, and clear, rather than as noise—chaotic, disordered, random, accidental, and inexplicable. The person high on the sense of comprehensibility expects that stimuli he or she will encounter in the future will be predictable, or at the very least, when they do come as surprises, that they will be orderable and explicable. It is important to note that nothing is implied about the desirability of stimuli. Death, war, and failure can occur, but such a person can make sense of them.

Meaningfulness—the extent to which one feels that life makes sense emotionally, that at least some of the problems and demands posed by living are worth investing energy in, are worthy of commitment and engagement, and are challenges that are "welcome" rather than burdens that one would much rather do without. This does not mean that someone high on meaningfulness is happy about the death of a loved one, the need to undergo a serious operation, or being fired, but rather that when these unhappy experiences are imposed on such a person, he or she will willingly take up the challenge, will be determined to seek meaning in it, and will do his or her best to overcome it with dignity.

Manageability—the extent to which one perceives that resources that are at one's disposal are adequate to meet the demand posed by the stimuli that bombard one. "At one's disposal" may refer to resources under one's own control or to resources controlled by legitimate others—one's spouse, friend, colleagues, God, history, the party leader, or a physician—who one feels one can count on—whom one trusts. To the extent that one has a high sense of manageability, will not feel victimized by events or feel that life treats one unfairly. Untoward things do happen in life, but when they do occur one will be able to cope and not grieve endlessly (Antonovsky, 1987, pp. 16–18).

Relationship to Successful Coping

Antonovsky stated that the SOC construct is the core of a theory of successful coping. It develops over time as the person successfully or unsuccessfully attempts to reduce tension from the stressors in life. In the salutogenic perspective, it is hypothesized that a person with a high SOC will use personal resources and the resources of others in the best possible way in dealing with the challenges of life. This is done by seeing the broader picture when dealing with a problem and searching for coping resources, taking into account cognitive, affective, and instrumental issues simultaneously. Using this approach, both the client and the health professional are encouraged to look for salutary factors in the situation—the negentropic or order-promoting forces—to facilitate coping. Antonovsky posited that the ability to manage tension is dependent on the person's access to "generalized resistance resources" (GRRs) that are the potential resources a person may use to reduce the tension created by a stressor. These resources include such things as membership in social and cultural groups, flexible coping strategies, intelligence, economic resources, a stable and personal value and belief system, and social support. Antonovsky found that a person with a higher SOC would be able to cope more successfully with a major stressor than a person with a lower SOC.

Antonovsky (1993a) described SOC as a stable underlying personality characteristic that is rooted in social structure and culture, referred to as the developmental environment in the Artinian Intersystem Model (AIM). The generalized SOC develops within the totality of one's life experiences. Antonovsky postulated that a person's SOC is stabilized by the end of young adulthood, thereafter showing only minor fluctuations "barring major and lasting changes in one's life situation" (p. 118).

Research in the area of crisis resolution has demonstrated that the adaptation level of people can change, as illustrated in Hill's (1949) angle of recovery concept in his crisis model. Hill's crisis model, the ABC-X Model, defines crisis as a period of disorganization following a stressor (A). Hill argued that if the individual and family have sufficient resources (B) and a favorable definition of the stressor event (C), they would be able to reverse the disorganization and begin to reorganize with the possibility of reaching a new level of reorganization. He diagrammed the process as a sharp line, the crisis response (X), from the organization of the steady state following the stressor event followed by an angle of recovery at some level—either lower than or exceeding the level the individual or family experienced prior to the crisis.

Even Antonovsky (1993b) suggested that some changes may be possible. He said that there are "minor fluctuations (in SOC) in response to a particular experience" and in response to a given mode of therapy there may be "small-scale, incremental change in the lives of people which lead to small-scale but significant and meaningful change in their SOC" (pp. 15–16). In fact, he has observed that the hospital is an institution that destroys a person's SOC because it provides no opportunities for choice and disregards the person's role. Antonovsky (1993c) agreed that he had not given sufficient thought to ways in which SOC could be increased and saw this as an area of weakness in his work, because if conditions that could facilitate the increase of SOC were known this information could be used in designing treatment programs.

SITUATIONAL SENSE OF COHERENCE

Because Antonovsky viewed the global SOC construct as stable over the life span, a new construct, the situational sense of coherence (SSOC), has been developed for guiding the therapeutic interaction between client and nurse during the time of crisis (Artinian, 1991). This narrower construct describes the response that occurs in the period of time in which a client is attempting to deal with an illness event. The relative strength or weakness of the SOC as well as the severity of the event influence how the person will respond to a life stressor and is reflected in the measurement of SSOC. The SSOC measures the integrative potential in the person's understanding of the situation, the way of looking at the situation, and the ability to marshal resources. It is measured on a scale of high = 3, medium = 2, and low = 1. The client's SSOC is measured early in the interaction between nurse and client in consultation with the client and the family (when appropriate) as a means of developing a mutual plan of care designed to increase the client's SSOC. The success of the intervention is measured by re-scoring on SSOC at the conclusion of the interaction.

Taylor (1997) supported the use of the SSOC construct in understanding a person's experience of his or her illness. He wrote:

> Artinian argued that a person's experience of treatment is a complex consequence of a series of processes occurring over time and between interrelated biological, psychological, and spiritual systems and the continuing, and changing, relationships between each of these systems, and the environment, including the environment in which a person is being treated. Artinian understood that implicit in the theory of sense

of coherence are ideas relevant to the design of treatment programs that could facilitate physical and psychological recovery and growth following an illness or trauma (Taylor, 1997, p. 33).

Description of the SSOC Construct

The SSOC contains the same three dimensions identified in the SOC, but they are defined by Artinian (1997) to reflect a present, specific orientation rather than a global orientation. The definitions are as follows:

Comprehensibility—the extent to which one perceives the stimuli present in the situational environment deriving from the internal and external environments as making cognitive sense, as information that is ordered, consistent, structured, and clear rather than disordered, random, or inexplicable.

Meaningfulness—the extent to which one feels that the problems and demands posed by the situation are worth investing energy in, are worthy of commitment, and are challenges for which meaning or purpose is sought, rather than viewed as burdens.

Manageability—the extent to which one perceives that resources at one's disposal are adequate to meet the demands posed by the stimuli present in the situation so that one does not feel victimized or treated unfairly (Artinian, 1997, p. 23).

The SSOC construct as used in the AIM identifies cognitions and behavioral responses to a specific illness situation. Burr (1991) suggested that processes that are specific, observable, and concrete are more amenable to change. Change can occur by introducing new coping strategies or presenting new information. However, because the changes are situation specific, the changes may not generalize to new situations. It is possible, though, that because crisis points are periods of time when normal life patterns are disrupted, individuals, families, institutions, or communities may be more open to suggestions for behavioral change that could translate into permanent change. Antonovsky supported this idea. In an unpublished manuscript, Antonovsky (1993b) wrote, "for any given person, a chance encounter, a courageous decision, or even an externally imposed change may initiate a considerable transformation of the level of SOC in either direction" (p. 15). The goal of the AIM is for a nurse or other healthcare provider to initiate a change in health behaviors in partnership with the client as measured by SSOC that will bring about an increased level of SOC.

SSOC Theory of Recovery

The relationship of SOC to SSOC is described in the SSOC Theory of Recovery. The straight line of normal life in the Hill Model is SOC. When a crisis event occurs that requires nursing assistance, the person and family enter a time of disorganization called SSOC. The response to the crisis event can be measured using the three constructs of comprehensibility, meaningfulness, and manageability. Any event occurring within the entire period of time of disorganization within the downward line of crisis and the angle of recovery can be measured by scoring on SSOC. The response of the person to nursing interventions and social support are measured at the end of the intervention by re-scoring the person on SSOC. The level of recovery may be lower or higher than the original level of SOC depending on the level of the adaptation made to the event that is measured by a score on SSOC. Those persons or families who achieve a higher level of SOC see themselves as more able to handle the challenges of life. These relationships are diagrammed in Figure 2.1.

SSOC and SOC in Chronic Health Conditions

The health care stressors that can be experienced range from acute short-term illness to stable disabling conditions to chronic illness to life-threatening illness. The SOC of a person with an acute illness would not change because the illness is seen as a temporary problem. Often the problem can be handled without the

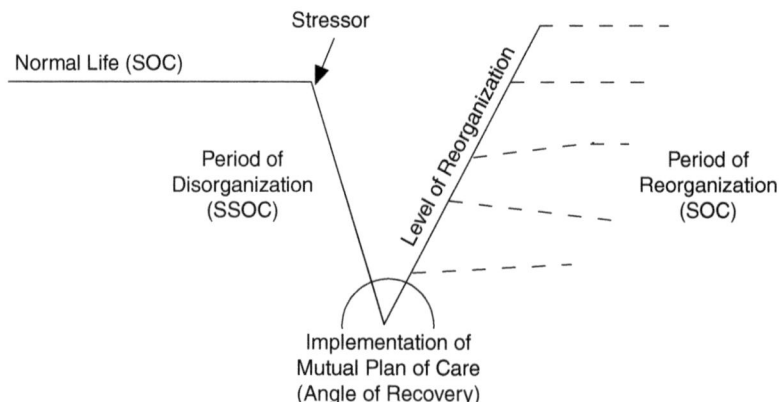

FIGURE 2.1 SSOC Theory of Recovery.
Copyright © 2011 B. Artinian. Adapted from Hill (1949).

TABLE 2.1 Conceptualization of Chronic Health Conditions

DIMENSION	SHORT-TERM CONDITIONS	LONG-TERM CONDITIONS		
		MODEL CASE	RELATED CASE	CONTRARY CASE
	ACUTE ILLNESS	CHRONIC ILLNESS	DISABLING CONDITION	LIFE-THREATENING ILLNESS
Cellular	Inflammation	Inflammation; degeneration	Destruction or atrophy	Proliferation
Time	Short	Long	Long	Short or long
Purpose of Treatment	Treatment to remove problem (e.g., cure)	Treatment to alleviate symptoms	Treatment to improve functioning	Treatment to kill cancer cells (i.e., cure)
Examples of immediate effect of treatment	Severe pain of surgery; immobility	Weight gain of prednisone therapy; dietary restrictions	Discomfort of splinting; pain of retraining muscles	Loss of hair; nausea; weight loss
Anticipated outcome	Cure expected	Cure not expected	Cure not expected	Cure hoped for or death
Trajectory	Short	Exacerbations and remissions; slow progressive decline; shortened life span	Steady	Remission or cure or death
Effect on ADLs	Severe during treatment; none after	Regimen required	Modifications required	Severe during treatment; none during remission or cure
Mental outlook	Temporary problem	Depression or challenge	Stigma or challenge	Fear or hope
Metaphorical interpretation	Temporary setback	Chain binding; a prisoner of uncertainty because body is unreliable	Obstacle to overcome	Sword hanging over head; a sentence

Source: Artinian (2011). Reprinted from *Community/Public Health Nursing: Promoting the Health of Populations* (p. 405), by M.A. Nies and M. McEwen, 2007, Oxford, UK: Elsevier. Copyright 2007 by B.Artinian. Reprinted with permission.

need for nursing intervention. When a long-term problem occurs, the impact on SOC is more pronounced. When the person experiences a disability such as blindness, deafness, or loss of a limb, the problem can be acute at first and the sense of being different affects the SOC of the person. If, over time, with effective interventions to aid in daily living, the person can develop a sense of self that integrates the disability and can view the disability as a challenge or obstacle to overcome. If the intervention is not successful, the person's precrisis level of SOC may not be achieved. Early intervention programs often assist in the integration of the disability into the self. The effects of chronic illness often appear slowly, and the person who uses appropriate denial can maintain a stable SOC over time. However, as the illness progresses, the person loses the sense of predictability of the body and therefore has a lower SOC. A team approach to partner with the patient during the SSOC event can provide continuity of care that can be of great help in restoring SOC. It is with a life-threatening illness that SOC is profoundly affected and the former way of life can no longer be maintained. With adequate assistance during the time in which SSOC is

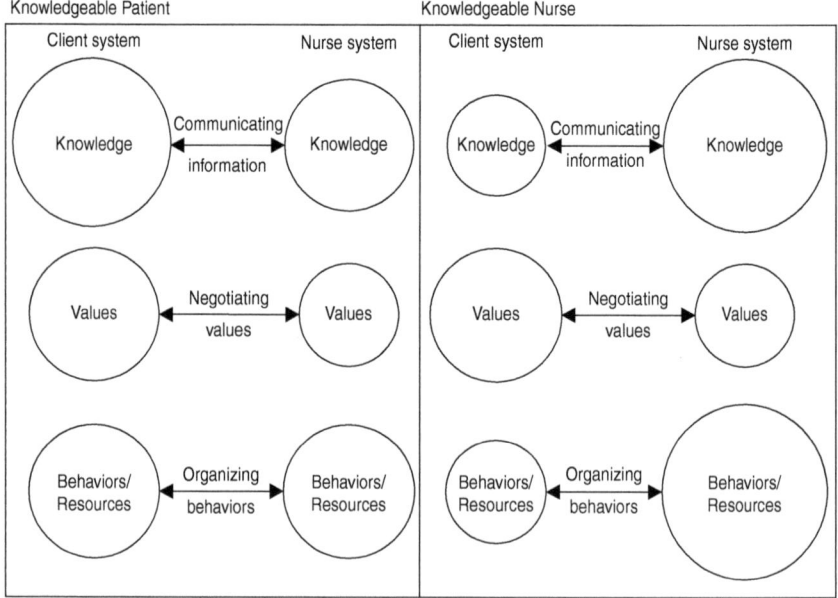

FIGURE 2.2 Knowledgeable client and knowledgeable nurse in the Artinian Intersystem Model.

Source: Artinian. Reprinted from *Community/Public Health Nursing: Promoting the Health of Populations* (p. 408), by M.A. Nies and M. McEwen, 2007, Oxford, UK: Elsevier. Copyright 2007 by B. Artinian. Reprinted with permission.

experienced, the person can move to hope and a renewed sense of self. The responses to each of these types of illness events are described in Table 2.1.

Different illness conditions provide different challenges for the nurse in attempting to increase the SOC of the patient. In acute illness, a person often draws on the knowledge of the nurse in an informal way. The nurse is often viewed as knowledgeable about a condition the person has not experienced before. In the case of a person with a long-term disability or chronic illness, the patient may view self as more knowledgeable than the nurse and may just need assistance with the manageability of the disability or chronic illness. A life-threatening illness usually is one that is outside of the experience of the patient and often of the family. Therefore, they rely on the knowledge of the nurse. The AIM acknowledges these differences in experience with a health care problem and provides a way for the nurse to examine his or her approach to the patient to enhance the patient's level of SOC. The relative shift in levels of knowledge that occurs between health care provider and patient with a long-term illness is illustrated in Figure 2.2.

Development of the SSOC Theory of Recovery

The SSOC theory of recovery was developed from the analysis of first person reports written by survivors of catastrophic life events. It was found that the person who experienced an adaptive response to the major life stressor went through the following stages.

1. Change from the normal SOC. There is an interruption of a normal, often unexamined life in which little thought is given to existential issues. For example, one cancer survivor said she was having a wonderful year in which she enjoyed her job and gave no thought to getting enough rest or eating properly, because she was living in the moment. This care free life changed abruptly when she was given the diagnosis of cancer.

2. Seeking comprehensibility. All attention is given to learning about the illness and finding the best treatment plan. Often this means enlisting the help of knowledgeable friends and family members. One mother reported that after her child was diagnosed with autism, she read everything she could find about autism and consulted leading specialists.

3. Accepting the meaningfulness of the treatment. The crisis is embraced as one that is worth the effort. In spite of the physical discomfort caused by the treatment or the time needed to overcome the problem, the survivor continues the treatment plan by focusing on the desired outcome,

such as being cancer free or the ability of a child with autism to function in society. The mother of the child with autism reported that she continued to work with her child over many years in spite of little initial response to her efforts.
4. Finding manageability. Outside resources and family members are enlisted to assist with the requirements for carrying out the treatment program. Emotional support is sought from health professionals, family, and peer support groups.
5. Resolution of the crisis. After experiencing the darkness of the crisis, survivors report that they look at life in a different way. They often report that their families become closer because of the crisis. One mother of a child with Down syndrome said "We were not really a family until Emily came". Cancer survivors often measure their success in overcoming the diagnosis by taking on new goals, such as running a marathon. The mother of the child with autism measured her success by her child's achievement of significant developmental markers, such as admission to university and getting a job.

This theory of recovery illustrates how it is possible to achieve a higher level of SOC following a major life event when appropriate support is available and there is determination to accept the challenges of the problem. For many persons who encounter a life event that dramatically changes the way life is managed, there is a need for planned intervention in order to bring about a positive change. The SSOC Theory of Recovery outlines the stages in the positive adaptation to a crisis event.

AN EARLY PREVENTION PROGRAM TO INCREASE SOC

Antonovsky believed that there is a need for treatment programs that are designed on salutogenic rather than on pathogenic assumptions. He suggested that an understanding of pathogenic programs would be useful in designing a treatment program based on salutogenic principles. Taylor (1997) summarized the characteristics of a pathogenic model of treatment based on his understanding of Trieschmann's ideas (1988, p. 32):

- There is an acute orientation in treatment.
- The person who is being treated is analyzed into parts.
- There is a fragmented approach to treatment.

- Only objective data are considered valid.
- The emphasis in treatment is on crisis intervention.
- Professionals are the only source of legitimate knowledge.
- Emphasis in the interpretation and diagnosis of behavior is on the abnormal.
- There is little coordination of services.
- Medical staff are the gatekeepers for all services.
- There is a focus on treatment in a hospital or in a clinic.
- The person who is being treated is the passive recipient of services.
- The emphasis is primarily on physical treatment. (Taylor, 1997, p. 180)

In addition, Taylor added more characteristics to this list based on his research. He found that the treatment staff held the power in the institution. He also found that staff members who provided physical care had more power than staff members who provided psychological or social therapy. He observed that patients had the least power. Because there was no input from patients, treatment team meetings, if held at all, were not effective. Therefore, there was little communication and coordination within the treatment team. He also observed that the emphasis of the treatment program was on the injured person rather than on the person as part of a family system that was also experiencing the trauma of the injury or illness. Therefore, the emphasis in follow-up was on the treatment of physical problems rather than on the psychological and social issues confronting the patient and the family. He found that boundaries between the different treatment disciplines were clearly defined and strictly enforced and that individual members of the treatment staff were only responsible for their defined area of expertise. He found that there was little emphasis on staff education training, particularly in the area of the psychological needs of the patient. Taylor summarized his observations in this way: "There was no sense of a broader shared responsibility within an integrated and systemic plan of treatment" (Taylor, 1997, p. 187).

In contrast to these characteristics of a treatment program based on a pathogenic model, a treatment program based on a salutogenic model has as entirely different perspective and is based on different assumptions. Some of the assumptions used in developing a salutogenic treatment program based on the Artinian Intersystem Model include the following:

- It is important to understand a person's experience of his or her illness.
- Stressors are always present in life, but they do not necessarily lead to physical and psychological pathology.

- The effect of a stressor depends on the person's perception of the stressor and on the ability to manage the stressor.
- A person's experience of treatment is a complex consequence of a series of processes occurring over time between interrelated biological, psychosocial, and spiritual subsystems and the continuing and changing relationships between each of these subsystems and the environment including the one in which a person is being treated.
- Increases in SSOC can facilitate recovery from illness.
- Treatment programs can be designed that facilitate increases in SOC by using salutogenic assumptions.

RECOMMENDATIONS FOR DEVELOPMENT OF INTERVENTION PROGRAMS TO INCREASE SOC

In 1997, Taylor published a series of recommendations for the development of an early intervention treatment program that would enhance the SOC of patients following a traumatic spinal cord injury. The recommendations grew out of his dissertation research experience as a clinical psychology student at the University of Wollongong, Australia. The focus of the research was on correlating the construct of SOC with other measurements of anger, state anxiety, trait anxiety, depression, and pain. The purpose was to identify the implications of SOC for the early treatment of people who had had a traumatic spinal cord injury. In addition to the psychometric measurements, Taylor also interviewed the patients about their experiences as patients in the program. Although his recommendations for a treatment program were based on the experience of spinal cord injured patients, they can be modified to provide direction for any rehabilitation program that is based on salutogenic principles. His recommendations for the treatment of the injured person (when appropriate) apply to family members as well.

Because Taylor based his recommendations for an intervention program on his understanding of the Artinian Intersystem Model, it is appropriate to use his recommendations in any person-to-person helping encounter when the goal is to develop a mutual plan of care. Taylor's (1997) recommendations integrate Antonovsky's ideas (1987) with those of Trieschmann (1988). They include a structure that is designed on the principles of the Intersystem Model (1991). Taylor's recommendations support the need for a paradigm shift in the design of treatment programs from the pathogenic model to the salutogenic model. The following characteristics of an Artinian Intersystem Model–based program have been abstracted from the discussion section of Taylor's dissertation and from the actual recommendations he made (Taylor, 1997).

Recommendation 1

Use the health care (or salutogenic) model rather than the medical (the pathogenic) model. "With the educational or health care model, rehabilitation is viewed as the process of teaching the person to live with his disability in his own environment. It is a learning process and everyone in the rehabilitation team functions as a teacher. The person must be an active participant in this process, and a rehabilitation program must be designed by the staff with, rather than for, the person in order to meet his needs. The emphasis is on partnership" (Trieschmann, 1988, p. 39).

Recommendation 2

Use a systems approach with a synthesis of parts into the whole. The focus in on interpersonal and environmental interactions.

Recommendation 3

Focus on problem prevention. "The emphasis in treatment is on education and training in health and wellness, activities of daily living, social skills and assertiveness, negotiation skills, financial survival, family, social, and sexual relationships, recreation and leisure, the management of personal care attendants, and vocational skills" (Trieschmann, 1988, p. 39). Both professionals and patients are the sources of knowledge.

Recommendation 4

Assume that the behavior of the patient is the normal consequence of the illness event and "care would be taken to understand, and not to place pathogenic interpretations on, normal processes such as anger grief, adaptive denial, and hope. Care would also be taken to help the injured person regain predictability, trust, and control" (Taylor, 1997, p. 196). The psychological consequences of a disability are considered to be normal rather than pathological or out of the ordinary. If emphasis is placed on pathology, it is possible to miss "positive psychological processes that are potentially invaluable in treatment and in recovery" (Taylor, 1997, p. 176).

Recommendation 5

Use a care manager to coordinate all services and provide for equal access to a variety of services in the community (Trieschmann, 1988).

Recommendation 6

Be sure that the person is an active participant in for planning for all health interventions. "The injured person would be given access to all information concerning him or her, including diagnoses and prognoses. Emphasis would be given to explaining this information so that it could be understood" (Taylor, 1997, p. 196).

Recommendation 7

Aim to strengthen the SSOC in the treatment process. Important physical and psychological consequences follow an emphasis on strengthening SOC during treatment. The person's SSOC can be determined early in the treatment program and the program can then be designed so that SSOC can be strengthened during treatment.

Recommendation 8

Identify level of SOC and strengthen it. Emphasis in treatment would be on identifying and strengthening important meanings in a person's life (meaning), on assisting the person to understand his or her illness or injury and its implications (comprehensibility), and on identifying and strengthening the person's skills and resources (manageability; Taylor, 1997, p. 192).

Recommendation 9

Distribute power within the treatment program so that the injured person is fully involved in decisions concerning his or her treatment. In addition, power should be distributed so that treatment decisions are not dominated by members of staff who are primarily involved in the physical or medical treatment of the patient, but the decisions are shared by patient and other staff members (Taylor, 1997, p. 196).

Recommendation 10

Educate patient and staff to reinforce patient self-care skills. Emphasis would be given to training the injured person. In addition, emphasis would also be given to the ongoing training of staff. This would include training in communication skills and in the skills of training and of teaching (Taylor, 1997, p. 197).

Recommendation 11

Obtain feedback about the treatment program. Emphasis would be given to obtaining ongoing feedback on all aspects of the treatment program. This feedback would be integrated into ongoing treatment. Emphasis would be given to encouraging discussion of the treatment program and its assumptions. At regular intervals, the assumption and aims of the treatment program would be reconsidered (Taylor, 1997, p. 197).

Recommendation 12

Create a long-term relationship with the patient. Emphasis would be given to creating a long-term (treatment) relationship with an injured person. In this relationship, emphasis would particularly be given to the integrated treatment of physical, psychological, and social issues, and to the preventative identification of potential problems at an early stage. Such a long-term emphasis would have implications for the selection of staff and for personnel policy (Taylor, 1997, p. 197).

Recommendation 13

Integrate acute and rehabilitation phases of treatment. Emphasis would be given to the development of an integrated relationship between the acute and rehabilitation phases of treatment. Emphasis would also be given to the development of long-term organizational memory and to the development of procedures to retrieve information from the organizational memory both for treatment and for research (Taylor, 1997, p. 198).

Recommendation 14

Design the treatment program to maximize the patient's successful adaptation. Emphasis would be given to treatment programs based on salutogenic assumptions to "maximize the person's possibility of adapting successfully to the disability and avoiding the iatrogenic problems that are inherent in a program designed on pathogenic assumptions" (Taylor, 1997, p. 199).

Recommendation 15

Collect data to direct the treatment program and allow for research. Taylor found that subtle changes occurred daily in the phenomenological experience of the participants. He wrote, "It would have been valuable, therefore, to have been able to record more interviews with participants, particularly at critical times during their treatment" (Taylor, 1997, p. 210).

TABLE 2.2 Summary of Taylor's Recommendations

TAYLOR'S RECOMMENDATIONS FOR DEVELOPING A SALUTOGENIC PROGRAM	
Recommendation 1	Use the salutogenic model
Recommendation 2	Use a systems approach
Recommendation 3	Focus on problem prevention
Recommendation 4	Assume that the behavior of the patient is a normal consequence of the illness event
Recommendation 5	Use a care manager to coordinate all services
Recommendation 6	Be sure that the patient is an active participant in planning for all health interventions
Recommendation 7	Aim to strengthen SSOC in the treatment process
Recommendation 8	Identify level of SOC and strengthen it
Recommendation 9	Distribute power so that the patient is fully involved in all decisions
Recommendation 10	Educate patient and staff to reinforce patient self-care skills
Recommendation 11	Obtain feedback about the treatment program
Recommendation 12	Create a long-term relationship with the patient
Recommendation 13	Integrate acute and rehabilitation phases of treatment
Recommendation 14	Design the treatment program to maximize the patient's successful adaptation
Recommendation 15	Collect data to direct the treatment program and allow for research

Source: Artinian (2011). Adapted from Taylor (1997).

DISCUSSION

Taylor's recommendations have been summarized by Artinian in brief statements that give the essence of each. These directives are shown in Table 2.2. The validity of these recommendations has been demonstrated by comparing the recommendations made by Taylor with the assumptions and practices of a very successful intervention program to prevent readmission of heart failure patients to the hospital that was developed by Laurie Carson and Louise Della Bella at the Saddleback Hospital, CA and is still in progress. Their heart failure management intervention program is based on the AIM. This program is described in Chapter 14. The validity of these recommendations has also been demonstrated in the development and management of the Ararat Nursing Facility resident-centered program for the elderly that is described in Chapter 15.

CONCLUSION

In this chapter, the concepts of SOC and SSOC have been explored. The work of Antonovsky, the SOC, has been expanded to measure a client's response in a time of crisis, SSOC. The SSOC Theory of Recovery is useful in the real world of nursing to describe how the client moves to a new level of SOC following effective interventions by the care provider. An example is given to show how a patient can move to a higher level of SOC through salutogenic interventions. Recommendations for a treatment program designed to increase SOC in patients with a spinal cord injury that were developed by Taylor (1997) are summarized. These recommendations can be used in any treatment program that has the goal of including the patient in planning of care.

REFERENCES

Antonovsky, A. (1987). *Unraveling the mystery of health: How people manage stress and stay well.* San Francisco, CA: Jossey-Bass.

Antonovsky, A. (1993a). The implications of salutogenesis: An outsider's view. In A. Turner, J. Patterson, S. Behr, D. Murphy, J. Marquis, & M. Blue-Banning (Eds.), *Cognitive coping, families, and disability* (pp. 111–122). Baltimore, MD: Brooks.

Antonovsky, A. (1993b). *The sense of coherence: An historical perspective.* Unpublished manuscript.

Antonovsky, A. (1993c). The structure and properties of the sense of coherence scale. *Social Science and Medicine, 36,* 725–733.

Artinian, B. (1991). The development of the intersystem model. *Journal of Advanced Nursing, 16,* 194–205.

Artinian, B. (1997). Situational sense of coherence: Development and measurement of the construct. In B. Artinian & M. Conger (Eds.), *The intersystem model: Integrating theory and practice* (pp. 18–30). Thousand Oaks, CA: Sage Publications.

Burr, W. (1991). Rethinking levels of abstraction in family systems theories. *Family Process, 30,* 435–452.

Hill, R. (1949). *Families under stress.* New York, NY: Harper & Row.

Nies, M. A., & McEwen, M. (2007). *Community/public health nursing: Promoting the health of populations* (4th ed.). St. Louis, MO: Elsevier Science.

Taylor, D. (1997). *The implications of sense of coherence for the early treatment of people who have had a traumatic spinal cord injury.* Doctoral dissertation, University of Wollongong, Wollongong, Australia.

Trieschmann, R. B. (1988). *Spinal cord injuries: Psychological, social, and vocational rehabilitation.* New York, NY: Demos.

3

DEVELOPING A SENSE OF COHERENCE: THE DEVELOPMENTAL ENVIRONMENT

Katharine S. West and Barbara M. Artinian

THE PERSON'S SENSE *of coherence* (SOC) as defined by Antonovsky (1987) strongly influences the orientation the person has to life as being comprehensible, meaningful, and manageable. This orientation to life constitutes the way in which the world is viewed. It is the "integrative and interpretative framework" for judging life events and "the standard by which reality is managed and pursued" (Olthuis, 1989, p. 29). As such, it has a major impact on the health beliefs and practices held by individuals and aggregates.

A worldview is socially acquired within a cultural community through the process of socialization and is shared by that community. Children learn this worldview during the process of socialization. In the Artinian Intersystem Model (AIM), the developmental environment is the term for the arena in which a person's worldview is acquired. The purpose of this chapter is to describe the formative processes by which a person transforms a social environment through his or her particular biological, psychosocial, and spiritual subsystems at each stage of maturational development to become the person who enters the health care delivery system.

Antonovsky has identified particular times of life that are more specific to development of SOC. The first of these is infancy and childhood. Erikson talks about the crises and challenges of this period as "a succession of potentialities" (1959, p. 52). Antonovsky says what is crucial in these potentialities is the "extent to which something happens and its consequences" (1987, p. 95). Antonovsky states that the child over time "may become persuaded that his or her world, physical and social, can be counted on not to be constantly changing" (1987, p. 52). To the extent that this happens, the child develops a view of the world as comprehensible. When an infant or child's actions bring about a desired outcome, it can be said that there is participation in decision making and this brings about a sense of meaningfulness. When the demands from the internal and external environment do not underload or overload the child, the child can view the world as manageable.

The next important period for the development of SOC is adolescence. Erikson says that at this time, "The central problem confronting an adolescent in all cultures is to put one's act together, to develop a defined personality within a social reality which one understands and to derive a vitalizing sense of reality from the awareness that his individual way of mastering experience is a successful variant of the way other people around him master experience and recognize such mastery" (1959, p. 89). Antonovsky identifies the three components of SOC in these statements. He says the crucial question is to ask to what extent "the cultural context and the social-structural reality impede or facilitate the life experiences" (1987, p. 102).

The final phase in the formation of SOC is young adulthood. The adolescent may have attained a tentative strong sense of SOC that is useful for short-range planning, but it is in the entry into adulthood with its long-range commitments that the experiences of childhood and adolescence are reinforced or even reversed. Antonovsky believes it is in this period that "one's location on the SOC continuum becomes more or less fixed" (1987, p. 107). By entry into the adult role, an identity and career choices provide the experiences that make the world comprehensible, manageable, and meaningful.

THE CULTURAL CONTEXT OF DEVELOPMENT

Leininger (1991) defines culture as the "learned, shared, and transmitted values, beliefs, norms, and life practices of a particular group that guide thinking, decisions, and actions in patterned ways" (p. 147). Because each culture is shaped by particular social, economic, and geographical realities, each has a different pattern of values, beliefs, norms, and life practices. It follows, therefore, that each cultural group has a different frame of reference for viewing health and health care. In addition, individuals within a culture also view health and health care differently from others within their own cultural group because of their unique characteristics. For example, socioeconomic status allows differential access to health care, and specific biological and social characteristics provide different experiences in social interaction.

The cultural orientation of both the client and the nurse influences the clinical encounter, either overtly or covertly, with implications for successful health outcomes dependent on the health care provider's awareness of and willingness to provide culturally competent care. The National Standards for Culturally and Linguistically Appropriate Services in Health Care Final Report define cultural and linguistic competence as "the ability to respect the beliefs, language, interpersonal styles, and behaviors of individuals, families and communities receiving services as well as the health care professionals who provide the services" (USDHHS OMH, 2001). The Cultural Competence Project (2010) Web site explains that cultural competence is important to nursing practice because, in order to eliminate disparities in health outcomes for all segments of the population, nurses must be able to communicate with their patients/clients, understand what constitutes illness within the background of their cultures, and mutually decide upon appropriate nursing care that is evidence-based and culturally competent. The AIM provides a framework for the assessment, planning, and delivery of health care that is congruent with the patient's cultural health beliefs and supports the needs identified earlier.

Patients are more likely to be compliant and adhere to a plan of care to resolve their main concern when their cultural health beliefs and their input are included when designing the plan of care (Adeniran, 2008, p. 124). Adeniran further emphasizes variables beyond the health care provider's willingness, knowledge, and skill in providing culturally competent care, because the employer organization or agency also has a major role to play by providing an infrastructure of policies, procedures, and resources to support and sustain clinical practice. When the organization provides the foundations and expectations for culturally competent care and the nurse engages the patient in a dialogue over health beliefs while providing consideration for these beliefs in the plan of care, studies show that health disparities can be reduced and outcomes improved (p. 124). Adeniran reported evidence-based research studies that linked providers' cultural competence with "better health outcomes, higher quality of health services, increased access to health care services, and more satisfied health care consumers" (p. 128).

THE SUBSYSTEMS OF PERSON

When a person enters the health care delivery system, the nurse evaluates the effects of the developmental environment by assessing the client's biological, psychosocial, and spiritual subsystems. Each of the subsystems will be described in terms of the components of the subsystem. For a depiction of the subsystems see Figure 1.3.

The Biological Subsystem

Conger (1997) states that the "human body is a unity of interrelated biological subsystems that corporately maintain all the physiological functions needed for life" (p. 64). A systems approach to understanding how each subsystem is controlled and how it interacts with both the internal and external environment is used in the AIM. The body's subsystems are divided into the following:

> Regulatory subsystem (includes neurological, endocrine, and immune subsystems)
> Circulatory and respiratory subsystem
> Musculoskeletal subsystem
> Gastrointestinal subsystem
> Renal subsystem
> Reproductive subsystem

Each subsystem functions under a series of control mechanisms so that a constant internal environment is maintained. When a control mechanism ceases to function, or has diminished function, homeostasis is disrupted and a pathological event can occur. In addition to responding to the internal environment of the body in order to maintain homeostasis in the body, many of the subsystems are open to inputs from the external environment. There are cultural values and practices associated with the biological subsystems and differences exist both between cultural groups and within groups.

The subsystems contribute to the overall vitality and appearance of the person. Because the response to visible physical characteristics forms the matrix of human interaction, personal appearance greatly influences the feedback a person receives from others and therefore the sense of self. Just as others respond to a person's biological makeup, the person also responds to self as a person. Mead (1934) describes this as the "I" reflecting on the "me" as the person learns to treat self as an object. For this reason, Kuhn (1974) considers the person's biological system to be his or her internal environment because "the individual learns and makes decisions about his own body by the same processes as for the world outside his skin" (p. 40). Cultural values of what is appropriate appearance are internalized and then person views self through the same lens as the dominant culture, even if that means devaluing of self. Thus, the child with an acceptable appearance grows up in a very different maturational environment from the handicapped or physically less appealing child.

The Psychosocial Subsystem

The psychosocial subsystem of the person is the social self of the person that relates to self and others. It includes the cognitive subsystem, which processes information, the affective subsystem, which "displays feeling and emotions mediated through values" (England, 1997, p. 83), and the interactional subsystem, which organizes behavior in established patterns. England (1997) writes

> The unique configuration of the psychosocial domain of human experience emerges from experience within and across all domains of experience. The interplay of experiences within other domains of experience provides feedback to the affected domain so that it can further pattern itself. (p. 83)

Through examining the "pattern of life experiences" that takes place within societal and historical conditions (Antonovsky, 1987, p. 91), the person develops self-awareness.

Self-awareness is made up of all of those things that we know about ourselves—where we invest our energies, where we devote our time, where we derive our satisfactions, where we meet out greatest frustrations, what we strive for, what we consider to be "us" (Furhmann & Carson, 1996, p. 154).

The development of the self and the self-concept begins in infancy and continues developing over the course of life resulting in the level of SOC experienced by the person. This development will be described in greater detail in the context of development within the family.

The Spiritual Subsystem

The spiritual subsystem lies at the heart of the description of person in the AIM. It is the spiritual center of the person that answers such questions as "Who am I? Where am I going? What's it all about" (Olthuis, 1989, p. 29). It is the center that allows the person to connect with God and find meaning in life's circumstances. Furhmann and Carson (1996) write

Within the spiritual self reside beliefs about the universe, our place in it, and feelings of transcendence, joy, hopefulness, and love. The spiritual self is expressed through behaviors of selflessness, commitment, moral decisions, choice, self-discipline, honesty, and reverence for God, or a higher power as defined by the person. (p. 164)

Spiritual beliefs develop in interaction with others within a particular culture and provide a basis for the person's fundamental decision-making process in life situations. They are expressed in specific religious practices. Life events are processed through the spiritual subsystem and produce either spiritual well-being or spiritual distress. In the AIM, spiritual is used as the descriptor for the inner center of the person. Emblem states that "religious practices will flow out of that center in expressions of the internal spiritual system" (1997, p. 107).

A series of questions have been developed to help the nurse assess the patient responses associated with the biological, psychosocial, and spiritual subsystems and also her own responses (Table 3.1). The answers to these questions may help the nurse clarify the main concern.

TABLE 3.1 Questions to Assess Biological, Psychosocial, and Spiritual Subsystems

PATIENT/CLIENT	NURSE
Comprehensibility What does client know about physical symptoms, treatment, prognosis, or resources available for management of the Main Concern?	*Comprehensibility* How much information does the nurse have about the client problem and the cultural, developmental, or role characteristics of the client and his or her significant networks?
Meaningfulness What attitudes, values, and beliefs does the client have that may influence a plan of care or provide strength to face the Main Concern?	*Meaningfulness* What biases does the nurse have that may affect the plan of care? What attitudes, values, and beliefs does the nurse have that provide strength to assist the client?
Manageability What coping strategies, role relationships, technical skills, or religious practices does the client have that will influence the carrying out of plan of care?	*Manageability* What behaviors does the nurse manifest that may affect the interrelation, such as fatigue, shyness, technical skills, religious beliefs, supportive role relationships?

Source: Adapted from Artinian, B. (1991). The development of the Intersystem Model, *Journal of Advanced Nursing, 8*, 202.

IDENTIFYING THE MAIN CONCERN

Bertalanffy (1968) described a system as being that which provides an overall structure so that parts that are not directly connected to each other can be integrated into an organized whole. When a person or family enters the health care system for assistance with a specific concern, the biological, psychosocial, and spiritual subsystems of that individual or family present themselves in a unique way. Nurses skilled in the use of the AIM can assess and incorporate this information into their client assessments and identify the main concern based on their analysis of the information. For example, by examining each of the subsystems, the nurse can correctly assess that the cause of distress for a particular patient is spiritual rather than psychosocial when the person is experiencing a challenge to a belief or value system.

After doing the initial assessment, through further interaction with the patient, the main concern is identified. When identifying the main concern of the interaction, the concern can be that of either the patient or the nurse. In some cases, the concern that the patient has may be based on an incorrect perception of the situation. In that case, the concern of the nurse forms the basis of the interaction that takes place in the situational environment so that resolution of the real concern is possible and the patient's SOC is enhanced.

DISCUSSION

The development of the individual is influenced by many factors at each stage of development. Some of these are the personal goals of individuals, their genetic makeup, their emotional and rational characteristics, their ethical or religious inclinations, their interactional processes within a culture, and the contextual constraints of the culture. These factors work together to form the individual who enters into interaction with the nurse or health care provider. It is through the process of living that individuals discover who they are and what is important to them. This is their worldview that gives "reason and impetus for deciding what is true and what really matters in our experience" (Olthuis, 1989, p. 20). Two outcomes of a particular worldview that are especially important in the health care delivery system are the orientation a person has to life as being comprehensible, meaningful, and manageable, and the formulation of a health belief system.

As children mature within a particular social community, their educational, work, and family experiences will shape how they view the world. If their life experiences have been consistent, they will view the world as comprehensible; if there has been a balance between responsibilities, they will view their world as manageable; and if there has been the opportunity to participate in important decision-making, their SOC will be strengthened. This view of the world shapes the appraisal of a particular illness experience and guides the person's response to it.

The health belief model offers an explanation of how health behaviors and attitudes toward health influence the delivery of care. It includes concepts such as perceived seriousness, perceived susceptibility, and cue to action (Becker, 1974). It incorporates many responses to the health-illness situation, such as how individuals conceptualize physical and mental health or illness; what their beliefs are about ways to prevent illness or promote health; what they think causes illness and their ideas about how to treat illness; their preferences for self-care and home remedies; their use of lay healers or professional health providers; and their ways of describing or expressing illness.

It is through an understanding of the factors influencing development experienced through the biological, psychosocial, and spiritual subsystems of the person, the family, the institution, the community, and state/nation/world that nurses are able to understand the worldview of the clients. Such an understanding helps them to provide culturally appropriate care. It helps them to understand aspects of culture such as the meaning of special verbal and nonverbal communication styles, the meaning of space and time to the client, the hierarchal organization of the culture, and an orientation to nature that is fatalistic, harmonious, or seeking to master it (Giger & Davidhizar, 1991). This knowledge makes it possible to mutually plan and implement health care with the client in a culturally perceptive manner.

INTRODUCTION TO ONLINE CARE PLAN

Mary Barkman has prepared a care plan that illustrates the integration of the biological, psychosocial, and spiritual subsystems. A patient who had been recently diagnosed with breast cancer needed to decide which of two radically different approaches to treatment she should follow. She was able to examine her alternatives through conversation with a nurse friend who was a member of her church and was able to come to a resolution of her problem. The full text of the care plan is available online (see Care Plan 3.1).

CONCLUSION

Although this chapter has focused primarily on the influences that have shaped the individual, the same influences shape the social groups within the culture because they are made up of individuals socialized within that culture who experience development over time. By focusing on an understanding of the developmental world of the clients from their perspective and on an understanding of the nurse/provider shaped by a particular culture, an ongoing process of negotiation is possible within the health care delivery situation that is carried out in the situational environment.

REFERENCES

Adeniran, R. K., & Watts, R. (2008). Developing cultural competence in long-term care nursing. In E. Sullivan-Marx & D. Gray-Miceli (Eds.), *Leadership and management skills for long-term care.* New York, NY: Springer Publishing.

Antonovsky, A. (1987). *Unraveling the mystery of health: How people manage stress and stay well.* San Francisco, CA: Jossey-Bass.

Becker, M. H. (Ed.). (1974). *The health belief model and personal health behavior.* Thorofare, NJ: Slack.

Bertalanffy, L. (1968). *General systems theory.* New York, NY: George Braziller.

Conger, M. (1997). Theoretical foundations for the biological subsystem. In B. Artinian & M. Conger (Eds.), *The Intersystem Model: Integrating theory and practice.* Thousand Oaks, CA: Sage Publications.

Cultural Competence Project. (2010). *Frequently Asked Questions.* Retrieved from http://www.cultural-competence-project.org/en/faq.htm

Emblem, J. (1997). Theoretical foundations for the spiritual subsystem. In B. Artinian & M. Conger (Eds.), *The Intersystem Model: Integrating theory and practice.* Thousand Oaks, CA: Sage Publications.

England, M. (1997). Theoretical foundations for the psychosocial domain of human experience. In B. Artinian & M. Conger (Eds.), *The Intersystem Model: Integrating theory and practice.* Thousand Oaks, CA: Sage Publications.

Erikson, E. H. (1959). Growth and crises of the healthy personality. *Psychological Issues, 1*(1), 50–100.

Furhmann, J., & Carson, V. (1996). Shared attributes of every traveler: The mosaic of self-concept. In V. Carson & E. Arnold (Eds.), *Mental health nursing: The nurse-patient journey.* Philadelphia, PA: W.B. Saunders.

Giger, J., & Davidhizar, R. (1991). *Transcultural nursing.* St. Louis, MO: C.V. Mosby Year Book.

Kuhn, A. (1974). *The logic of social systems: A unified deductive system-based approach to social science.* San Francisco, CA: Jossey-Bass.

Leininger, M. (Ed.). (1991). *Culture care diversity and universality: A theory of nursing.* New York, NY: National League for Nursing Press.

Mead, G. (1934). *Mind, self, and society*. Chicago, IL: University of Chicago Press.

Olthuis, J. (1989). On worldviews. In P. Marshall, S. Griffioen, & R. Lieuw (Eds.), *Stained glass, worldviews, and social science*. New York, NY: University Press of America.

US Department of Health and Human Services Office of Minority Health (USDHHS OMH). (2001). *National standards for culturally and linguistically appropriate services in health care: Final Report*. Washington, DC: Government Printing Office. Retrieved from http://minorityhealth.hhs.gov/assets/pdf/checked/finalreport.pdf

4

THE CONTEXT OF INVOLVEMENT: THE SITUATIONAL ENVIRONMENT

Barbara M. Artinian

It is in the situational environment that nurse and patient/client meet. All the unique characteristics of the nurse and of the client as well as the characteristics of the setting interact to make the experience what it is. Different nurses with differing life experiences would make the encounter a different type of experience for a particular client, as would different characteristics of the client or the setting. Using the Artinian Intersystem Model (AIM), each nurse would attempt to understand the concerns that the client is experiencing and work with him or her within the constraints of a particular setting to resolve the main concern. This is done as nurse and client work together to communicate information, negotiate values, and organize behaviors. The goal is to enhance the client's *sense of coherence* (SOC). This goal is influenced and modified by the quality of intersystem interaction in the situational environment.

The situational environment, as defined in the AIM, encompasses all the details of the encounter between the nurse and the client. Included in these details are the time, place, circumstances, resources available, and the rapport and trust between the nurse and client. Awareness of the needs of others, the ability to do active listening, and the degree of ambiguity in the situation influence the encounter. Situational constraints of the particular environment also influence the repertoire of behaviors that a person uses and limit the outcomes available. The AIM provides a systematic way for nurse and client to come together to explore the definitions of the present situation to negotiate a plan of care for the client that is acceptable to both client and nurse. Resolution of the main concern is measured by changes in the client's *situational sense of coherence* (SSOC).

CHARACTERISTICS OF CLIENT

Although each client brings a different mindset to the interaction, some characteristics are especially important to consider. Glaser and Strauss (1965) have found that the social value of a client greatly influences the interaction. For example, an infant is seen as having greater social value than an elderly person or a person with celebrity status has greater social value than an indigent client. The level of SOC of the client also influences the interaction. Antonovsky (1987) states that a client with a high SOC is better able to manage stress than a person with a low SOC. The level of self-esteem of the client is also important.

How the client approaches the main concern is very important. Some clients are very knowledgeable about the concern whereas others have little knowledge. Some clients come to the interaction with firm opinions about how it should be handled whereas others are willing to accept guidance. Clients may experience a stressful health event as one of uncertainty or danger or alternatively, may deny its existence. In addition, the mental ability of the client greatly influences the type of interaction that is possible. Family support and cultural and religious practices must be considered in any interaction.

CHARACTERISTICS OF CHANGE AGENT

To carry out intersystem interaction, the nurse or change agent must be an effective communicator. Arnold (1996) identifies several characteristics of an effective communicator. Among the most important is the ability of the nurse to be aware of his or her personal communication style and its effect on rapport with the client so that information about the main concern can be gathered. Included in this is an awareness of the needs of others. Arnold (1996) writes "Reaching another human being through a therapeutic conversation involves not simply talking to the other about a problem, or need, but actually being with the other in understanding and resolving the barriers to successful realization of the journey's potential" (p. 194).

Another important factor in the negotiation of values carried out by the nurse and client is recognition of the inequality of power between them. Knickrehm (1994) has developed a theory of inequality in social interactions within the perspective of symbolic interactionism. Because symbolic interaction is "an on-going process involving actors who are communicating their interpretations of the meaning of whatever is being communicated, and their definitions of the situation of the interaction" (Blumer, 1969, p. 66), it is apparent that each actor will have a different definition. Actions taken by the actors are based on their interpretation of their own definition of the situation and on their interpretation of the perception of the other party's definition of the situation. Knickrehm (1994) refers to the synthesis of the definitions brought to and emerging from an interaction as the staging of the interaction process. The factor affecting the staging is the awareness context of the participants, which Knickrehm says is derived from their identities that are developed prior to the interaction (i.e., in the developmental environment). These are "structural properties of social interaction which circumscribe the range of possibilities for human behavior available in any interaction...and shape the interaction" (Knickrehm, 1994, p. 11).

The outcome of the interaction process is a mutual definition of the situation that Knickrehm calls a negotiated awareness context. Because each person has a unique self, no two persons have the same awareness context. Knickrehm (1994) writes, "Their awareness contexts will differ on the basis of their prior experiences, as these experiences have come to shape their selves" (p.13). Through manipulations of the awareness context, a mutual definition emerges. Because of the differing ability of each to manipulate the resultant definition, however, one person may have more input into the mutual definition than the other. In other words, one person may be more powerful than the other if power is defined as the ability to do something. Knickrehm writes, "power is rooted in the differential abilities of actors to manipulate the mutual definition of the interaction situation" (p. 14). Power must be considered as a dimension of interaction. Knickrehm further states:

> A person's position in a status hierarchy has an effect on that person's interactions, because definition of the interaction situation status is based on that person's status as perceived by others. This serves to mobilize the ways in which the persons respond to each other. Thus, power, and so inequality, is not only derived from the process of the formation of self. It is an interactive part of this formation. Inequality, that state in society in which one status is relatively lower than another status, is indeed a quality inherent to social life. (p. 16)

This is an important consideration in attempting to develop a mutual plan of care in the AIM. The nurse, because of a greater knowledge of the medical aspects of care and institutional polices as well as a more dominant position within the care giving environment, will have a greater ability to steer the mutual definition of the situation. The purpose of the model is to make it possible to participate in the planning of care on a more equal basis. This is done by reducing the inequality of power distribution and promoting equality by attending to the values of the patient through giving information and by providing the patient with the skills and resources needed to resolve the main concern.

CHARACTERISTICS OF THE SETTING

Although the interpersonal factors in an interaction are important, it is no longer sufficient to merely examine the patient's and nurse's attitudes about a situation without examining the institutional structure and environmental climate of the surroundings in the setting in which care is administered. Strauss (1978) identified three factors that affect the outcomes of negotiation between individuals: (a) structure (the larger societal level within which negotiations take place; (b) process (the ways of getting things accomplished); and (c) the negotiation context (the "relevant features of the setting which directly enter into negotiations and affect their course") (p. 101).

The structural context includes the stable features of an organization that are the background through which people interact, such as organizational size, type of leadership, rules and policies, organizational goals, degree of professionalization of staff, and focus of resource allocation. Process includes the types of interactions used by persons in the setting, such as bargaining, compromising, fighting, and colluding. The actual negotiation context includes those aspects of the situation that directly affect the negotiation, such as the extent to which information is shared, personal goals, hidden agendas, limited budget, amount of time available, the participants' emotional state and relative power position, and the immediate situational context. Each of these factors will influence the outcome of the negotiations and produce what Strauss (1978) has called the negotiated order. The societal expectations for the particular structural context influence how each of the persons in the setting will react. The relationships between the individuals in negotiation and the structural organization have been diagrammed by Artinian and depicted in Figure 4.1.

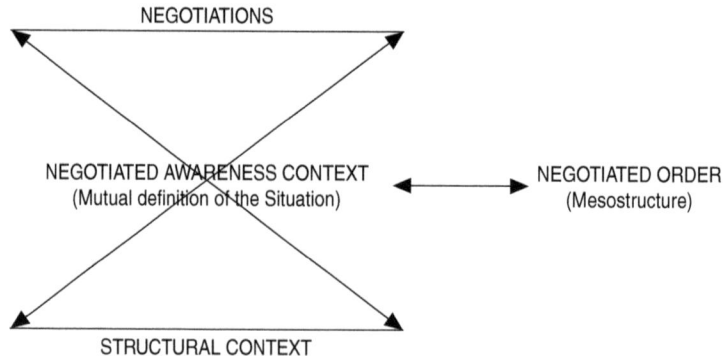

FIGURE 4.1 Negotiated order.
Source: Artinian (1997). Adapted from Strauss, A. (1978). *Negotiations*. San Francisco, CA: Jossey-Bass.

Maines (1979) has extended the concept of negotiated order to show how negotiation contributes to the formation of social order and how social order influences the negotiation process. He used the term *mesostructure* to describe the domain in which the dialectical activity takes place between subject and object (negotiation and social order) to form the domain of subject–domain unity. He says that the mesostructure (or negotiated order) is the domain in which the negotiation process takes place that mediates between the organizational structure and interacting person. It is the domain between the interactional and the structural aspects of the situation.

Because the workplace is the context of the negotiated order, it can be seen that the work setting in which nurses practice can possess great power to enhance or inhibit practitioner function. The particular management style and the level of bureaucracy and technology can inhibit the ability of the nurse to understand and communicate with the patient so that they can identify the main concern in the patient situation and work on resolving it. The negotiated order can only be achieved when there is an awareness of the power differential between nurse and patient and the nurse seeks to minimize its effect.

The environment of a specific health care setting has considerable effect on the nurse–patient interaction. Because health care today has shifted its focus from acute care to outpatient or community-based care, nurses need to learn to function in environments in which the nurse–patient interaction has very different dynamics. A few examples of the effect that differences in the clinical setting have on interaction will be given:

- Nurses working in home settings work in an environment in which the patient is in control and often families of patients base their care on their own best judgment and the resources available to them. This shift in power from a hospital setting requires an adjustment that the nurse must make.
- In contrast, nurses working in an intensive care unit (ICU) have a disproportionate amount of power because of the patient's vulnerability and health status and the nurse's knowledge and familiarity with the setting.
- Nurses working in an oncology setting are faced with the many physical and emotional needs of the patient and family and see themselves as being on the front line against death and suffering.
- In a forensic hospital, nurses see themselves as working with patients who may be unpredictable and sometimes not able to manage their care. Nurses have the keys to locked wards and must enforce control and adherence to rules and policies while attempting to maintain a therapeutic caring environment in which patients can be healed.

CHARACTERISTICS OF INTERACTION IN THE SITUATIONAL ENVIRONMENT

The characteristics of the client, change agent, and the setting come together at a particular point in time for a particular health-related concern. These characteristics influence the ability of the client and change agent to resolve the main concern.

Each situation has its own set of meanings to the persons involved that cannot be anticipated by another. Blumer (1969) developed the theory of symbolic interaction to study the interaction between two or more persons that takes into account the meaning they have assigned to it. He has identified the following three premises.

1. People act on the basis of the meaning a situation has for them.
2. Meaning is not absolute; it is socially derived.
3. Social symbols are interpreted through the person's thought process. (Kollock & O'Brien, 1994, p. 54)

The personal concerns of the individual will determine the issues of importance in any given situation (Benner & Wrubel, 1989). The meaning of an illness is more than just the immediate situation that the illness brings. It is the responsibility of the change agent to gain information about the whole context of the situation precipitated by the illness. Benner and Wrubel say that the impact that the illness will have on the person's expectation, goals, and dreams will have an impact on the response to it (p. 15). In addition, the person's understanding of the situation, the meaning attached to it and the resources available will determine the lines of action and possibilities that are available to the patient. The nurse must understand these possibilities from the patient's perspective in order to negotiate values with the patient. Operating from a position of power, the nurse must be careful not to impose personal attitudes and values in the negotiation process.

NURSE–PATIENT INTERACTION TO RESOLVE THE MAIN CONCERN

Use of the AIM in interaction between client and nurse provides a process to encourage mutuality. The nurse and client may meet for the first time as strangers or they may have an established relationship. In either case, the main concern of the patient/client must be explored by assessing the knowledge, the values and beliefs, and the behaviors the patient/client has in relation to the main concern. The situational constraints of the particular environment determine the repertoire of behaviors that can be used and limit the outcomes available as nurses attempt to resolve the main concern of the patient or nurse. Friesen (1999) found this to be true in her study of caregiving behaviors of intrapartum nurses. She found that nurses formed resistive, restrictive, or involved relationships with their patients depending on factors in the situational environment (see Care Plan 16.5). Friesen's study is reported in the book Glaserian grounded theory in nursing research: Trusting Emergence (Artinian, Giske, & Cone, 2009).

The nurse has the primary responsibility for establishing a relationship with the patient. The patient approaches the interaction because of a need for assistance and it is important for the nurse to assess the coping strategies the patient has for resolving the main concern. It is also important for the nurse to assess what the patient knows about the concern, the interpretation of the situation, and what the patient believes an appropriate treatment would be.

When the nurse has completed the intrasystem analysis of the intrasystem mindset for both patient and nurse and the main concern has been identified, the nurse assesses the ability of the client and nurse to work together to resolve the main concern. Factors that can affect this ability include the nature of the main concern, the interpersonal climate between the nurse and client, and barriers in the setting. If the nurse determines that the client and nurse can work together to resolve the main concern, intersystem interaction begins. By communicating information and negotiating values, goals and strategies are developed and a mutual plan of care is determined. After the strategies are implemented, the plan is evaluated by rescoring on SSOC. If the main concern has been resolved no further intervention is needed for that concern and the nurse and client can work on a new concern if it occurs. On the other hand, if the concern has not been resolved, the nurse must do a new analysis of the intrasystems as a basis for new intersystem interaction. In either case, the interaction that took place to resolve the main concern becomes part of the developmental environment for both the client and nurse.

CONCLUSION

When the AIM is used to direct nursing practice, the nurse and patient come together to clarify their understandings of the situation and negotiate mutually agreed upon goals. In this highly symbolic, meaningful interaction, values are negotiated and behaviors are organized to develop a joint plan of care. This process leads to increasing the SOC of the patient, thus enhancing the patient's health.

The patient may be unaware of the nature of the stressful health event and may view the main concern to be something that is peripheral to the problem. For example, in the care plan presented in Chapter 1 (see Care Plan 1.2), the patient's main concern was to prevent addiction to narcotics whereas the main concern of the nurse was pain management so that the patient could ambulate and do deep breathing exercises. The nurse used the process of the AIM to educate the patient about the benefits of pain alleviation and to negotiate an acceptable plan. The cognitive state of the patient may also disrupt his or her capacity to adequately understand and manage the situation, particularly when patients are uncertain about outcomes. In this case, their ability to make plans for their life situation may be hindered. Therefore, all the skills of the nurse in communication and negotiation must be used so that a plan of care that is mutually acceptable can be worked out that can increase the SSOC of the patient. When a trust relationship develops, the patient and nurse can work together so that the patient can regain or increase the prior level of SOC and maintain an optimal level of health in the context of the threatening illness.

REFERENCES

Antonovsky, A. (1987). *Unraveling the mystery of health: How people manage stress and stay well.* San Francisco, CA: Jossey-Bass.

Arnold, E. (1996). Points of intersection: Therapeutic communication. In V. Carson & E. Arnold, *Mental health nursing: The nurse-patient journey.* Philadelphia, PA: W. B. Saunders.

Artinian, B. (1997). *The Intersystem Model: Integrating theory and practice.* Thousand Oaks, CA: Sage Publications.

Benner, P., & Wrubel, J. (1989). *The primacy of caring.* Menlo Park, CA: Addison-Wesley.

Blumer, H. (1969). *Symbolic interactionism.* Englewood Cliffs, NJ: Prentice Hall.

Friesen, M. (1999). *Intrapartum nurses' perceptions of their care-giving behaviors with laboring patients.* Unpublished master's thesis, Azusa Pacific University, Azusa, CA.

Friesen, M. (2009). Caregiving behaviors of intrapartum nurses. In B. Artinian, T. Giske, & P. Cone, *Glaserian grounded theory in nursing research: Trusting emergence* (pp. 95–106). New York, NY: Springer Publishing.

Glaser, B. G., & Strauss, A. (1965). *Awareness of dying.* Chicago, IL: Aldine Publishing.

Kollock, P., & O'Brian, J. (1994). *The production of reality.* Thousand Oaks, CA: Pine Forge Press.

Knickrehm, B. (1994, August). *The origins of inequality: A theoretical synthesis.* Paper presented at the 1994 American Sociological Association Meeting, Los Angeles, CA.

Maines, C. (1979). Mesostructure and social process. *Contemporary Sociology, 8,* 542–547.

Strauss, A. (1978). *Negotiations.* San Francisco, CA: Jossey-Bass.

PART

II

INCREASING SENSE OF COHERENCE IN AGGREGATES

Barbara M. Artinian

PART II DESCRIBES how the *sense of coherence* (SOC) can be increased in aggregates. In Chapter 5, the family is described as a system of interacting persons who develop their SOC through family interaction. Family theories are presented, which have an effect on SOC. Characteristics of the biological, psychosocial, and spiritual subsystems of the family are described. A care plan is described, which illustrates the use of the model with a family in a long-term interaction with a community health nurse.

The client is described in Chapter 6 as institution. Institutional theories are presented, which impact SOC. In addition, the characteristics of the biological, psychosocial, and spiritual subsystems of an institution are described. The development of a program to prepare nurses from other countries for the registered nurse licensure examination is described. A care plan illustrating the resolution of an institutional problem of inadequate staffing is presented.

Chapter 7 describes public health settings where the focus is on the community as client and on health promotion at the community, state, or national level. The focus is on how community health nurses and public health nurses use the Artinian Intersystem Model to guide the Core Functions of Public Health (Assessment, Assurance, and Policy Development) with aggregate and vulnerable populations. An example of a multidisciplinary program for newborn hearing screening and student vignettes illustrate how the public health nurse negotiates with the client to increase SOC in health promotion programs at Primary and Secondary Levels of Prevention.

5

FAMILY AS CLIENT: AN INTERACTIVE INTERPERSONAL SYSTEM

Barbara M. Artinian

ALTHOUGH MOST NURSING care is directed toward the individual, the Artinian Intersystem Model (AIM) provides a format for assessing and intervening with the family as a whole. Because it is possible to think about a member of a group at one level and think about the group itself at a more abstract or second level, it is possible to consider individuals to be members of a family and also the family itself (Watzlawick, Weakland, & Fisch, 1974). This makes it possible to provide nursing care to the individual, and at another hierarchical level, to the total family system, recognizing that change in an individual is a different type of change from change in a family group.

The family can be defined as a system of interacting persons who live together over time developing patterns of kinship and who hold specific role relationships to each other, characterized by commitment and attachment, and who have economic, emotional, and physical obligations to each other. This definition includes the traditional two-parent family as well as alternative forms.

The term "family" can also be used to describe the informal family relationships that are developed in some institutions. This is illustrated in the research study done by Winter (2010), "Family Making," which focuses on staff relationships in a nursing home institution. The staff members saw themselves as family and exhibited many of the characteristics of a family as defined previously. Through interaction, any type of family develops its own unique paradigm, which Reiss (1981) defines as "the enduring, fundamental, and shared assumptions families create about the nature and meaning of life, what is important, and how to cope with the world in which they live" (pp. 2–3). This shared paradigm allows pattern and predictability to occur in families that enable families to allocate resources to attain family goals.

Just as the individual has subsystems, so does the family. They are the biological, psychosocial, and spiritual subsystems of the family (Table 5.1). When the family encounters a stressor, the stressor is processed through these subsystems. In the biological subsystem of the family, the stressor interacts with

TABLE 5.1 Family Subsystems

BIOLOGICAL SUBSYSTEM	PSYCHOSOCIAL SUBSYSTEM	SPIRITUAL SUBSYSTEM
Developmental stage Gender composition Role function Genetic factors Illness trajectory Age-related health changes Availability of food, shelter, and medical care	Family themes Marriage forms Family type Coping strategies Family strengths Family liaisons (coalitions) Culture and ethnicity Decision-making patterns Parenting skills Family rituals and traditions Family secrets	Church affiliation (beliefs) Spirituality (values) Faith development (practices) Worship (affective response)

Source: Adapted from Artinian (1997).

family characteristics such as developmental stage, gender composition, role function, genetic factors, illness trajectory, age-related health changes, and availability of food, shelter, and medical care. In the psychosocial subsystem, the stressor is influenced by family themes, marriage forms, family type, coping strategies, family strengths, family coalitions, culture and ethnicity, decision-making patterns, parenting skills, family history of rituals and traditions, and family secrets. These reflect the cognitive, affective, and interactional climate of the family. The stressor is also processed through the spiritual subsystem in which the family belief system as expressed in church affiliation, the religious values expressed in spirituality, the religious practices expressed in rituals, and affective responses expressed in the form of worship interact to provide meaning and purpose during the time of stress.

When a family experiences a health-related problem, the level of health knowledge about the concern, the orientation to health care, and the health practices and skills exhibited mediate health stressors and are seen as generalized resistance resources (GRR) or coping resources in the salutogenic model developed by Antonovsky (1987). Antonovsky proposes that individuals, over time, develop a global orientation to life that expresses the extent to which they see the world as comprehensible, manageable, and meaningful. He calls this orientation, a sense of coherence (SOC). As an ongoing interdependent system, the family also develops a global orientation to life. In an experience of stress, the family' global appraisal of the overall situation leads to the actual response of the family to the stressor. When coping resources are adequate, the family manages the stressor without the need for nursing intervention. However, when the stressor cannot be managed without nursing intervention, the family enters a period of disorganization and seeks assistance from the nurse. The level of comprehension about the stressor, the willingness to confront the stressor, and the resources to manage it can be measured as the family situational sense of coherence (SSOC) that is scored as high, medium, or low. This measurement of the family reality expresses the actual coping ability of the family system. The effectiveness of the intervention is evaluated by rescoring on SSOC.

A number of family theories assist in understanding the development of the SOC of the family. Among these are family developmental theory (Duvall & Miller, 1985), Kantor and Lehr's (1975) description of family types, and the family stress theory developed by Hill (1949) and expanded to a theory of adjustment and adaptation by McCubbin and McCubbin (1987). These theories form the background for the SSOC theory of recovery developed by Artinian. An understanding of these theories will enable the nurse to more adequately assess family SSOC to assist families to plan for their health care needs. An example from a community health case study will illustrate the process of providing care to a family system using the AIM framework.

FAMILY DEVELOPMENTAL THEORY

For more than 40 years, family developmental theory has taken a life cycle approach toward understanding how families function and relate over time. In this conceptual frame of reference or general orientation, families pass through obvious stages over the course of life. The functions commonly attributed to the family development perspective have changed over time and currently focus on the emotional support and socialization needed for living in the extended environment. These functions include:

- Giving affection
- Providing personal security, nurturance, and respite
- Giving satisfaction and purpose to life
- Assuring continuity of companionship, acceptance, and communication
- Providing socialization and status
- Teaching values and beliefs. (Duvall & Miller, 1985; Janosik & Green, 1992)

The life course perspective best represented by the family development theory of Duvall and Miller (1985) follows the family across hierarchical and universal stages. The stages are based on the establishment of a marital or couple relationship and then follow the birth and transition events of the first child. Duvall and Miller have identified factors pertinent to family life cycle stages such as number of children in the family, the age and school placement of the oldest child, and the functions and status of the family during the child rearing and launching periods.

The family developmental perspective recognizes the importance of structural roles and positions within the family. At each advancing stage in the cycle, an ever-changing number of roles are added. The family begins as a couple with roles of husband and wife or partners and expands at its peak to include roles of wife, mother, husband, father, son, daughter, sister, brother, grandmother, grandfather, aunt, and uncle. This conceptualization of family development shows the variation of the family over time and reveals the significant amount of time the couple spends in a dyad without children in the home.

Although Duvall and Miller (1985) focused on the intact family, others have studied the family life cycle events of separating or divorced families (McGoldrick & Carter, 1982). McCown (1997) has identified the different patterns of expansion, contraction, and realignment of relationships and the additional stages and tasks that separated families go through (Table 5.2). Neither Duvall and Walker's nor McCown's lists of functions or tasks takes into account the many other variations of families relative to culture, poverty, and nontraditional forms of marriage.

Antonovsky (1987) has noted the effect of social class and societal and historical conditions in determining the development of the GRR available to families. These resources determine the location of the family on the SOC continuum. He says that "being male or female, black or white, upper or lower class, Canadian or Kampuchean, Cuban, or Costa Rican—with all that these social categories imply—is decisive in determining the particular patterns of life experiences that engender a stronger or weaker SOC" (p. 91). Antonovsky emphasizes the predictable responses and feedback of experience in terms of a "characteristic, phenomenon, or relationship...that provides extended and continued experience in making sense of the countless stimuli with which one is constantly bombarded" (p. 121). Antonovsky states that the most important periods for the development of the SOC of the person are infancy and childhood, adolescence, and young adulthood. He says that it is with entry into adulthood that the experiences of childhood and adolescence are reinforced or reversed. "Consistent experiences provide the basis for the comprehensibility component; a good load balance, for the manageability component; and...participation in shaping outcomes" as the meaningfulness component (p. 92). After entering into adulthood, Antonovsky "believes that one's location of the SOC continuum becomes more or less fixed" (p. 107).

TABLE 5.2 Divorced Family Developmental Cycle

STAGE/STEPS	EMOTIONAL/DEVELOPMENTAL TASKS
Decision to divorce	– Acceptance of inability to resolve marital conflicts – Acceptance of one's own part in the failure of the marriage
Planning the breakup of the marriage	– Supporting workable arrangements for all parts of the family – Working cooperatively on problems of custody, visitation, and finances – Dealing with extended family and friends
Separation	– Mourn loss of intact family – Maintain cooperative co-parental relationship – Resolve attachment to spouse and restructure relations with extended family – Adapt to living separately and restructure parent-child relationships
Divorce	– Overcome feelings of hurt, anger, and guilt – Relinquish hope for reunion and marriage – Maintain contact with extended families
Entering new relationship	– Recover from loss of first marriage and establish openness in new relationship
Decision to remarry	– Accept one's own fears and those of new partner and children about forming a new family – Accept need for time for adjustment to (a) new roles; (b) boundaries of time, memberships, space, and authority; and (c) affective issues of guilt, loyalty, conflicts, mutuality, and past hurts
Remarriage and establishing a new family	– Resolve attachment to previous spouse and ideal intact family – Accept a new model of family with permeable boundaries – Establish attachment to new partner and inclusion in family system – Realign relationship throughout subsystems to permit interweaving of several systems – Share memories and histories across systems

Source: McCowan (1997). Combined and adapted from McGoldrick and Carter (1982) and Ransom, Schlesinger, and Derdeyn (1979).

The family developmental life course framework builds on several main features. It assumes that the members interact within the unit and within the external environment on the basis of roles. The members fulfill specified tasks pertinent to the life of the family whether it is in the expanding or contracting cycles. Developmental tasks are those that arise at a specified time in an individual's life when, if accomplished successfully, they will contribute to success and advancement in later tasks. Although the developmental task originates from within the system, social and cultural pressures encourage appropriate developmental tasks. At times, within the family, developmental tasks of the various subsystems may be congruent or in conflict. For example, the adolescent's task is to establish independence. The parent, however, may still feel a need for close supervision and ongoing parental control, thus resulting in continuing struggle between them. As the family makes transitions and moves from one stage to the next, these moves are attended by a new set of tasks and role expectations. Successful accomplishment of the tasks and goals brings a sense of confidence, satisfaction, and success to the family (Rodgers & White, 1993).

The family development cycle has changed over time in response to multiple factors. Increased mobility has distanced generations of families and altered the space dimension. Delayed childbearing has extended the first stage and has increased the number of babies born at risk. Decreasing family size has reduced the number of relationships required in the family. Increasing rates of divorce, however, have complicated parenting roles and required alternative household arrangement. Longevity frequently enables extended families to the fourth generation and has added responsibilities for care of elderly members. Overload can occur when a family is dealing with health problems at both ends of the life cycle.

FAMILY STRUCTURES AND THEMES

The family as a system of interacting individuals is an open, semipermeable system. The family exchanges energy internally within its subsystems and also with the external environment and changes and adapts according to the forces involved. Kantor and Lehr (1975) described three basic structural arrangements or family types for regulating distance and processing information and adapting to change. The major family types are open, closed, and random.

Open, closed, and random family types can be distinguished by the kind of boundaries they form. Boundaries are defined as the rules and norms within the family that develop over time and guide family behaviors. Individual boundaries serve to establish and protect the self of individual member. Interpersonal subsystem boundaries may also be established between spouses to protect the parenting system. Boundaries—the rules defining who participates and how—surrounding the family and its subsystems need to be strong enough to protect the systems but also permeable enough to allow an exchange of information between the individual members and the family within the community. If boundaries between members are weak, the development and sustenance of individuality is threatened and members become enmeshed. When boundaries

TABLE 5.3 Kantor and Lehr's Family Types and Access and Target Dimensions

DIMENSION	FAMILY TYPE		
	CLOSED	OPEN	RANDOM
Goal	Stability through tradition	Adaptation through consensus	Exploration through intuition
Access distance regulation			
Space	Fixed	Moveable	Dispersed
Time	Regular	Variable	Irregular
Energy	Steady	Flexible	Fluctuating
Target distance regulation			
Affect (joining–separating)	Durability Fidelity Sincerity	Responsiveness Authenticity Latitude	Rapture Whimsicality Spontaneity
Power (freedom–restriction)	Authority Discipline Preparation	Resolution Allowance Cooperation	Interchangeability Free choice Challenge
Meaning (sharing–not sharing)	Certainty Unity Clarity	Relevance Affinity Tolerance	Ambiguity Diversity Originality

Source: Kantor and Lehr (1975), *Inside the Family* (p. 150). Used with permission from Meredith Winter Press.

between members become rigid, such as may occur between parents and children, disengagement from each other may result (Janosik & Green, 1992). In either case, the SOC of both the child and family will be lower.

Each family type presents unique ways of focusing on the family access and target dimensions that maintain it as a system. Specific strategies are used by the family to help to interpret, protect, and maintain family traditions. Kantor and Lehr (1975) identified various other ways in which families control access to space, time, and energy (Table 5.3).

Closed-type families establish fixed constant feedback systems. The core purpose of the closed family is to create stability in the family process. These families admit only information, events, and ideas that are congruent with their own norms, values, and beliefs. They keep external traffic and input to a minimum. This type of family may be identified by external evidence of tight security systems and rigid scrutiny of visitors and credentials. Pace in closed families is fixed. Reading and viewing materials and school activities are carefully evaluated and controlled. In closed families, interactions of family members are governed by authority figures.

The purpose of the open-type family is to create a system that is adaptive to the needs of the individual and society. Emotions and affection are overtly expressed. Consent of members is sought in decision making. Persuasion rather than coercion is a mode of operation. Autonomy and negotiation are encouraged and cooperation is fostered. New ideas are incorporated into the system. Communication in open families is authentic and informal.

The random family as described by Kantor and Lehr (1975) is identity seeking. Reasoning is predominantly inspirational and intuitive. Variant views and ambiguity are acceptable. Communication is flexible and variant. Creativity is encouraged and valued. Diversity and originality are ideals of the random family system.

Each family type has flaws and strengths. In reality, families do not rigidly follow a single type and may mix strategies across types. Families that exhibit the traits of a healthy family as described by Curran (1983) are more able to provide an environment that increases the SOC of its developing members regardless of the type of family organization. However, as the family seeks to adapt and maintain family stability through balancing the forces of equilibrium and disequilibrium, many different strategies may be used. Tension in the family helps to generate energy to foster growth. However, excessive tension may strain the system and requires mechanisms for discharge of the tension. Any of these family types can contribute to a high sense of SOC if there is consistency. It is when the type moves from the ideal type to an extreme form of type, problems arise. For example, a closed family may take on the dysfunctional characteristics of the psychosomatic family as described by Minuchin, Rosman, and Baker (1978, pp. 30–32). These characteristics include enmeshment, over protectiveness, rigidity, conflict avoidance, and using the child as regulator. A random family may not offer the consistency to maintain a prescribed treatment and medication schedule that is needed by a family member.

FAMILY STRESS THEORY OF ADJUSTMENT AND ADAPTATION

Over 50 years ago, Hill introduced the theory of family stress. In his theory, Hill (1949) attempted to explain the response of families to stressor events generated by war separation and reunion. He developed a basic pattern described as the ABCX model of family stress. Traditionally, A is defined as the stressor event, B is the family crisis-meeting resources, C is the definition the family makes of the event, and X represents the crisis. The stress theory of Hill has been expanded. Recent scholars have recognized the importance of family types, family strengths and capabilities, and the number of stressors. McCubbin and McCubbin (1987) developed the T-Double ABCX model of adaptation. This model is divided into two phases: the adjustment phase and the adaptation phase. In the adjustment phase, the stressor event interacts with the family vulnerabilities, family type, and family's problem-solving and coping responses. If the family makes a favorable adjustment, there is no crisis. However, the family enters the adaptation phase when it is considered to be in crisis since it is not able to handle the stressor without outside intervention. In the adaptation phase, the family's strengths and resources interact with outside resources to resolve the crisis.

Antonovsky and Sourani (1988) have studied many of the same factors and have reported that individuals and families with a strong family SOC as measured by the perception of spouses that family life is comprehensible, manageable, and meaningful are more likely to be well adapted and are more likely to have reached a high level of reorganization after a period of crisis. This is measured by the satisfaction with family fit, internally and vis-à-vis the social environment. They write:

> A tendency to expect the world to be ordered, or orderable, facilitates cognitive clarification of the nature of the problems stressor pose. A tendency to expect the demands posed by these problems to be manageable leads one to search out the appropriate resources potentially available to one. And a tendency to see life as meaningful provides the motivational drive to engage in confrontation with the problems. It should be noted that the SOC is not at all a specific coping style, active or otherwise. Its hallmark, rather, is flexibility in selecting coping behaviors that are judged to be appropriate. These may vary radically according to the situation and the culture. This approach proposes that if one has a strong SOC, the motivational and cognitive bases exist for transforming one's potential resources, appropriate to a given stressor, into actuality, thereby promoting health. (p. 80)

SSOC THEORY OF RECOVERY

When a family experiences a health-related stressor, the crisis generates an immediate disruption in the level of SOC previously held. If the stressor can be managed using the coping strengths of the family, the family is able to handle the disorganization brought about by the stressor and does not need to seek

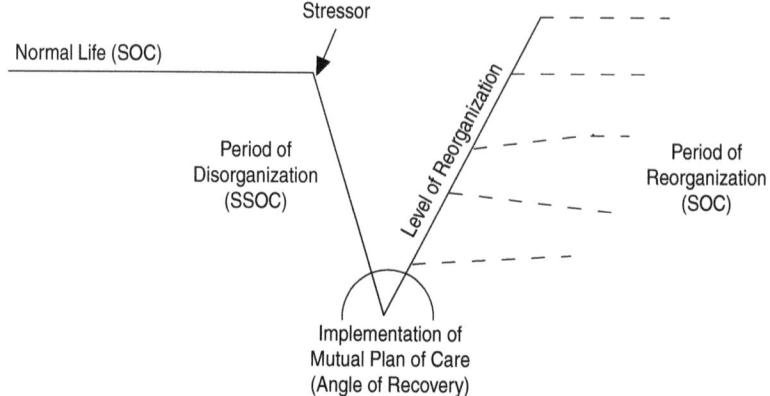

FIGURE 5.1 SSOC Theory of Recovery.
Copyright © 2011 B. Artinian. Adapted from Hill (1949).

nursing intervention. In this case, the family would experience a momentary change in SOC but the overall level would remain the same. This corresponds to the adjustment phase described by McCubbin and McCubbin (1987). However, when the stressor is of a magnitude that cannot be resolved using family resources, the person and family enter a period of disorganization. Using the concept of angle of recovery developed by Hill (1949), the person and family plunge into a sharp decline from the SOC state experienced in ordinary life. The period of time in the angle of recovery is called the SSOC. Depending on the resources, assistance, and support available to the person and family, they can emerge from the experience with a lower or even higher level of reorganization. This would be expressed as the new normal level of SOC (see Figure 5.1), corresponding to the adaptation phase described by McCubbin and McCubbin (1987). The difference between the SSOC theory of recovery and the T-Double ABCX Model is that the SSOC theory relates only to stressors resulting in the need for nursing intervention whereas the T-Double ABCX Model identifies all stressors, both those that can be met with family resources (the adjustment phase) and those for which nursing assistance is needed (the adaptation phase). Successful adaptation would correspond to the resolution of the main concern using the AIM.

Interaction occurs within the system and between the system as a whole and the environmental context. When a family encounters a stressor that must be resolved using nursing intervention, the stressor is the event that begins the interaction. The stressor is processed through the biological, psychosocial, and spiritual subsystems of the family. The subsystems are assessed to identify the main concern of either the family or the nurse. To the extent that the family acts as a unit, it is possible to analyze its behavior with respect to a main concern through an intrasystem assessment of knowledge about the main concern, values regarding it, and behaviors used to address it. The nurse also assesses her intrasystem in relation to knowledge about the main concern, values about it, and behaviors associated with it. This analysis of the intrasystems of both nurse and family is especially useful because there are often major discrepancies between the fit of the family and the value system of the nurse.

Following intrasystem analysis of all data, the nurse makes a nursing diagnosis and develops goals to increase SSOC. If the nurse and the client have the ability and willingness to work together to resolve the main concern, intersystem interaction begins by communicating information and negotiating values (Kuhn, 1974). If there is an agreement on values, a mutual plan of care is outlined and implemented. The effectiveness of the intervention at the aggregate level can be measured by rescoring on SSOC as the level of health knowledge about the main concern, the orientation to health care, and the health practices and skills exhibited by family members. All the characteristics summarized in Table 5.1 mediate health stressors that are experienced and can be seen as GRR or coping resources in the salutogenic model developed by Antonovsky (1987).

INTRODUCTION TO ONLINE CARE PLAN

A care plan was developed illustrating a long-term relationship with a family. It is based on one part of a 6-week case study written by Beverly Brownell when she was a graduate student at Azusa Pacific University. It illustrates how a community health nurse and the family can develop a mutual plan of care to relieve the pain of a decubitus ulcer by using the AIM. The full text of the care plan is available in the online adjunct manual.

CONCLUSION

The theories presented in this chapter provide insight for the nurse/provider about various types of family structures. These theories are useful in assisting a family during a time of disorganization following a crisis event. Through interventions directed at both the client and the family, the SOC of the family system can be strengthened.

REFERENCES

Antonovsky, A. (1987). *Unraveling the mystery of health: How people manage stress and stay well.* San Francisco, CA: Jossey-Bass.

Antonovsky, A., & Sourani, T. (1988). Family sense of coherence and family adaptation. *Journal of Marriage and the Family, 50* (February), 79-92.

Curran, D. (1983). *Traits of a healthy family.* Minneapolis, MN: Winston.

Duvall, E., & Miller, B. (1985). *Marriage and family development* (6th ed., pp. 3-64). New York, NY: Harper & Row.

Hill, R. (1949). *Families under stress.* New York, NY: Harper & Row.

Janosik, E., & Green, E. (1992). *Family life: Process and practice* (pp. 3-66). Boston, MA: Jones & Bartlett.

Kantor, D., & Lehr, W. (1975). *Inside the family.* San Francisco, CA: Jossey Bass.

Kuhn, A. (1974). *The logic of social systems: A unified, deductive system-based approach to social science.* San Francisco, CA: Jossey-Bass.

McCown, D. (1997). The family as client. In B. Artinian & M. Conger (Eds.), *The Intersystem Model: Integrating theory and practice* (p. 135). Thousand Oaks, CA: Sage Publications.

McCubbin, M., & McCubbin, H. (1987). Family stress theory and assessment. In H. McCubbin & A. Thompson (Eds.), *Family assessment inventories for research and practice* (pp. 3-33). Madison, WI: University of Wisconsin Center for Excellence in Family Studies.

McGoldrick, M., & Carter, E. (1982). The family life cycle. In F. Walsh (Ed.), *Normal family processes* (pp. 167-195). New York, NY: Guilford Press.

Minuchin, S., Rosman, B., & Baker, L. (1978). *Psychosomatic families: Anorexia nervosa in contest.* Cambridge, MA: Harvard University Press.

Reiss, D. (1981). *The family's construction of reality.* Cambridge, MA: Harvard University Press.

Rodgers, R., & White J. (1993). Family development theory. In P. Boss, W. Doherty, R. LaRossa, W. Schumm, & S. Steinmetz (Eds.), *Sourcebook of family theories and methods* (pp. 225-254). New York, NY: Plenum Press.

Watzlawick, P., Weakland, J. H., & Fisch, R. (1974). *Change: Principles of problem formation and problem resolution.* New York, NY: Norton.

Winter, V. (2010, October). *Family Making: A grounded theory study.* Paper presented at the Joint Southern California Sigma Theta Tau International Chapters' Conference—Nursing Odyssey 2010, San Diego, CA.

6

INSTITUTION AS CLIENT: INSTITUTIONAL INTERACTION

Margaret M. Conger and Lourdes Casao Salandanan

THIS CHAPTER WILL examine how the Artinian Intersystem Model (AIM) can be applied to the functioning of an institution because an institution consists of two or more parties engaged in some type of intersystem interaction (Kuhn, 1974). The ability of the system to develop mutually agreed upon goals will affect the success of the institution. Like an individual or family, institutions can be assessed to identify issues of concern to their functioning. Because both the well-being and the efficiency of the institution are important to its success, such assessment is necessary to promote optimal function. The AIM process of assessing the institution's biological, psychosocial, and spiritual subsystems and the situational sense of coherence (SSOC) can be used to identify problems within the organization. The interventions negotiated between employees and management of the institution can be used to improve its sense of coherence (SOC). The goal of the entire process is to improve the SOC of the organization. In doing so, the members of the organization will have a better understanding of the organization, learn to manage better, and alter the organization's practices to better meet its goals.

The application of the AIM is especially useful to an analysis of a health care organization because there can be major discrepancies between the values of the institution and those of the employees. An examination of these value systems, and how they relate to one another, is vital to the achievement of institutional goals. If the value systems are not congruent, the institutional goals may not be achieved. The AIM provides a structure for analysis of the values of the intrasystems of an institution and its employees and facilitates the development of goals for organizational planning.

INSTITUTIONAL LEADERSHIP THEORY

Institutions are undergoing radical changes in leadership styles. The 21st century is bringing a total transformation in how institutions operate

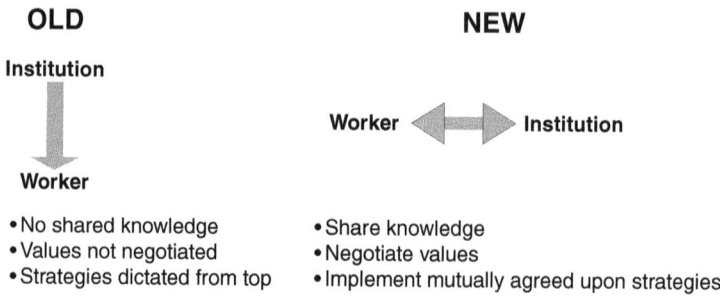

FIGURE 6.1 Management styles.
Copyright © 2011 M. Conger.

(Porter-O'Grady & Malloch, 2003). The style that is reflected in many of the management strategies of the past was based on a vertical pattern of management at the top and the worker (client) below with little or no interactive communication between them. Rather the communication came from the top management in a one-way fashion. There was no sharing of knowledge between the management and the worker. The values of each were different and not negotiated and work strategies were dictated from the top (Figure 6.1).

The old management type of structure is shown on the left side of Figure 6.1. Successful institutions including many health care facilities have now moved to a more horizontal pattern in which the management and worker interact cooperatively as shown on the right side of Figure 6.1. This mode of interaction exemplifies the principles of the AIM in which the knowledge, values, and behaviors of each are shared. When all are working together to implement mutually agreed upon strategies, the organization is able to be more successful in achieving its goals.

An organization can meet its goals only through the people involved in the organization. As the values of both the organization itself and the people within the organization are explored, differences can be clarified. New ways to bridge differences in the value systems can be negotiated leading to improvement in the output of the organization.

ASSESSMENT OF THE DEVELOPMENTAL ENVIRONMENT

The AIM provides a structure that can be used when assessing the management practices of an institution. It begins with review of the biological, psychosocial, and spiritual subsystems of the institution. Using this information, an understanding of the institution is developed, and problems that can hinder the success of the organization can be identified.

Biological Subsystem

Because organizations are composed of people, the biological subsystem must be considered. In an organization, health policies that affect the well-being of the workforce such as sick leave time, wellness programs, and health insurance benefits should be examined. Work schedules such as shift work, rotation of work schedules, vacations, and other benefits that affect the health of employees as well as the predominant gender of the workforce are important. If the workers are primarily of one gender, the effects of work policies on that gender need to be considered. In addition, employee safety programs that relate to sex should be examined. The actual structure of the building housing the organization can also have an effect on the health of employees.

Psychosocial Subsystem

Much of the interaction within an organization lies at the social level thus making this area vital to understanding the working of the organization. Each organization has its own unique cultural climate often expressed by a number of "unwritten" rules that become part of how the organization functions. The presence of employee unions or other employee groups may have a strong voice in determining institutional policies. In other institutions, upper management may tightly control employee groups. The level of morale of the employees will be affected by the degree of input employees have in determining workplace policies.

The environment of an institution is directly affected by the leadership style of the managers within the organization. The role of the workers and their ability to interact with the managers in setting organizational policies set a tone for the entire functioning of the institution.

For some institutions, empowerment of the workers is a key concept in achieving its mission and goals (Tebbitt, 1993), a paradigm shift from organizational control to that of participation of the workers in decision-making functions. However, this focus has not been the norm for most health care institutions. The leadership style in many health care institutions has long been one in which the focus has been on the task rather than the personnel. Current leadership theory suggests that a more person-centered style will achieve the desired organizational goals more effectively. Some leadership experts suggest that this should not be an either or situation, rather one's style should vary based on the situation.

Task-oriented leadership is bureaucratic or pyramidal. The power is centered at the top of the organization with an emphasis on accomplishing a specific task. The worker is viewed as a means to an end and easily interchanged with other workers. Taylor (1911) was one of the earliest theorists in leadership. His focus was improvement of productivity through improvement of techniques. This view persisted for many years. McGregor (1960) described this type of leadership as Theory X in which the worker was viewed as unmotivated and in need of close supervision. Gilbreth (1973) continued with this view by conducting time and motion studies to perfect a work process. This type of leadership has been very prevalent in hospital management where decisions affecting the workers are made by top management with little input from the workforce.

Many management experts have advocated a more person-centered leadership style. McGregor (1960) in his Theory Y concept described the importance of a human relationship in which the workers were self-directed. He advocated taking into consideration the feelings and attitudes of the workers as central to good management. He believed that self-control in the worker is indispensable to accomplishing organizational goals. Argyris (1971) further explored this concept.

The concept of situational leadership has been advocated by a number of theorists (Fiedler, 1967; Hersey, Blanchard, & Johnson, 1996; House & Mitchell, 1974; Stinson & Johnson, 1975; Tannenbaum & Schmidt, 1958; Vroom & Yetten, 1973). In this approach, the effective leader is able to alter his/her style to fit the needs of the worker. Emphasis is placed on identifying worker behavior and then utilizing an appropriate management style. Thus, the effective leader is the one who can adapt to the workers needs rather than relying on the style that may be most comfortable to the leader. When working with a person with low motivation, emphasis on a task-oriented approach will provide the most effective outcome. When managing a highly motivated worker, a more person-centered approach will be most effective.

Porter-O'Grady and Malloch (2003) suggest that these old models of leadership are not effective for the coming century. Their model *Quantum Leadership* is based more on the person rather than the leader. The employee needs new skills to function in the current technology age. The Internet has changed the way knowledge is obtained. It is no longer in the control of the leader but is now accessible to all. This places greater emphasis on the individual and management behaviors must change. In health care, there is movement away from the hospital-based sickness model. Prevention services based in the community are becoming the focus of health care. With this shift, a top-oriented management system is no longer effective. The role of the leader has changed from a planning and organizing function to that of adapting to the ever-changing environment.

The purpose of a health care organization is to provide services to achieve specific outcomes rather than adhere to a series of processes. The central point of the organization is where service is provided. Thus, changes must start at this point of service rather than from top leadership. This is a radical change from old hierarchal models of leadership. The AIM method of examining shared values is a useful tool for managing in this new organizational environment. As the employee at the point of service senses what is needed to meet the common goal of the organization, this information can be shared with the leader. Joint decision-making can then follow.

Spiritual Subsystem

When looking at a health organization, the spiritual subsystem must also be considered. Does the organization have a mission statement that articulates its belief system? Are there policies on organizational ethics and values? Does the organization have any religious affiliations? For instance, an institution representing a particular religious group will display many of the value systems of that group and will affect how decisions will be made within the organization. Even if the institution has no direct religious affiliation, the presence of a religious program such as a chaplain program will indicate something about the religious values of the institution.

Assessment of the Situational Environment

After the developmental environment of an institution is examined, an analysis of the data obtained is done. This analysis includes the knowledge level, the values, and the behaviors of both the leadership of the institution and the employees. Areas that can hinder the institution's success are identified.

Personal Cultural Values

Interaction within an institution takes place within the cultural values of an organization. These are especially important to the social well being of an institution. If there is conflict between the cultural values of management and the employees, progress toward institutional goals will be affected. Schein (1985) suggests that there are three levels of organizational culture: (a) the physical environment, (b) the values held by members of the organization, and (c) the basic underlying assumptions held by the members of the organization. The values and underlying assumptions of the organization result in expectations for group member behaviors forming a means of internal control over them. Such expectations have generally arisen out of a need to solve work-related problems and provide for the survival of the group (Coeling & Simms, 1993). As new members come into the group, most quickly adapt their behaviors to fit those of the group. Shibutani (1994) calls the group culture a "reference group" and it is used by newcomers to make changes in their behavior. He suggests that new members will often adopt behaviors of the group that are quite inconsistent with their former behavior. However, members of an organization come to the workplace with their own religious, ethnic, and family cultural norms. If these are in opposition to the organizational culture, conflict may occur.

Cultural Values of the Organization

In addition to differences in the personal culture that each member brings to the workplace, differences in cultural values can exist between groups within the organization. Hospitals have been described as having three distinct cultural values espoused by members of the organization. The management espouses a business culture in which profit and loss, efficiency of workers, and other business values are stressed. Nurses bring the value of caring for the individual, including advocacy for the client and a concern for open access to health care for all persons (Cooper, 1991; Gadow, 1985; Leininger, 1984; Peter & Gallop, 1994; Watson, 1988). Physicians, although often not a part of the employee contingent, also have an important cultural impact on the organization. They view the hospital as their workshop where they espouse a culture of cure. These three divergent cultural values often lead to dissension.

An example of this type of dissension has been called "the doctor–nurse game" in which the doctor has a superior role over the nurse (Stein, 1967). The nurse role was to make recommendations for client care in a manner that made it look like the suggestion came from the physician. This relationship is no longer considered to be in the best interest of the client. Stein, Watts, and Howell (1990) suggest that the rules of the game have changed. Nurses are increasingly becoming specialists in their chosen area and are seeking independence in practice. This can bring real conflict between the nurse and doctor.

Using data from the review of the knowledge, values, and behaviors of the organization, stressors within the organization can be identified. Often these stressors arise from varying cultural beliefs among both the management staff and the employees. Differences in approach to ethical concerns also can cause stress in the organization. Resources for coping with these differences can also be identified at this time.

INTERSYSTEM INTERACTION

It is not sufficient to just collect information and identify areas that are hindering an institution from achieving its goals. Positive actions need to be implemented to bring resolution to problems identified. In nursing, the current movement is to decentralize management so that decisions are made closer to the people who will be affected by them. Providing all staff members a communication chain so that their concerns are heard has been shown to be a way that motivates members to support organizational goals. The development of professional governance models has done much to promote this type of communication. In this model, all members of the organization give input in the decision-making process. For example, staff nurses have control over decisions that directly affect client care, while the unit manager has control of decisions concerning how the unit is organized. In such a structure, the organizational chart appears to be more of a multi-armed centipede rather than the typical ladder approach of the hierarchal structure. For nurses to be effective in communicating within a more horizontal organizational structure, they need to learn negotiating strategies.

Negotiation

The art of negotiation is necessary for all workers in an organizational setting because of conflicting needs, wants, and desires of the members of the group. The values of the employees are often not accordant with the organizational values. In this case, strategies are needed to resolve the differences. Smeltzer (1991) has described negotiations that can occur as either cooperative or competitive. In cooperative negotiation, everyone wins; in competitive negotiation, only one party wins. To retain harmonious work relationships, cooperative negotiation will be far more effective.

The term cultural brokering has been suggested to describe the type of negotiation that occurs when there is a gap between two cultural groups (Jezewski, 1993). It is effective in situations in which two groups are of unequal status such as the staff nurse and hospital management or staff nurse and physician. In such situations, it is necessary to know how to circumvent the barriers that are present in preventing the group with less power from being heard. Three aspects of brokering are needed: (a) the ability to mediate when the two groups are in conflict; (b) the ability to negotiate to reach an agreement; and (c) the ability to be innovative when new solutions to the problem are needed.

A strategy to use in successful negotiation of conflict in an institution has been described as *polarity management* (Johnson, 1996; see Figure 6.2). In this strategy, the manager recognizes that there are two opposite, conflicting opinions about a situation. These are referred to as "poles." On both sides of the conflict, there are both positives and negatives. If you focus on only one side of the conflict, you will experience the negative aspects of that side. Rather you need to explore both sides of the conflict. Johnson recommends that you start the negotiation by exploring the negatives of one side of the conflict and then moving to explore the positives of the other side of the conflict. Then you move to examining the negatives of that pole and then positive aspects of the opposite pole. By exploring the negatives of both poles, the value of positive aspects of both sides of the conflict can be identified. It is then the task of the manager to recognize the strengths of both sides of the conflict and support practices that incorporate both. There is no "right" answer to the conflict, just recognition that both sides have valid points that need to be appreciated.

This process is shown in Figure 6.2, where one starts by examining the negatives of the position on the left side of the diagram. One then moves to examining the positives of the opposite viewpoint as shown on the right side. From there, the negative aspects of the issue on the right are examined. Finally, the positives on the left side are considered. By recognizing that there are both positive and negative aspects of any conflict, it is easier to negotiate a common goal. People on both sides of the conflict have been allowed to express their opinions and see the

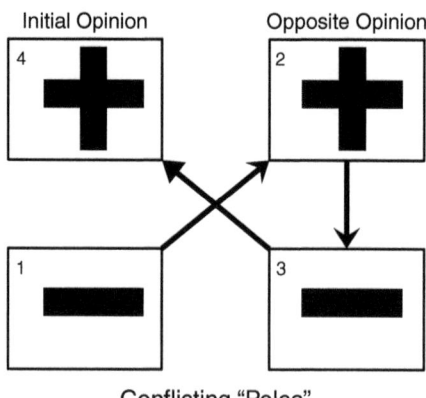

FIGURE 6.2 Polarity management.
Copyright © 2011 M. Conger. Adapted from Johnson (1996).

value of all opinions. In this arena of mutual sharing, a common goal can often be developed. A negotiation using a system such as Polarity Management can only work if all parties are willing to be open to discussion. If one of the parties is adamant in holding to the viewpoint, "just say no," the system cannot work.

Ethical Concerns

Another hindrance to this type of negotiation is a problem involving ethical concerns. All institutions face ethical issues that arise from differences between corporate policy, the values of the workers, and the public served. Hospitals face increased ethical responsibility because of their service to the public in situations that are often life threatening. The values of the institution will have some bearing on how each issue is evaluated.

Ethical decisions are never made easily. White (1991) states that, "No matter what you do in the case of an ethical dilemma, there is no satisfactory answer or solution. Each situation has unique considerations that must be evaluated on its own merits. Often, the ethically correct action is not economically expedient" (p. 21). Values concerning life, definition of person, and religious beliefs of the institution will affect the decision.

An example of how a family's health care decision is affected by an institution's moral values is that of a set of conjoined twins born with a shared liver and heart. The twins were born at a Catholic hospital where the value of each individual life was supreme. After months of agonizing discussions and study, the hospital staff made their decision based on the ethical principle of futility to encourage the parents to keep the twins "warm, fed, and cuddled" until they died (Brandon, 1994a). The ethical principle of futility anticipated the surgical outcome that one baby would definitely die and the other would probably die anyway, and so the surgery would be futile.

The parents did not accept this opinion and had the twins transferred to a large children's hospital for possible separation surgery. A decision was made there to proceed with the surgery, knowing that one of the twins would definitely die, but the other had a very marginal chance for survival. The ethical decision made at this hospital was based on the principle of beneficence where the emphasis was placed on "If somebody thinks he can save the life of one baby, shouldn't he try?" (Brandon, 1994b).

Each of these institutions viewed the situation from different ethical perspectives. The Catholic hospital staff embraced a value in which extraordinary means to sustain life were considered futile. On the other hand, the children's hospital staff focused on the technical capabilities available in their institution and their belief that a surgical intervention could possibly be beneficial to at least one twin. The belief systems of the staff were congruent with their institutional values, but it was the ethical principle of parental autonomy that led the parents to seek a hospital with a value system congruent to their own that guided the decision-making process.

APPLICATION OF THE AIM TO INSTITUTIONAL CHALLENGES

To demonstrate the application of the AIM to institutional challenges, the following examples are given: a rehabilitation program, the Budding RN (B-RN) program, and the MAP program.

A Rehabilitation Program

An in-service educator was concerned that there was a lack of consistency in the care being provided to rehabilitation patients. To resolve this problem, she developed a program using the AIM to provide a systematic way to deliver care to all patients. Instruction in the use of the model was given to all staff followed up by performance evaluations based on the successful use of the model. The model was taught to all levels of nursing staff as well as to the social workers and other team members. Although the program was fully implemented, the program did not continue after an administrative change. An information sheet about the model that had been prepared for the rehabilitation organization has been updated to make it useful in any clinical setting. It is given in Table 6.1 and is available in the online adjunct manual.

Programs to Address the Nursing Shortage

Innovative programs to meet the challenge of the nursing shortage have been developed by Citrus Valley Medical Center (CVMC). Two of these will be discussed in the following section. The first of these is the B-RN program that was initiated as a solution to the nursing shortage that affected the ability of the Medical Center to provide holistic nursing and medical care to the community it serves. By 2020, the national nursing shortage is projected to increase to more than one million registered nurses (RNs). As the nursing shortage becomes more severe, one can expect to see market and political forces create pressures that will increase the need for more RNs. During an acute nursing shortage, institutions must continue to develop optimal measures to ameliorate the situation.

TABLE 6.1 Worksheet for In-service Education

INTRODUCTION TO THE ARTINIAN INTERSYSTEM MODEL (AIM)

What is the AIM?
The model is described as a communication system that focuses on sharing information and negotiating values on a clinical problem between the nurse/provider and patient/client which will result in organizing a mutually agreed upon plan of care.

Why is the model needed?
The model provides a framework for the practice of nursing, which is consistent with the mission and values of health care organizations. All organizations need a framework of reference that makes sense on which to build practice and provide guidance to the staff in their work.

What are the benefits of the model?
The model provides the staff a sense of direction, application, and evaluation of the interventions provided to patients and clients. It will help increase patient satisfaction and job satisfaction by fostering positive outcomes. It is highly applicable to all health care settings and supports patients and clients in achieving their health care goals.

What are the risks of the model?
The application of the model may not work for all patient situations. When considering the best interest of the patient, some problems encountered by staff and patients may be non-negotiable.

Who participates in the model?
The focus of the model is primarily directed toward nurses providing patient care; however, it is also inclusive of the interdisciplinary team process. To maximize the benefits of the model, all members of the interdisciplinary team need to participate in the model. The model exemplifies the team building approach.

What are the key components of the model?
1. One patient, one problem, and one plan.

   | Patient A | Problem: incontinent bowel | Plan: bowel program |
   | Patient B | Problem: acute fracture | Plan: mobility and cast care |

2. It is a goal oriented process rather than a task-oriented process.
3. It includes the patient's decisions in the plan of care.
4. It is a nurse-active/patient-active process.
5. The patient value system can be superseded by the nurse value system when necessary (e.g., *self-inflicted harm*).

What is the process?

1. Communication of information between individuals
2. Negotiation of values

What is the outcome?

1. Organization of the plan of care
2. Mutual plan of care for the problem identified
3. Exemplars in nursing practice
4. Highly efficient and effective treatment plans
5. Highly satisfied staff, patients, and family caregivers

(Continued)

TABLE 6.1 (Continued)

Questions to ask the patient.
What does the patient know about his/her problem?
What does the patient want to achieve?
What skills does the patient/caregiver have to manage the problem?

Questions to ask yourself.
What do I know about the problem?
What do I want to achieve?
What skills do I have to work with the patient's problem?

ACTION POINT: Set a mutually agreed upon goal and set up a plan of care to resolve the main concern.

Source: Artinian (2011). Adapted from unpublished inservice worksheet.

According to Citrus Valley Health Partners (2010a, 2010b), "Through its three hospital campuses and hospice, [they] serve a community of nearly one million people in the San Gabriel Valley. The Inter-Community Campus offers a complete range of inpatient and outpatient services... with the only open heart surgery program in the ESGV. The Queen of the Valley campus is renowned for its family-centered maternity services and Level IIIB Newborn Intensive Care Unit (NICU). This campus also offers The Geleris Family Cancer Center, a Robotic Surgery Program, and a full range of rehabilitation services" (About Citrus Valley Health Partners, para 1–2). The CVMC Mission Statement is "to help people keep well in body, mind and spirit by providing quality health care services in a compassionate environment" (Our Mission, para 1). CVMC was confronted with the challenges presented by the nursing shortage and the need for ongoing professional development of RNs. Numerous programs were initiated at CVMC to address the problem.

One of these programs, the B-RN program, was designed, using the AIM, to revisit the educational preparation of current non-RN staff and identify those who were qualified to take the RN licensure examination, but had either not attempted it or had previously failed. The B-RN program assisted these potential RNs to achieve success on the exam. The AIM was used to develop educational activities to prepare these staff members to pass the National Council for Licensure Examination for Registered Nurses (NCLEX-RN). A 9-week course focused on preparation for the exam was developed in collaboration with a local community college. Thirty-one staff were identified as potential candidates for taking the NCLEX-RN. Twenty-one of these employees (67%) participated in the program. Seventeen of the participants (80%) were subsequently successful in passing the exam and became RNs on staff.

The AIM was also used in the implementation of another program based on the COPE Health Solutions' Mentoring & Professional Development (MAP^{SM}): Residency and Preceptor Training program. With the aid of a Unihealth Foundation Grant, a local version of the program, the Citrus Valley Health Partners, Mentorship, and Professional Development Program (CVHP MAP^{SM}), began in 2005. The CVHP MAP^{SM} Coordinators and nursing staff developers planned the program to support and properly prepare new graduate nurses for the complexity and reality of their chosen careers. The CVHP MAP^{SM} Program had three major components: (1) Enhanced Preceptor Workshop; (2) Cultural Competency Workshop; and (3) the only RN Residency program in the East San Gabriel Valley.

The CVHP MAP^{SM} coordinators found the Residency program to be very helpful for re-entry nurses, internationally trained, and foreign-born nurses since all of these nurses come with diverse backgrounds and experience. As of summer 2010, the Residency program has graduated 18 cohorts of nurses with a total of 355 participants, and 31 enhanced preceptor workshops have been given with 403 participants. One outcome of the Residency program is that the turnover rate has decreased from 32% to 4% for new graduates employed by CVHP (2010a).

AN ANNOTATED CARE PLAN FOR THE B-RN PROGRAM

The AIM describes the interactional process that takes place between a provider and client. In the care plan that follows, the provider is the staff developer, and the B-RNs who were board eligible staff members are the client group. In this process, the two systems come together for intersystem interaction characterized by the specific sets of relationships that connected them to one another in both the developmental and situational environment.

THE DEVELOPMENTAL ENVIRONMENT

The developmental environment is the milieu that provides the cultural and social background of the clients and forms the worldview of the clients. This worldview interacts with the other constraints of the situation and provides the context for the interaction at the time of a specific encounter. In this case, the interaction focused on the need to have more RNs to staff the hospital and the unsuccessful attempts of the board-eligible staff members to pass the examination.

Focus of Interaction

CVMC was confronted with the challenges presented by the nursing shortage and the need for professional development of the RNs. While they continued to prepare for the NCLEX-RN, 31 employees worked as licensed vocational nurses, unlicensed assistive personnel, and unit secretaries. Many of them had been unsuccessful in previous attempts to pass the NCLEX-RN. However, they were B-RNs who were board eligible staff members.

Assessment of Client Subsystems

Biological Subsystem

These 31 employees had had training as professional nurses and were eligible to become RNs but had been unsuccessful in previous attempts to pass the NCLEX-RN. Many of these were immigrants who had had received their nursing education in their country of origin.

Psychosocial Subsystem

The potential candidates for the B-RN program expressed embarrassment and discouragement because of earlier unsuccessful attempts to pass their licensure examination. For many of them, English was their second language. All members of the group had families that they supported.

Spiritual Subsystem

The personal values and beliefs of the individuals were not assessed. Two participants were Catholic nuns trained in India. The religious affiliation of the others was unknown.

Tentative Identification of the Main Concern

The CVHC was experiencing difficulty in meeting its staffing needs and saw the development of a program to assist its board-eligible staff members to pass the licensing examination as a means to increase the pool of RN's for the hospital to meet its staffing needs.

Intrasystem Data Collection About Client Related to Main Concern

Knowledge

The potential RN participants expressed a lack of full understanding and awareness of methods and resources for preparation for the NCLEX-RN.

Values

The B-RNs realized that they needed the assistance of knowledgeable individuals who could guide them through a preparatory program such as the B-RN program. The potential B-RN participants viewed the passing of the examination as a high priority.

Behaviors

The potential B-RN program participants had family members, friends, managers, and coworkers who had vowed to support them through the educational activities. Because of work and family responsibilities, this support would be vital to their success.

Intrasystem Data Collection About Provider Related to Main Concern

Knowledge

Although the nurse/provider (B-RNC) who was responsible for the B-RN program had never developed an NCLEX-RN preparatory class, she had a sufficiently strong clinical and educational background to provide guidance for the program.

Values

The staff developer was an internationally trained nurse who empathized with the group and believed that the group's continuous commitment to a well-developed educational activity would help them to succeed. Although the B-RN Coordinator (B-RN) was enrolled in a nursing master's program, she was committed to providing time and energy to mentor and tutor the group. Moreover, because she was foreign-born, she could serve as a role model for the group.

Behaviors

The B-RNC had strong working relationships with a local community college with a nursing program that could provide assistance. It was anticipated that the nursing faculty from that college could provide educational assistance for the program.

Validation of Main Concern of Client and Provider

The main concern of the client is to become licensed as an RN, and the main concern of the hospital (provider) is to increase RN staff from the current employee pool.

THE SITUATIONAL ENVIRONMENT

Analysis of Intrasystem Information by Nurse

The situational environment includes all the details of the encounter such as the place, time, circumstances, motivational state, and receptivity of the B-RNC and the B-RNs. Intersystem interaction is mutually influencing. It includes how information is communicated, how values are negotiated to develop a joint plan of care, and how the behaviors are organized to increase the SOC of the B-RNs. The SOC contains three dimensions that reflect the specific orientation of the B-RNs in terms of comprehensibility, meaningfulness, and manageability.

Identify Stressors of Client

- Acculturation to the Western lifestyle of the United States was difficult for the participants.
- English was their second language.
- They had families or other individuals who relied on them for support.
- NCLEX-RN preparatory programs were usually three 8-hour days and cost approximately $500. This is time they could spend working and earning money instead of preparing for the examination.
- The majority of the staff members worked at night and some did not drive.

Identify Coping Resources of Client

- The organization, community college, families, friends, unit managers, and coworkers expressed support of the group's endeavors.
- The staff developer's record of accomplishment in developing new programs and mentoring was a benefit for the group.
- The community college was located 5 miles away from the medical center making it easy to access.
- The college could apply for funds for this pilot program.

Score on SSOC (1 = Low, 2 = Medium, 3 = High)

Comprehensibility = 1

The B-RNs understood the situation they were in and understood that they would have to sacrifice much of their time and energy to reach their goals, but they were unfamiliar with the resources available and how to access the resources.

Meaningfulness = 2

The B-RNs felt that they really wanted to reach their goals for the sake of the families they were supporting, but they were uncertain about spending so much time in preparation for the examination.

Manageability = 1

To achieve their goals, the B-RNs felt they needed assistance in the form of guidance and instruction from outside sources. There was no program available that would meet their individual needs.

State Nursing Diagnosis

Potential for enhanced community coping related to increased number of RNs.

Identify Goals to Increase SSOC

Provide support to program participants to enable their success in passing NCLEX-RN.

Assess Ability of Client and Provider to Resolve Main Concern Together

The strong commitment of both the B-RNs and the staff coordinator overseeing the program indicated that this would be a worthwhile endeavor. The benefits to the B-RNs were immeasurable. Their job potential and self-esteem for achieving success on the nursing licensing examination would be increased. The institution would benefit from a new pool of RNs to meet critical nurse staffing needs.

INTERSYSTEM INTERACTION TO RESOLVE MAIN CONCERN

Communicate Information

The B-RNC provided information about the program by phone and personal meetings to potential program participants. They were told that they would attend classes at the community college and that the Regional Health Occupation Resource Center (RHORC) had funds available to assist internationally trained health care professionals. Potential program participants were told that the program would take 9 weeks but that the B-RNC would be available to assist them with work schedules, transportation problems, emotional and psychological support, and special learning needs.

Negotiate Values

The participants felt that they were at a disadvantage because English was a second and perhaps a third language for them. Many of them had graduated more than 5 years before and felt that they needed a program that was longer than the average 4-day review program currently available within the community. Some of them felt uncomfortable using computers. They all had had experience working in acute care facilities where their practice might not have been congruent with standard textbook procedures. In addition, all of the staff members were embarrassed that they had been unsuccessful after numerous attempts to pass the NCLEX-RN. Some were concerned about the financial impact of the program and the time they would have to sacrifice, time that they would have used to work or spend with their families. They were advised that their success would be based on their commitment but that the B-RNC would also commit to their learning during their preparatory program.

Develop Mutual Plan of Care

The B-RNC and potential program participants developed joint goals and strategies. They included the following:

1. The program would take into account the following factors: (a) international training, (b) ESL, (c) immigrant status, (d) length of time since completion of RN program, (e) work schedules, (f) gender of participants, and (g) computer skills.
2. B-RNC would agree to attend didactic sessions and would be available for tutoring.
3. Staff members would register at the RHORC and community college, pay for their study materials ($50), lab fees ($8), and parking fees ($35), and attend all scheduled classes.

Implement Strategies

Negotiation was held between the B-RNC and the nursing faculty at the local community college. Since the educational activities' target audience was not composed of current community college nursing students, the involved faculty

TABLE 6.2 NCLEX-RN Preparation Course

NURSING CONTENT	PSYCHOSOCIAL CONTENT	BIOLOGICAL CONTENT
Overview of NCLEX-RN	Test-taking techniques for the international graduate	Cardiopulmonary
Nursing process		Endocrinology
Obstetrics	Leadership	Gastrointestinal
Pediatrics	Mental health	Musculoskeletal
Pharmacology		Neurology
		Renal

Source: Salandanan (2011).

members were contracted with the RHORC to provide instruction over and beyond their usual teaching load. The faculty members were very eager to assist the institution because of the existing strong working relationships that the two institutions already had.

After many weeks of assessment and communication with RHORC, a 9-week program was developed. Two 5-hour didactic sessions were scheduled on Thursdays and Fridays from 5 p.m. to 10 p.m. Topics for the didactics portion are shown in Table 6.2.

The funding of the program was approved through the RHORC. Instructors, post-test fees, classrooms, and the computer laboratory were provided by the community college. Many instructors agreed to participate according to their specialty, including internationally trained and male instructors. The participants were required to complete 6 hours of computer laboratory sessions each week. Laboratory instructors for the program were present in the computer lab every Saturday from 8 a.m. until 4 p.m. Computer lab assistance was also available Monday to Friday for participants who were not able to come on Saturday.

The B-RNC scheduled herself to attend all of the didactic sessions and posttests. She was present during the didactic sessions to listen to content, provide insight into disparities between current practice and what was being taught, thereby assisting participants and instructors. The staff developer positioned herself in front of the classroom to observe class and individual reactions to the content presented. She was available before, during, and after the program for tutoring. The program providers strongly suggested that participants take the NCLEX-RN immediately after the review. In fact, every day the class met, the program providers and staff developer encouraged them to secure an application, and they assisted participants in their reapplication for licensure.

Evaluate Resolution of Main Concern by Rescoring on SSOC

Comprehensibility = 3

The B-RN had a stronger understanding of the didactic portion of the NCLEX-RN, including content and computer skills. This was evidenced by 17 of the 21 participants passing the NCLEX-RN exam.

Meaningfulness = 3

The B-RNs felt that they received significant support and mentoring from loved ones, faculty, and CVHP and believed this had been a worthwhile project.

Manageability = 3

B-RNs during and after the program reported a sense of increased control over the results of their exams.

Plan Further Interaction

- 21 NCLEX-RN eligible staff members participated in the program; 17 have passed NCLEX-RN at the time of this writing.
- A second cohort of students was admitted to a preparatory course for NCLEX-RN.
- Unsuccessful program participants were admitted to a second iteration of the program.
- Internationally educated health professionals in the community were recruited for the second iteration of the program.

DISCUSSION

The success of this program was brought about the unwavering commitment of each of the providers and the participants. Constant communication and respect for the identified learning and psychosocial needs of the participants were important elements in the program. Persistent supervision and reassurance were valuable elements that may not be necessary for nurses who receive their nursing education in the United States, but these programs made a difference for these foreign-educated adult learner.

Although many institutions face the challenge of the nursing shortage, the focus of this discussion has been on the innovative programs developed by the CVMC. The strategies for meeting the goals developed by the institution are only tools. For them to be successful, there must be an awareness of the underlying values of all parties. The care plan presented describes a program that illustrates the strategies used for mutual decision making in developing a plan of action. The care plan shows how the underlying values of the participants and the institution were respected. Clear communication occurred between all parties involved in the decision-making process. Successful problem strategies can be applied only when the communication between the parties is clear and the values of each are identified and respected.

CONCLUSION

In this chapter, strategies to utilize the AIM in an institutional setting are presented. The model emphasizes the need for valuing the concerns of both the client and provider; in this case, the employee and the manager of an institution. Successful problem-solving strategies can be applied only when the communication between both parties is clear and the values of each are identified and respected. As health care institutions move toward a more horizontal management style to meet the needs of the 21st century, the AIM provides a structure to both assess the organization and implement programs to meet the goals of the institution.

REFERENCES

Argyris, C. (1971). *Management and organizational development: The path from XA to YB.* New York, NY: McGraw-Hill.

Brandon, K. (1994a, February 20). More than just life—or death—decision. *Chicago Tribune,* pp. A1, A20.

Brandon, K. (1994b, February 21). For survivor, "What are we really creating?" *Chicago Tribune,* pp. A1, A6.

Citrus Valley Health Partners. (2010a). *About Us.* Retrieved from http://www.cvhp.org/About_Us.aspx

Citrus Valley Health Partners. (2010b). *Our Mission.* Retrieved from http://www.cvhp.org/Our_Mission.aspx

Coeling, H., & Simms, L. (1993). Facilitating innovation at the nursing unit level through cultural assessment, part 1. *Journal of Nursing Administration, 23,* 46–53.

Cooper, M. C. (1991). Principle-oriented ethics and the ethics of care: A creative tension. *Advances in Nursing Science, 14,* 22–31.

Fiedler, F. (1967). *A theory of leadership effectiveness.* New York, NY: McGraw-Hill.

Gadow, S. (1985). Nurse and patient: The caring relationship. In A. H. Bishop & J. R. Scudder (Eds.), *Caring, curing, coping* (pp. 31–43). Tuscaloosa, AL: University of Alabama Press.

Gilbreth, F. (1973). Applied motion study: A collection of papers on the efficient method to industrial preparedness. In F. B. Gilbreth & L. M. Gilbreth (Eds.), *Hive management history series no. 28.* Easton, PA: Hive.

Hersey, P., Blanchard, K., & Johnson, D. (1996). *Management of organizational behavior: Utilizing human resources.* Upper Saddle River, NJ: Prentice Hall.

House, R., & Mitchell, T. (1974, Autumn). Path-goal theory of leadership. *Journal of Contemporary Business,* p. 81.

Jezewski, M. (1993). Professional governance: The missing link. *Nursing Management, 22*(8), 26–30.

Johnson, B. (1996). *Polarity management: Indentifying and managing unsolvable problems.* Amherst, MA: HRD Press.

Kuhn, A. (1974). *The logic of social systems: A unified, deductive, system-based approach to social science.* San Francisco, CA: Jossey-Bass.

Leininger, M. (1984). *Care: The essence of nursing and health.* Thorofare, NJ: Slack.

McGregor, D. (1960). *The human side of enterprise.* New York, NY: McGraw-Hill.

Peter, E., & Gallop, R. (1994). The ethic of care: A comparison of nursing and medical students. *Image: Journal of Nursing Scholarship, 26,* 47–51.

Porter-O'Grady, T., & Malloch, K. (2003). *Quantum leadership: A textbook of new leadership.* Sudbury, MA: Jones & Bartlett.

Schein, E. (1985). *Organizational culture and leadership.* San Francisco, CA: Jossey-Bass.

Shibutani, T. (1994). Reference groups as perspective. In N. J. Herman & I. T. Reynolds (Eds.), *Symbolic interaction: An introduction to social psychology.* Dix Hills, NY: General Hall.

Smeltzer, C. H. (1991). The act of negotiation: An everyday experience. *Journal of Nursing Administration, 21*(7–8), 26–30.

Stein, L. L. (1967). The doctor-nurse game. *Archives of General Psychiatry, 16,* 699–703.

Stein, L. L., Watts, D. T., & Howell, T. (1990). The doctor-nurse game revised. *New England Journal of Medicine, 322,* 546–549.

Stinson, J. E., & Johnson, T. W. (1975). The path-goal theory of leadership: A partial test and suggested refinement. *Academy of Management Journal, 18*(2), 242–252.

Tannenbaum, R., & Schmidt, W. H. (1958, March/April). How to choose a leadership pattern. *Harvard Business Review,* pp. 95–102.

Taylor, F. W. (1911). *The principles of scientific management.* New York, NY: Harper & Brothers.

Tebbitt, B. V. (1993). Demystifying organizational empowerment. *Journal of Nursing Administration, 23*(1), 18.

Vroom, V. H., & Yetten, P. W. (1973). *Leadership and decision making.* Pittsburgh, PA: University of Pittsburgh Press.

Watson, J. (1988). Human caring as a moral context for nursing education. *Nursing and Health Care, 9,* 423–425.

White, G. (1991, October). Students, too face ethical issues. *The American Nurse,* p. 21.

7

COMMUNITY, STATE, OR NATION AS CLIENT: PUBLIC HEALTH NURSING

Katharine S. West

THE PUBLIC HEALTH Nursing Section of the American Public Health Association (APHA, 2010) describes public health nurses (PHN) as nurses who "integrate community involvement and knowledge about the entire population with personal, clinical understandings of the health and illness experiences of individuals and families within the population" (Public Health Nursing Section, para. 1). To accomplish this, attention must be paid to the interpersonal interactions taking place within the community and between community members. In addition, all the structural resources available to and constraints impinging on the community, such as economic, religious, political, and legal factors, must be considered. The Artinian Intersystem Model (AIM) provides a model for assessing and working with the community that takes into account community definitions and knowledge of health (*comprehensibility*), community values regarding health (*meaningfulness*), and community behaviors carried out to promote health (*manageability*). It also provides direction for assessing the community's needs using standard public health approaches and tools. With this information, the public health nurse partners with the community to identify its main concern and develops a mutual plan of care for resolving it.

This chapter will discuss three broad aspects of public health nursing: (a) dimensions of public health nurses, including the distinctions between community health nurses and public health nurses working with communities as clients, (b) the availability and use of practice models in public health with the applicability of the AIM across all levels of public health nursing, and (c) several case study vignettes using the AIM demonstrating health promotion with different population aggregates and across community levels.

DIMENSIONS OF PUBLIC HEALTH NURSING

In 1978, the World Health Organization (WHO) and UNICEF hosted, at Alma Ata, Kazakhastan, the International Conference on Primary Health Care for the world's nations. The Alma-Ata Declaration emerged from that meeting as a major public health milestone of the 20th century, identifying primary care as the key to attaining Health for All (Bryant, 2010). The US response to Health for All was the Healthy People initiatives beginning with the 1979 US Surgeon General's Report, *Healthy People.* The Office of Disease Prevention and Health Promotion (n.d.) website states that the Healthy People national health objectives serve as the basis for states, communities, professional organizations, and others to help develop programs to improve health. Public health nurses are uniquely poised to contribute to, guide the planning of, and implement programs to improve community health. The APHA Public Health Nursing Section website describes these roles of the public health nurse. The steps of the AIM model can be discerned in their description of these roles.

Public health nurses translate and articulate the health and illness experiences of diverse, often vulnerable individuals and families in the population to health planners and policy makers and assist members of the community to voice their problems and aspirations. Public health nurses are knowledgeable about multiple strategies for intervention, from those applicable to the entire population to those for the family and the individual. Public health nurses translate knowledge from the health and social sciences to individuals and population groups through targeted interventions, programs, and advocacy. Also guiding public health practice for public health nurses today are the *Core Competencies of Public Health Nursing* (Association of State and Territorial Directors of Nursing, 2003) and the *Ten Essential Services of Public Health* (Center for Disease Control [CDC], n.d.).

Community Health Nursing and Public Health Nursing Compared

There has been considerable debate about what to call the practice of nurses outside of the hospital. Unfortunately, *community health nursing* and *public health nursing* are terms that have been used interchangeably, leading to confusion by the public and even among health care workers themselves. Despite this confusion, there is basic agreement that the defining characteristic of public health nurses is that their focus is on the health and wellness of populations. Even though public health nursing is usually delivered to individuals, one person at a time, the

TABLE 7.1 Distinctions Between Community Health Nursing and Public Health Nursing

NURSING SPECIALTY	PUBLIC HEALTH NURSING	COMMUNITY HEALTH NURSING
Education requirements (varies by state)	<ul><li>BSN (generalist/staff PHN)</li><li>MSN (Manager/CNS/Consultant/Program Specialist/Executive)</li><li>RN license</li><li>Public Health Nurse certificate</li></ul>	<ul><li>RN license</li></ul>
Level of prevention	<ul><li>Primary and Secondary prevention</li></ul>	<ul><li>Secondary and Tertiary prevention</li></ul>
Client of focus	<ul><li>Populations (City, State, Nation as client)</li><li>Aggregate populations</li><li>Vulnerable populations</li></ul>	<ul><li>Families</li><li>Individuals</li></ul>
Focus of care	<ul><li>Health promotion</li><li>Wellness</li><li>Disease prevention</li><li>Screening for asymptomatic disease and conditions</li></ul>	<ul><li>Restoration to health</li><li>Acute</li><li>Subacute</li></ul>
Predominant practice	<ul><li>Health education</li><li>Health promotion</li><li>Surveillance</li></ul>	<ul><li>Restoration support</li><li>Rehabilitation support</li><li>Maintenance support</li></ul>
Examples of roles	<ul><li>Public Health Department Nurse</li><li>Corrections Facility Nurse</li><li>School Nurse</li></ul>	<ul><li>Home Health Nurse</li><li>Community-based Nurse Educator (Lactation Consultant, Asthma Nurse Educator)</li><li>Hospice Nurse</li><li>Parish Nurse</li><li>Skilled Nursing Facility</li><li>Rehabilitation Facility</li></ul>

Source: West (2011).

beneficiary of the public health nurse's efforts is the community or population. In contrast, the community health nurse's ministrations primarily benefit individuals or their families. The efforts of the nurse usually do not make an impact on the overall health of the community. As can be seen in Table 7.1, distinctions between public health nursing and community health nursing show that public health nurses focus primarily on primary and secondary prevention to target the health of aggregates or population groups. Public health nurses focus on assurance of, access to and advocacy for health care advocacy on behalf of populations.

Populations and Communities as Clients

When defining the client or recipient of care of the public health nurse, the accepted concept is "community as client." Community, however, is a generic term and can be used to refer to public health nursing population groups, aggregate populations, or geopolitical communities. Webster's Third New International Dictionary (2000) defines *community* as (a) "the body of individuals organized into a unit or manifesting usually with awareness some unifying trait," (b) "the people living in a particular place or region and usually linked by common interests," or (c) "simply an aggregation of mutually related individuals in a given location." Public health nurses provide care for communities they care for people "organized into a unit...with a unifying trait" (homeless, school children, adult women), "living in a particular region" (distinct neighborhoods or states), or "aggregates...in a given location" (correctional inmates, third graders enrolled in a particular school).

Although most public health nursing care is ultimately delivered to an individual member of a group, the AIM provides a format for assessing, planning, and intervening with the defined community. Because it is possible to think about a member of a group at the level of the individual and think about the group itself at a more abstract level, it is possible to consider individuals to be members of a population group and also of the population group itself (Watzlawick, Weakland, & Fisch, 1974; see Figure 7.1). This makes it possible to deliver nursing care to individuals on behalf of the targeted population, recognizing that a change in the individual is a different type of change than a change in the targeted group, but at the same time, a change in the individual is what drives change in the group.

For public health nurses to deliver care that reflects joint goals and strategies for the targeted population, the nurse can develop a population-focused plan of care using the AIM. The first step is for the nurse to address the Developmental Environment, which includes the reason why the client needs

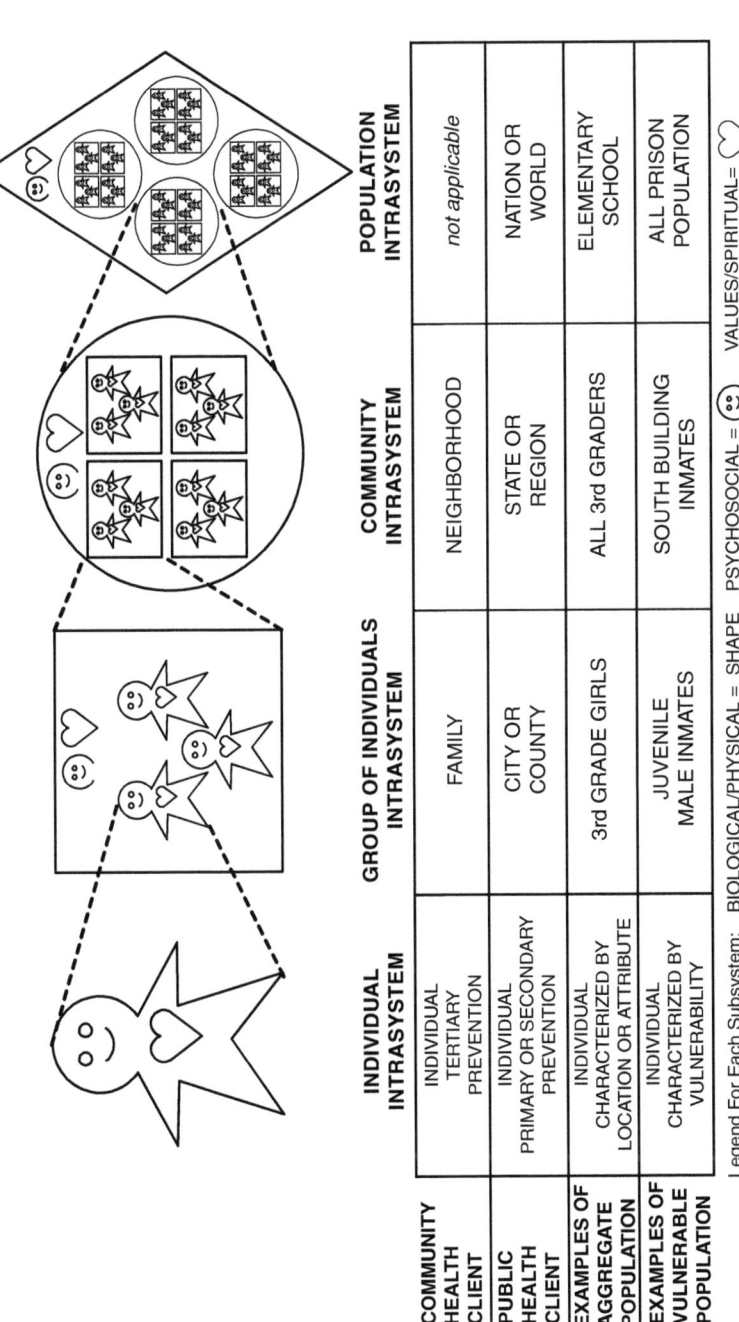

FIGURE 7.1 Hierarchy of intrasystems.
Copyright © 2011 K. S. West.

TABLE 7.2 Examples of Intrasystem Functions of Community Health Clients

FUNCTIONS	INDIVIDUAL HAS…	FAMILY HAS…	NEIGHBORHOOD OR LOCAL COMMUNITY HAS…	HEALTH CARE INSTITUTIONS HAVE…
Knowledge	■ Knowledge about the health care concern or condition ■ Knowledge about own body and responses ■ Knowledge of resources	■ Knowledge about the health care concern or condition ■ Knowledge of resources ■ Family history	■ Health agencies ■ Health care clinics ■ Special interest groups ■ Libraries	■ Policies ■ Procedures ■ Clinical Practice Guidelines ■ Connections to libraries and health care content databases
Beliefs and values	■ Personal beliefs and values of health ■ Spiritual orientation ■ Personal world view	■ Family belief system of health and wellness ■ Spiritual orientation ■ Family world view	■ Spiritual groups (churches, temples) ■ Neighborhood Watch charters	■ Mission Statement ■ Corporate philosophy of caring
Behaviors, physical resources, and support systems	■ Skills and abilities to respond to main concern ■ Use of resources to support behavior change	■ Skills and abilities to respond to main concern ■ Social Network, including extended family members and agencies to support the family	■ Cultural networks ■ Aggregate population networks (school PTA, Senior Centers, Homeless shelters) ■ Gyms and health spas ■ Schools ■ Farmers Markets	■ Experienced professional providers with skills to educate and treat the main concern (nurses, physicians) ■ Ancillary and support staff

PHN services and the assessment of the client subsystems leading to a tentative identification of the main concern of the PHN or client. The PHN may start with an initial assessment using secondary data sources about the targeted community and identify one or more topics for the potential main concern. To confirm this main concern with a community client, a needs assessment, using primary data collection such as direct interviews with members of the targeted group, helps validate the PHN's assessment. This additional assessment of the knowledge, values, and behaviors of the intrasystem leads to validating the main concern.

Community clients, whether geopolitically defined, such as cities or nations; population defined, such as school-aged children; or defined by their vulnerability, such as homeless, all have the same three intrasystem functions as the individual client: knowledge, values, and behaviors. For example, a family's knowledge is held by the members of the family. In family stories, the values and beliefs are expressed in the family's belief system of health and wellness and their spiritual worldview, while the family's behaviors are supported by their social network and specific skills and abilities that can be brought to bear on resolving the main concern (see Table 7.2).

In a similar manner, when the client is defined geopolitically such as the United States, the nation's knowledge about the health of its citizens is held by agencies such as the Department of Health and Human Services (DHHS) and the Center for Disease Control and Prevention (CDC). The nation's values can be determined by reading the US Constitution, federal laws, and the mission statements of government programs such as the Healthy People Goals and Objectives. National behaviors and resources are carried out by agencies such as the US Public Health Services commissioned corps, the Environmental Protection Agency, Medicare, and emergency preparedness through the Federal Emergency Management Agency (FEMA) (see Table 7.3).

PUBLIC HEALTH NURSING PRACTICE MODELS

In the late 1990s, nurse theorists began conceptualizing models for community health nursing. Their works were influenced by the fields of sociology, anthropology, epidemiology, occupational health, and health education. Public health nurses adapted theoretical models for nursing in an attempt to guide their management of care of populations. For example, the Community–as–Partner Model was developed by Anderson and McFarlane based on Betty Neuman's Health Systems model (Anderson & McFarlane, 2000). Other models have been developed to answer this need of PHNs. Because public health nursing has had

TABLE 7.3 Examples of Intrasystem Functions of Public Health Clients

FUNCTIONS	CITY OR COUNTY HAS…	STATE HAS…	NATION HAS…	GLOBAL ORGANIZATIONS HAVE…
Knowledge	<ul><li>Public Health Departments and Agencies</li><li>Health care entities (for profit, not-for-profit, HMO, religious-based)</li><li>Health care clinics</li><li>Vital records (county)</li><li>Libraries</li></ul>	<ul><li>Public Health Department and health-related agencies</li><li>Vital Statistics Branch</li><li>Community Colleges, Colleges, and Universities</li></ul>	<ul><li>Department of Health and Human Services programs</li><li>National Institutes of Health</li><li>Center for Disease Control and Prevention (state health statistics, health surveys, MMWR)</li></ul>	<ul><li>World Health Organization (leadership on global health matters; setting norms and standards, evidence-based policy, statistics, data)</li><li>United Nations</li><li>Center for Disease Control and Prevention: Global Health and travel information</li></ul>
Beliefs and Values	<ul><li>City Mission Statements</li><li>County Charter</li><li>County Code</li><li>Healthy People programs (City level)</li><li>Local publications and media</li></ul>	<ul><li>State constitution</li><li>Laws and regulations</li><li>Healthy People Goals (State level)</li><li>Regional publications and media</li></ul>	<ul><li>Declaration of Independence</li><li>Bill of Rights</li><li>Constitution</li><li>Laws and regulations</li><li>Healthy People Goals and Objectives 2010/2020</li><li>National publications and media</li></ul>	<ul><li>Alma-Ata Declaration of 1978 of "Health for All"</li><li>UN Declaration of Human Rights</li><li>Ministerial Declaration on Global Public Health (UN, 2009)</li><li>WTO (World Trade Organization) Rules (patents, intellectual property, emergency drugs, emerging cultures)</li></ul>

| Behaviors, Physical resources, and Support systems | - Healthy Communities Project
- Public health protection
- Public social services
- Public safety
- Property assessment
- Law enforcement
- Emergency services
- Environmental safety inspection
- Food safety inspectors | - State Public Health Programs
- Clean air and water services (state epidemiologist)
- Health insurance (Medicaid, Healthy Families)
- State Disability Insurance
- Worker's Compensation
- Services for workers (OSHA)
- Services for disabled
- Services for veterans
- Services for Seniors
- Children's Services
- Early Start programs
- Lobbyists and Advocates for health and wellness
- Emergency preparedness and support to counties and cities | - US Public Health Service commissioned corps
- Indian Health Services
- Department of Health and Human Services
- Environmental Protection Agency
- Food and Drug Administration
- Health insurance (MediCare)
- Social Security
- Port inspections
- National safety
- Federal law enforcement
- Emergency preparedness and support to the states (FEMA)
- Center for Disease Control and Prevention (support state and local health departments) | - World Health Organization programs and commissions (provide technical support to nations)
- World Bank
- International Monetary Fund (IMF)
- NGO (non-governmental organizations) programs
- Non-profit organizations and initiatives (Gates Foundation, Central Asia Institute, aka Pennies for Peace, Partners in Health)
- USAID Global Health Bureau |

Source: West (2011).

challenges finding models that accurately reflect the unique aspects of population care, there have been many attempts to create an appropriate model. Los Angeles County public health nurses developed a model that combines the 10 Essential Public Health Skills with the Nursing Process, essentially combining content and process (LA County, 2007). By contrast, the AIM is process-oriented but content-free, which allows greater flexibility in its application to any health setting with any health care client. Because the AIM addresses the interplay of systems, it can be used at any level of public health nursing practice, from individuals to nations. The focus of the AIM is on participation of the clients in the decision-making process. This is foundational for creating partnerships with the community; it is the cornerstone of quality public health practice.

When using the AIM to plan for care of communities or aggregate populations, just as when nurses use it to plan care for individuals or families, the nurse must be aware of the power differences between the public health nurse and the clients. For a true partnership to occur, the interactional process must be carefully monitored to be sure that input from both groups is honored. The problem of inequality of power is further complicated in the public health setting because the socioeconomic, political, and legal bases for problems are more evident and the clients often do not have the resources or skills to challenge the system. Although community participation is a major goal in public health through the fostering of community partnerships, public health nurses are sometimes conflicted in how to include the community. Without community participation, goals may be vague, unrealistic, or simply ignored with the result that planners act from their own perspectives or from secondary data sources with no real input from the community and miss the true main concern. The PHN must guard against rhetoric that claims community ownership without evidence of mutual goal setting and planning interventions with the community. The AIM provides a framework to bring together the "public, private, voluntary, and community sectors united under the common purpose of promoting health for city residents" (Yan, 1993, p. 185). Only through an awareness of the main concern as defined by the community and a concerted effort to honor those values and input from the community's members will it be possible for PHNs to engage in mutual interaction to resolve the main concern of their community clients.

HEALTH PROMOTION ACROSS COMMUNITY LEVELS

Not only can the AIM be used to guide practice among the hierarchy of public health clients, it can also be used as a framework to review the roles of the various agencies as they provide health care services across the levels of prevention. An example of the intrasystem functions of public health clients and how their particular roles complement each other in a comprehensive national effort can be discovered through a review of the Early Hearing Detection and Intervention (EHDI) programs at different geopolitical levels (see Table 7.4).

Health Promotion in a Multilevel Comprehensive Integrated Program

In late 1969, the Joint Committee on Infant Hearing (JCIH) was established and composed initially of representatives from audiology, otolaryngology, pediatrics, and nursing. The JCIH was charged with two responsibilities: first, to make recommendations concerning the early identification of children with or at-risk for hearing loss, and second, to make recommendations regarding newborn hearing screening. In 1970, the committee's first statement issued was that mass hearing screening could not be justified at that time because there were no appropriate test procedures. The statement, however, encouraged ongoing research and acknowledged the need to detect hearing loss early in life (JCIH, n.d., para. 1). Over the years, the Committee's primary activity has been to publish position statements summarizing the state of science for and the art of infant hearing screening and care and to give recommendations for action by health care providers and the government. By the mid-1990s, technology had advanced sufficiently to make universal newborn hearing screening feasible and efficacious. Every state responded to the JCIH 2000 Position Statement to implement universal newborn hearing screening programs. The current 2007 JCIH Position Statement provides this goal:

> ...early hearing detection and intervention (EHDI) is to maximize linguistic competence and literacy development for children who are deaf or hard of hearing. Without appropriate opportunities to learn language, these children will fall behind their hearing peers in communication, cognition, reading, and social-emotional development. Such delays may result in lower educational and employment levels in adulthood. To maximize the outcome for infants who are deaf or hard of hearing, the hearing of all infants should be screened at no later than 1 month of age. Those who do not pass screening should have a comprehensive audiological evaluation at no later than 3 months of age. Infants with confirmed hearing loss should receive appropriate intervention at no later than 6 months of age from health care and education professionals with expertise in hearing loss and deafness in infants and young children.

TABLE 7.4 Intrasystem Functions to Support EHDI Programs

FUNCTIONS	FAMILY HAS…	STATE OF CALIFORNIA HAS…	NATIONAL EHDI PROGRAMS HAVE…	GLOBAL PROGRAMS HAVE…
Knowledge source	▪ Family without deaf experience: dependent on health care providers for knowledge initially ▪ Family with deaf experience: lived experience	▪ Hearing Coordination Centers (HCC) ▪ HCC Screening Coordinators ▪ State consulting audiologists ▪ Department of Education Deaf-Blind Unit	▪ CDC EHDI ▪ Boy's Town Infant Hearing Web site ▪ Gallaudet University ▪ National Association for the Deaf ▪ National Association for Hearing Assessment and Management (NCHAM) ▪ National Institute on Deafness and Other Communication Disorders (NIDCD)	▪ International Working Group on Childhood Hearing (annual surveys)
Statements of beliefs and values	▪ Communication with newborn is important	▪ Article 5 (commencing with Section 123800) of Chapter 3 of part 2 of Division 106 of the Health and Safety code, as amended by Assembly Bill (AB) 2780, Chapter 310, statues of 1998 ▪ Health And Safety Code Sections relating to Newborn Hearing	▪ Joint Committee on Infant Hearing (JCIH) Statement 2000, 2007 ▪ American Academy of Pediatrics (AAP) Policy Statement "Newborn and Infant Hearing Loss: Detection and Intervention" 1999, rev 2000 ▪ ASHA Guidelines for the "Audiologic assessment of children	▪ 1998 European Consensus Statement ▪ GPOD (Global Coalition of Parents of Children who are Deaf or Hard of Hearing) 2010 Position Statement and recommendations for Family Support in the Development

		Screening with amendments required by (AB) 2651, Chapter 335, Statutes Of 2006	of Newborn Hearing Screening Systems (NHS)/Early Hearing Detection and Intervention Systems (EHDI) Worldwide
Behavioral response	• Follow through on the 1-3-6 Plan • CA Department of Developmental Services, Early Start Programs: Individualized Family Service Plan (IFSP) for home speech and language services • California Children's Services financial support for hearing aids • Support for families from specific communication option organizations	• Communication Disorder Centers—Type C (audiologists specializing in newborn care) • House Ear Institute CARE Center • John Tracy Clinic, Los Angeles, CA (Southern California free evaluations and services)	• NIH Consensus Statement 1993 • IDEA (special education law) • NCLB (general education law) • Section 504—Americans with Disabilities Act • American Society for Deaf Children • Alexander Graham Bell Association for the Deaf and Hard of Hearing • BEGINNINGS (non-profit organization) • Boys Town • Cued Speech Association • Hear Now • Listen-Up Web site	• EU Projects on Universal Newborn Hearing Programmes [sic] • John Tracy Clinic, Los Angeles, CA (world-wide parent-centered services to young children with a hearing loss)

Source: West (2011).

Regardless of previous hearing-screening outcomes, all infants with or without risk factors should receive ongoing surveillance of communicative development beginning at 2 months of age during well-child visits in the medical home. EHDI systems should guarantee seamless transitions for infants and their families through this process (JCIH, 2007).

In 1998, California passed the Newborn and Infant Hearing Screening, Tracking and Intervention Act. This law mandated that the California Department of Health Care Services (DHCS), Children's Medical Services (CMS) Branch, implement a statewide comprehensive Newborn Hearing Screening Program (NHSP). Integral to the success of this program are the regional Hearing Coordination Centers with nurses in the roles of the RN Screening Coordinators, state case managers, who facilitate communication between families, health providers, and educational professionals and ensure successful transition for the families between the stages of services in a timely manner (PH core services of *assurance* and *access*). The Screening Coordinators engage in intersystem interactions with the families as clients, as well as various health care providers and the state of California as clients. Working with the state as client, the Screening Coordinator works to resolve the main concern that newborns and infants complete the 1-3-6 plan on time. When an infant does not pass the birth hearing screening, the Screening Coordinator collaborates with the family to resolve the main concern which is to communicate with the baby (Table 7.5).

Not all families need a nurse or a plan of care. One newborn identified with hearing loss in the CA NHSP had been admitted to the well-baby nursery. When he did not pass his initial hearing screening, the mother said she knew intuitively that the baby was deaf because he had not responded to sounds *in utero*. For her, it was very important to immediately determine his level of hearing loss. Her baby was diagnosed with a moderate hearing loss and fitted with hearing aids by 4 weeks of age. The family was integrated with Early Start services well before the 6-month EHDI goal.

Conversely, there were parents who were themselves deaf and eager to have their newborn daughter screened for hearing loss. When the baby did not pass the initial screening, they pursued a diagnostic audiological evaluation because it was also very important to them to determine her level of hearing loss. They were pleased with the confirmation of profound hearing loss because, as they explained to the Screening Coordinator, "Our daughter is like us!" But, at that point, they refused any further services for their baby, as they said, "Who better than us who have experienced this to introduce a deaf baby to a hearing world?" As their SOC was adequate, they had no need for a nurse—they already knew what to do. The AIM is designed for people who need assistance from nursing. When working with these parents who were confident with their ability to manage the situation, the Screening Coordinator used the information from the Developmental Assessment of the family's subsystems and concluded there was no need to mutually negotiate a plan of care. In concept, this proved a dilemma, initially, for the Screening Coordinators working with deaf families. Indeed, it took some time and adjustment before the nurses could trust in the situation before them: SSOC did not apply in this situation because the family was not in crisis; their SOC was not impaired because the family knew what to do. The AIM process enables PHNs to determine when care can be discontinued even after the initial assessment. The Screening Coordinators became comfortable concluding care at any point of the AIM that matched the client's needs.

Health Promotion at the Local Level

The AIM can be used to facilitate resolution of the main concern of community clients at local neighborhood and city levels. When I teach Public health nursing courses, I spread the community teaching assignment for the students over a 4-week period, staging their efforts according to the AIM process. Students submit their first report on the Developmental Environment assessment phase: Intrasystem Data Collection, Tentative Identification of a Main Concern, and Validation of the Main Concern. Their second report describes their Analysis of the Intrasystem, the Development of Joint Goals and Strategies, and the Mutual Plan of Care. Their final paper recounts their Implementation Strategies and Evaluation of Resolution of the Main Concern. I expanded the AIM Block Care Plan Template (see Appendix A) for Community Health to include identification of the corresponding Healthy People Goal(s) and Objective(s) and a Community Nursing Diagnosis (see Appendix B, AIM Community Health Care Plan Template).

Below are five case study vignettes of public health nursing students addressing the main concern of each of their community clients. Each one highlights a different aspect of the AIM in helping the PHN navigate the resolution of the main concern. The first vignette illustrates the need for an iterative collection of data in order to validate the main concern. The next two vignettes showcase aspects of the Intersystem Interaction, one on Communicating Information and the other on Negotiating Values. The fourth vignette focuses on the readiness for change in an aggregate population. The final vignette shows the use of the AIM in facilitating the PHN Core Competency of Advocacy.

TABLE 7.5 Intersystem Interactions in the Stages of the California Newborn Hearing Screening Program

STAGE	BIRTH ADMISSION SCREENING	FOLLOW-UP SCREENING	DIAGNOSTIC AUDIOLOGY EXAM	EARLY INTERVENTION
Timeframe	At birth	By 1 month of age	By 3 months of age	By 6 months of age
Recipient	Family and newborn	Family and infant	Family and infant	Family and infant
Services provided	Hospital birth admission hearing screening results in a "Refer"	Out-patient hearing re-screening results in a "Refer"	Diagnostic Audiologic Evaluation (DAE) results in diagnosis of hearing loss with type and configuration	Coordinated services: ■ Early Start ■ Individualized Family Service Plan (IFSP) ■ Audiology ■ Speech pathology ■ Otolaryngology ■ Hearing Aid vendor
Transition facilitated	Inpatient hearing screening provider schedules outpatient re-screen appointment	Out-patient hearing screening provider schedules audiology appointment	Audiology provider reports infant status to Early Start Services (Department of Education) and California Children's	Early Start provider initiates an individualized Family Service Plan (IFSP) on behalf of infant and family, to help families be aware of all communication options

			and available hearing technologies (presented in an unbiased manner). Informed family choice and desired outcome guide the decision-making process.
Supportive funding	Health insurance coverage for inpatient hearing screening (MediCal, Healthy Families, HMO, PPO)	Health insurance coverage for outpatient hearing screening (MediCal, Healthy Families, HMO, PPO)	Health insurance and referral to state funding (CCS) for audiology and ancillary services (MediCal, Healthy Families, HMO, PPO)	Health insurance coverage for ongoing medical services as indicated (MediCal, Healthy Families, HMO, PPO)
Actions to resolve the main concern of the state	Inpatient screening result sent by hospital to regional state HCC for tracking	Outpatient screening result sent by outpatient provider to regional state HCC for tracking	DAE results sent by audiologist to regional state HCC for tracking	Initiation of Early Start Services confirmed by state HCC

Source: West (2011).

Case Study Vignettes

Case Study 7.1

Reducing Dietary Sodium for Indonesian Seniors[1]
Antonius Hardianto, BSN, RN

In this community health example, Antonius Hardianto identified a Nichiren Buddhist Indonesian-speaking group with ages between 60 and 75 years old. They frequented a local senior center and were interested in learning about healthy choices in nutrition. Originally, he thought he would offer education on whole nutrition based on his initial needs assessment of a secondary review of data from the CDC, State of California Vital Statistics, and US Census Bureau.

To validate his tentative Main Concern, he interviewed the group leader. It was reported that the senior citizens followed a diet that Antonius knew was not very good for their health problems. They liked to eat red meat such as beef and lamb, believed that drinking whole milk was good for them, and liked to use soy sauce, a product very high in sodium. They also liked to eat animal intestines, an ethnic delicacy, and to cook with coconut milk. They liked to do "pot luck" when they met two or three times a week at the senior center. From this interview, Antonius identified three potential main concerns he thought would be of interest to the group: healthy nutrition choices related to saturated fat intake, sodium intake, and carbohydrate intake, with a focus on prevention or reduction of chronic heart diseases.

To validate the main concern of the group leader with the group members, he next interviewed the group members, one by one to learn about their health problems and their typical eating patterns. Five were on medications for high blood pressure and high cholesterol, one was on diabetes medication, and one had high blood pressure, high cholesterol, and osteoporosis. They reported that they frequently ate at restaurants and food courts, citing ease and frugal costs. For $5.00, they could have 3 or 4 different foods and rice, but foods that were greasy, salty, or sweet but tasty, and they did not have to cook. When he challenged them asking, "How could you eat like

---

[1] Used with permission from Antonius Hardianto, BSN, RN.

that every day?" they laughed, shrugged their shoulders, and said "Well ..."

He discovered in these interviews that they believed that they did not eat much salt, because they thought the salt shaker was the only source of salt; they rarely added table salt to their cooked foods. Thus, when Antonius analyzed all the data, it became clear to him that his main concern was to provide information in a culturally sensitive manner about reducing dietary sodium. He was able to link the main concern to Healthy People Focus Area 19, Nutrition and Overweight, Objective 19–10: *Increase the proportion of persons aged 2 years and older who consume 2,400 mg or less of sodium daily* (Healthy People, n.d. a).

The educational care plan was developed, resulting in a lesson plan, using culturally and linguistically appropriate handouts, to teach awareness of sodium content in traditional Indonesian foods with acceptable alternative food choices, and how to read packaged food labels to calculate daily sodium intake.

To implement the care plan, Antonius presented some of the popular foods often consumed by the group. "It got their attention when they saw their favorite foods," he reported. He showed them how much salt was in a standard serving of soy sauce, by measuring table salt on a kitchen gram scale. The group was surprised to see how much 180 g of salt was, for instance, and made them realize there was salt "hiding" in their foods. This type of visual demonstration worked well for the group. "They kept saying, 'Oh my God! I didn't know there is so much sodium in that food!'" he recounted, "because foods such as oyster sauce tastes sweet even though it is 40% salt from MSG." He also distributed packaging from their favorite foods, such as milk, tofu, Hochin sauce, black bean sauce, curry powder, and miso. He had them each find the sodium content on the label, and showed them how to add up the numbers to determine daily sodium intake. Even though many of the foods were imports with labeling in another language, the FDA requires nutrition labeling to be in English for foods sold in the United States. Learning how to locate the sodium content in English was appreciated by the seniors. In a follow-up session, he met the seniors at their favorite ethnic grocery store and took them on an aisle-by-aisle tour to compare favorite high-sodium foods with healthy alternatives.

What started as an obvious need for general nutrition teaching, based on secondary data sources, became fine-tuned to reducing

(Continued)

dietary sodium as Antonius looped back in the Intrasystem Data Collection phase to validate the main concern. The end result was that the seniors became more aware of monitoring sodium intake with healthy options for change. "Really," he said, "it is all about education. It requires a lot of work and help with this generation. You cannot teach them one time; you must go back in 2 or 3 months to give them reminders, or they will go back to their previous routine."

Case Study 7.2

Management of Hypertension for Chinese Seniors[2]

Michelle Song-Howe, BSN, RN

This vignette illustrates the aspect of Communicating Information with an ethnic population group. As a Chinese-English speaker, Michelle was well able to provide language-appropriate interactions for the group. The initial request from the Chinese Senior Center was to provide education and health promotion with a nutrition focus. Their morning Tai Chi group believed they were all healthy because they exercised regularly and were motivated to improve their diet. The nurse performed a needs assessment using secondary data sources. She then interviewed 19 women and 11 men ranging in age from 65 to 85. Her tentative identification of the main concern was that the elders wanted to hear about healthy food choices or reducing fat in the diet. She collected additional information by distributing Chinese-language questionnaires. However, when the needs assessment was completed, she discovered that 70% of the larger group had hypertension and were using hypertension medications. The others who were not on medication were nonetheless interested to learn more about how to manage blood pressure. They all were interested in learning how to use a blood pressure machine and wanted to understand what blood pressure readings mean. She validated the Main Concern with the group leader to be hypertension management and developed a mutual plan of care with input from the group leaders.

---

[2] Used with permission from Michelle Song-Howe, BSN, RN.

It was determined that she should provide her education prior to the 8:30 a.m. morning session in the park. Weekday participants of the Chinese Tai Chi Chuan Senior Group numbered around 30 seniors with as many as 40 seniors during the weekend. Most spoke Chinese, and a few spoke English very well. Michelle identified the appropriate Healthy People 2010 Objective 12–11: *Increase the proportion of adults with high blood pressure who are taking action (for example, losing weight, increasing physical activity, or reducing sodium intake) to help control their blood pressure* (Healthy People, n.d. b). In order to tailor her communication methods to her audience, she determined their stage of psychosocial development according to Erikson as Wisdom: Ego integrity vs. despair. She used Bloom's Taxonomy levels of *knowledge* (list, identify, or recall information) and *application* (exhibit, demonstrate, or practice) to develop her lesson plan.

"I chose demonstrations of the use of hands-on equipment such as a home blood pressure monitor and anatomical models of arteries, so the learner could physically manipulate these objects," she reported. "On the day I was set to teach, I arrived an hour before the Tai Chi class with a blood pressure monitor, my models, some alcohol gel, and colorful handout materials. The leaders of the group helped me set up everything on the table. The people all came around the table. They started to put their hands on my model, blood pressure monitor, and the other things I had brought along, and everyone got a brochure. I started a brief opening speech. I demonstrated how to monitor blood pressure correctly by checking the group leader's blood pressure. It showed 130/84. I asked everyone what did this blood pressure mean? Some people said that it was high. Some people answered that it was okay. I asked them to look at the brochure, and then tell me what it indicated. Now they all answered that the reading was pre-hypertension. 'That is very correct', I responded."

Michelle quickly realized that her success at communicating information with the participants was directly related to giving everyone a chance to use the monitor and manipulate the models. She let everyone use the equipment to check each other's blood pressure, reinforcing correct placement of the cuff, and reinforcing best practices of checking every day at the same time with the same equipment. There were 18 blood pressures checked. Seven of them were either prehypertensive or high enough to require same day

(Continued)

treatment. This surprised the group because they thought their practice of Tai Chi would protect them from hypertension. Even after rechecking, a few seniors had elevated blood pressures. For several, this was new information, and they agreed to contact their primary care provider that day for further evaluation and treatment. "We thought exercise was good enough. We thought high blood pressure and stroke is an old person issue," was their comment.

Michelle used every opportunity to stimulate the recall of her instruction by asking questions. She found that demonstration, return demonstration, and a role-playing learning format was an effective method of teaching, suitable for the elderly, and appropriate for the Chinese culture. By the end of the educational session, the seniors were able to define in their own words high blood pressure and name three steps they could take to improve their blood pressure. They were able to share in their own words the signs and symptoms of heart disease and stroke. Michelle summarized this in her final report of her student teaching experience:

> The American Hospital Association passed A Patient's Bill of Rights mandating client education as a right of all clients in 1992. Being a public health educator is an important role for nurse. As a nurse, I am in a position to promote health through education. Clients have the right to have health education in order to make informed decisions about their health. The Joint Commission on Accreditation of Healthcare Organizations (JCAHO) recently expanded standards of client education by nurses to include evidence that patients and their significant others understand what they have been taught. This requirement means that providers must consider the literacy level, educational background, language skills, and culture of every client during the education process. From this teaching project, I learned that teaching involves not only health promotion, but increasing a person's level of wellness also. (M. Song-Howe. May 5, 2010. [Teaching Project Phase 3 Report: Evaluation of Teaching Effectiveness]. Copy in possession of author.)

Case Study 7.3

Dating Safety Education for a Catholic Youth Group[3]
Abigail Evangelista, BSN, RN

This vignette highlights the importance of Negotiating Values with a community client and adapting the educational objectives of the nurse to match those of the client. After performing a needs assessment of a Catholic youth group, ages 12–16, the group indicated they would rather talk to a nurse about their main concern of sex and sex safety. However, when Abigail approached the youth group leaders for their approval of the topic, she found that the church was diametrically opposed to approving a topic that violated the church's values of celibacy before marriage. Abigail met with the youth group leaders several times, to negotiate values for an appropriate topic that would nonetheless satisfy the identified main concern. In these meetings, the youth leadership clarified that she must not cover birth control or safe sex practices, but could teach about date rape, date abuse, and physical violence against women. Finally, joint goals were developed for a mutual educational plan of care on the topic of safe dating. This confirms the importance of the needs assessment, validation of the main concern, and the importance of the intersystem interaction to develop a mutual plan of care.

After the joint goals were determined, Abigail re-evaluated the teens for this revised topic. During her re-evaluation of the group, she found that 12 of the 18 teens in the group were dating in one form or another (group dates, individual dates), with 3 reporting physical assault by their dating partner. She identified an applicable Healthy People 2010 Objective 15–34: *Reduce the rate of physical assault by current or former intimate partners with a target of 3.3 physical assaults per 1,000 persons aged 12 years and older* (Healthy People, n.d. c).

The implementation strategies for her educational plan of care were to host a teaching forum to teach the teens the warning signs of physical violence, how to get and give help to those who suffer from physical violence, and how to stop physical violence. Participating

(Continued)

---
[3] Used with permission from Abigail Evangelista, BSN, RN.

teens were required to obtain approval from their parents and submit a permission slip to the church office. Abigail also had to secure approval from the church office for all materials used in the teaching.

The teaching project was well received. Abigail used a skit as an ice breaker to get the students involved. As the student arrived at the class, two of the volunteers acted out a violence skit. A male was being verbally and physically abusive to the female in the skit. All the lights in the room were off with only a spotlight focused on the actors. When the skit was over, the students were asked how they felt about what they had just seen, and an open dialogue started. As the students became more comfortable discussing the topic, they were asked if any of them had witnessed or experienced violence first hand with an intimate partner. Again, open dialogue ensued. The teens next participated in an exercise called Stand Up and Have a Voice. In this exercise, the girls stand up and declare "NO" in a loud strong voice, then sit down. The boys then stand and state "I am listening to you, and I have heard what you said." Brochures and community resource information handouts were distributed.

The evaluation of the class showed the students stated that they enjoyed the class and would like Abigail to return to teach more topics. They indicated a positive rescoring on the Situational Sense of Coherence (SSOC), in that the information presented was comprehensible to them, very meaningful, and demonstrated behaviors they believed they could do (manageability).

One student in the class approached Abigail after the teaching to say she wanted to get out of an abusive relationship, but didn't know how to do that safely. She had learned a lot from the class, but was not ready to end her relationship at that time. As a result of the course, the youth leaders were now aware of the problem and could be more available to help her.

Abigail reflected on the challenges initially presented by the constraints of the values of the church. "It felt so restrictive at first. But then I realized that the PHN needs to be creative and inventive and honor the client's preferences that I could say this but not that." In her position as a public health educator, she said, "I need to remember that although I would like to teach everything, I need to keep focused on the 'must knows' according to the client's values. I would love to go back and teach additional classes. The evaluation of this teaching is ongoing at this time. I cannot change the way others act, but I can influence their behavior with good teaching."

Case Study 7.4

Smoking Cessation Program in a Homeless Shelter[4]

Darya Ratliff, BSN, RN

The fourth vignette focuses on evaluating the Resolution the Main concern and the need for further intervention. This teaching project focused on providing smoking cessation education at a community homeless shelter, using the Healthy People 2010 Objective 27–5: *Increase smoking cessation attempts by adult smokers.* The community homeless shelter hosts an average of 80 persons visiting daily with an average age of 40 years. The needs assessment was performed with the administrator of the shelter, who stated that smoking was a big problem in that particular homeless population; however, there was no funding for smoking cessation in their budget. Additional needs assessment was done by observing the clients, talking to them, and analyzing their responses. The Main concern was validated with the shelter administrator and case managers and plans were made to provide a class on smoking cessation. To reach the maximum numbers of clients, the class was planned for eight in the morning during breakfast while clients were getting ready for their day.

The teaching plan did not work as Darya planned. She found the clients were not able to stay at one place; they walked around talking to each other. She found that information was missed due to their short attention span and their continuous moving around the shelter.

"People kept coming and going all the time," she reported. "Some of them were reluctant to learn and refused to listen to me." However, after seeing the interest of others, the reluctant clients started walking through the teaching area, where she caught their attention by giving free candies, offering samples, and reading a few brochures out loud. The posters that she hung on the walls and the free candies she brought got their interest. Many were not interested in the brochures. However, one flyer showing the time nicotine stays in the body captured their attention. Nicotine candies and gum were popular as well. They were willing to try them and talk about

(Continued)

---

[4] Used with permission from Darya Ratliff, BSN, RN.

them. The small information cards that looked like credit cards quickly got their attention. She reported, "I had to adjust my teaching to constantly 'go with the flow.' It was a constant challenge. They were very sarcastic and reluctant to receive my teaching."

Nonetheless, Darya was able to have short discussions with a few clients. Some of them sat quietly and listened. They accepted written information and tried out the samples. Three people were very interested in quitting smoking. They took all the resources and information about smoking cessation. The supervisor took their names for follow-up. One week later, one of the clients phoned Darya to tell her that she had stopped smoking.

Evaluating the Resolution of the Main concern was initially very hard. It was difficult to assess the learning outcomes from the clients. Based on the success of only one client who stopped smoking as a result of the teaching, it looked like a poor outcome. Using another model to supplement the AIM allowed Darya to make a different assessment of the outcome. The Transtheoretical Model of Change, or Stages of Change Model, describes different stages of readiness for change. It may be more accurate to assess the stage of each participant before the teaching and measure movement to the next phase as evidence of success from the teaching, rather than assess measures of the ultimate desired outcome, cessation of smoking. In the Stages of Change model, clients can be in one of five stages: precontemplation, contemplation, preparation, action, maintenance, and relapse (Zimmerman, Olsen, & Bosworth, 2000). From the various behaviors of the clients observed at the time of the teaching, it appears as if many clients were in precontemplation or contemplation stages. Those who became interested and accepted the handouts and other materials moved into the preparation stage. Only the three clients who expressed interest and listened to the teaching were clearly in the preparation phase, and one of them moved into the action phase within the week by actually quitting smoking.

As a PHN educator, Darya learned that her own self confidence is very important when working with people who seemed not to care about their health. She also determined that evaluating behaviors of change may need to reflect several parameters along a continuum of readiness for change and incorporate insight from additional models or theories. Helping at least one person's life improve is still a success that provided encouragement to the other homeless clients, and the person served as a role model showing that smoking cessation is possible, even while homeless.

Case Study 7.5

Advocacy for Food Security: The WIC Program in a Farmer's Market[5]

Katerina Perez, BSN, RN

The final vignette shows the use of the AIM in facilitating the PHN Core Competency of Advocacy. In this case, the student was concerned with facilitating the Healthy People 2010 Objective 19–5: *Increase the proportion of persons aged 2 years and older who consume at least two daily servings of fruit* and as a corollary, Objective 19–18: *Increase food security among US households and in so doing reduce hunger* (Healthy People 2010. n.d. b). Food security is defined in the Healthy People 2010 Objective 19–18:

> Food security means that people have access at all times to enough food for an active, healthy life. It implies that people have nutritionally adequate and safe foods and sufficient household resources to ensure their ability to acquire adequate, acceptable foods in socially acceptable ways—that is, through regular marketplace sources and not through severe coping strategies like emergency food sources, scavenging, and stealing.

During her intrasystem data collection about her assigned community, Katerina discovered that four of five health food stores, and also the local farmer's market, did not accept the California Electronic Benefit Transfer (EBT) debit cards for the Women, Infants, Children (WIC) food supplement program. She also determined that food stamps households had increased 25.8% between February 2009 and February 2010 (California Department of Social Services, 2010). Her conclusion was that participants in these food supplement programs were limited in their access to fresh food and certainly not able to purchase food at the farmer's market with WIC funds.

Katerina reported, "I really enjoyed talking to owners and managers of health food stores. One proudly informed me that he

(Continued)

---

[5] Used with permission from Katerina Perez, BSN, RN.

does accept EBT in his store; others, who did not have the capability and equipment to process EBT cards, were really interested in starting. They felt like it was a great idea from a business point of view as well as a good idea for the whole community from a human prospective. They were pleased that somebody was looking into it."

Katerina's intrasystem analysis of the community led her to conclude that although she was unable to assess what the community at large knew about the problem and potential solutions, she was able to assess the city council's awareness, attitudes, and ability to respond to the issue at their monthly council meeting. Her intrasystem analysis of herself showed that her own convictions had become aroused through her assessment of the community. She found that she had strong feelings about advocating for people who were dependent on state-funded sources of food and that they should be able to access fresh local food.

Stressors in the community were identified as the economic crisis, rising unemployment, and more households dependent on supplementary food programs. Coping resources available were food stamp and WIC programs available from the county Department of Public Services for those who qualified. However, there was a lack of stores in the immediate community that accepted food stamps or WIC EBT cards. Upon further investigation, Katerina discovered that the state provided a "token" economy for farmer's markets to enable EBT cards be used to purchase fresh, local produce. The farmer's market needed to apply for the program. Then a booth could be set up where the WIC recipient could swipe the EBT card in exchange for tokens. The tokens could be used to purchase produce from the farmer merchants. At the end of the market, the farmers could exchange the tokens back into cash at the booth.

Katerina determined a unilateral community nurse goal, which was to raise awareness about the lack of acceptance of food stamps/EBT cards by the local health food stores or local farmer's market. She decided to offer a solution to the city council to encourage adoption of the "token" exchange at the farmer's market as a "first step" toward food accessibility. She completed a Speaker's Card to address the city council and prepared a 3-minute speech with supportive printed materials and references to support her argument.

Katerina reported, "When I was presenting my EBT card idea in front of council members, I was little shy and felt that perhaps I did not have the authority or credentials to do so. I could have done a better job 'selling the idea' to the councilors." Yet her credentials as an RN and as a public health nursing student afforded comprehensibility for the council. Her proposed solution, to implement the state's 'token' booth at the local farmer's market, was both manageable and meaningful. The city council had been unaware of the program and responded favorably to Katerina's presentation. "I guess," she mused afterward, "that's what advocacy in public health is all about—standing up for people in a community who cannot stand up for themselves."

CONCLUSION

Dr. Halfdan Mahler, Director General Emeritus of WHO, summarized the essence of the nature of public health care as described in this chapter. He said "Health is not a commodity that is given. It must be generated from within. Health action should not be imposed from the outside, foreign to the people; it must be a response of the communities to problems they perceive, supported by an adequate infrastructure. This is the essence of the filtering inwards process of primary health care" (Bryant, 2010, para. 4).

REFERENCES

American Public Health Association. (2010). *APHA: Public Health Nursing Section*. Retrieved from http://www.apha.org/membergroups/sections/aphasections/phn/

Anderson, E. T., & McFarlane, J. (2000). *Community as partner* (3rd ed.). Philadelphia, PA: Lippincott Williams & Wilkins.

Association of State and Territorial Directors of Nursing. (2003). *Quad Council PHN Competencies*. Retrieved from http://www.astdn.org/publication_quad_council_phn_competencies.htm

Bryant, J. H. (2010). *Alma Ata Declaration: Encyclopedia of Public Health*. eNotes. Retrieved from http://www.enotes.com/public-health-encyclopedia/alma-ata-declaration

California Department of Social Services. (April, 2010). *Federal food stamps program*. Retrieved from http://www.cdss.ca.gov/research/res/pdf/foodtrends/FS03.pdf

Center for Disease Control [CDC]. (n.d.). *National Public Health Performance Standards Program*. Retrieved from http://www.cdc.gov/od/ocphp/nphpsp/essentialphservices.htm

community. (2002). *Merriam-Webster's third new international dictionary unabridged*. Springfield, MA: Merriam-Webster, Inc.

Healthy People 2010. (n.d. a). *12 Heart disease and stroke*. Retrieved from http://www.healthypeople.gov/document/html/volume1/12heart.htm

Healthy People 2010. (n.d. b). *19 Nutrition and overweight*. Retrieved from http://www.healthypeople.gov/document/html/volume2/19nutrition.htm

Healthy People 2010. (n.d. c). *27 Tobacco use*. Retrieved from http://www.healthypeople.gov/document/html/volume2/27tobacco.htm#_Toc489766221

Joint Committee on Infant Hearing [JCIH]. (n.d.). *History of the Joint Committee on Infant Hearing*. Retrieved from http://www.jcih.org/history.htm

Joint Committee on Infant Hearing [JCIH]. (2007). Year 2007 position statement: Principles and guidelines for early hearing detection and intervention programs. *Pediatrics, 120*(4), 898–921.

LA County. (2007). *Public Health Nursing Practice Model*. Retrieved from http://www.lapublichealth.org/phn/docs/PracticeModelfinal2.pdf

Office of Disease Prevention and Health Promotion. (n.d.). *Healthy People 2010*. Retrieved from http://www.healthypeople.gov/About/history.htm

Watzlawick, P., Weakland, J. H., & Fisch, R. (1974). *Change: Principles of problem formation and problem resolution*. New York, NY: Norton, W. W. & Company, Inc.

Yan, J. (1993). *Community participation and the California healthy cities: A grounded theory study*. Unpublished doctoral dissertation, University of Southern California, Los Angeles, CA.

Zimmerman, G. L., Olsen, C. G., & Bosworth, M. F. (2000). A "Stages of Change" approach to helping patients change behavior. *American Family Physician, 61*, 1409–1416.

PART

III

THE ARTINIAN INTERSYSTEM MODEL IN EDUCATIONAL SETTINGS

Barbara M. Artinian

L EARNING THEORIES THAT are useful for students in developing clinical reasoning and critical thinking skills are presented in Chapter 8. In addition, a method of using evidence-based data to guide practice is given.

Chapter 9 describes the use of the AIM at Azusa Pacific University (APU). The congruence of the philosophy of the APU School of Nursing and the AIM is discussed. Boyers' priorities for quality schools are demonstrated in the APU curriculum. Case studies at the freshman, junior, and senior levels are presented. The introduction of the AIM at the graduate level through the use of personal philosophies of nursing is illustrated by two examples of philosophies written by graduate students. The templates for preparing care plans using the AIM is identified (see Appendices A, B, C, and D).

Chapter 10 describes an emerging nursing program in Burundi, Central Africa, that is based on Antonovsky's *sense of coherence* and the Intersystem Model (1997). The first students at the baccalaureate level have graduated, and a master's level program is being started. A course syllabus outlines the knowledge base the advanced practice nurse needs to effectively use the Intersystem Model (1997).

Mutuality in the patient/nurse interaction is the focus of Chapter 11. Vignettes of examples of mutuality in which student nurses were effective in identifying client value systems and developing nursing interventions based on mutually agreed upon goals are given.

8

LEARNING THEORIES TO ENHANCE CLINICAL PRACTICE

Margaret M. Conger and Rosalinda Haddon

How can nursing students be taught to think like a nurse? This is the question many nurse educators are asking. Tanner (2009) suggests that there are three skills nurses need to develop to think as a nurse: (1) using evidence-based research effectively; (2) skill in critical thinking; and (3) development of clinical reasoning. Benner, Sutphen, Leonard, and Day (2010) stress the need for clinical reasoning and use of evidence-based knowledge in nursing education. They also suggest that students need to develop habits of critical thinking to support the development of clinical judgment. Another needed skill for nurse students to learn is how to prioritize clients' needs so that they can differentiate between critical items of care and those aspects that are good but not critical. Benner et al. (2010) call this a "sense of salience" (p. 94).

Evidence-based practice (EBP) has become a byword of health care professionals. But the process is more than just how to develop research skills to ferret out the best practice; one must also be able to judge if that best practice is really best for the individual being treated. So an additional analysis must be done to match the practice with the individual. Development of critical thinking skills is a goal for most university curricula. It is closely tied to the development of clinical judgment. However, the path to acquire these two skills is different. How nursing students learn to develop clinical reasoning will be explored in this chapter.

THEORIES USED IN CLINICAL LEARNING

A number of theories about how learning occurs have been developed over the years. However, the type of learning that is associated with the level of thinking required to function effectively as a nurse is more limited. For example, behaviorist learning theories that are associated with a stimulus-response conditioning are not relevant to the critical analysis required for expert nursing. Cognitive learning theory that incorporates the management of learning as described by Gagne (1984, 1985) is more relevant. Cognitive learning theory incorporates the following five separate domains of learning: the use of verbal information, intellectual skills, motor skills, cognitive skills, and attitude. It is the higher order intellectual skills and management of learning such as remembering, thinking, and critical analysis that are important to developing clinical judgment in nursing.

Bevis and Watson (1989) believe that higher levels of learning are needed to advance the practice of nursing. Syntactical learning that focuses on analysis of a given situation and adaptation of care to meet its unique characteristics is expected at the baccalaureate level. At the highest level of learning, generation of new knowledge as it affects a given client situation is also expected. A typology of learning that consists of six distinct stages was developed by Bevis and Watson (1989). These stages are not necessarily sequential. Included in the typology are:

- Item learning—in which pieces of a information are learned to assist in performing tasks or procedures such as those found in a fundamentals of nursing course.
- Directive learning—in which rules, expectations, and the exceptions to the rules are used. Much of novice nurse learning is at this level (Benner, 1984).
- Rationale learning—in which reasons for what is done are learned. This stage provides a foundation for what is known about nursing practice at the novice learning level.
- Contextual learning—the stage in which the cultural framework for nursing is learned throughout student clinical experience, including the mores, rituals, and accepted ways of being a nurse.
- Syntactical learning—in which data are arranged into meaningful wholes. This stage allows the learner to vary from the rules or ordinary expectations to provide nursing care based on the unique qualities of the situation during clinical experiences.
- Inquiry learning—in which the art of investigation or theory generation is learned during graduate education level and in advanced practice.

Although all of these stages of learning are important at various points of nurses' development, the syntactical stage is necessary to develop clinical judgment skills. It is also important in evaluating information derived from best evidence practice sources as applied to a particular clinical situation of a specific client. Bevis and Watson (1989) suggest that at least 15% of the baccalaureate level of nursing curriculum should be planned at this level. They also suggest that this type of learning best takes place in the clinical area where rationale learning can be applied and modified to meet a particular client situation using syntactical learning strategies. In this arena, the student can be guided to search for and find new meaning in a client–nurse interaction. This clinical learning provides an opportunity to crystallize insights and to evaluate, project, predict, and intuit meanings to the situation.

Critical thinking is a vital skill for nurses. In the clinical environment, client conditions can rapidly change requiring a change in nursing priorities. The expert nurse is able to respond to these changes rapidly as the result of past experiences that have been reflected on. The new nurse needs to learn how to make these judgments. Both learning to think critically and creatively (Benner et al., 2010) are important to this process. When working with a preceptor, the student nurse needs to learn to question the preceptor about the "whys" of the situation to gain insight in how nursing decisions are made. A spirit of inquisitiveness is vital to the critical thinking process. Strategies that develop a nurse's ability to critically analyze a client situation and make nursing judgments about required actions are essential to the development of the nurse from the beginner stage to that of the expert as defined by Benner (1984).

The need for critical thinking in cognitive learning is emphasized in the work of both Gagne (1980) and Bevis and Watson (1989). The constructs incorporated in critical thinking are applicable to both evaluating EBP and developing clinical judgment. A recent definition of critical thinking (Facione, 2010) reflects the work of a number of educators using a Delphi process. It states:

> We understand critical thinking to be purposeful, self-regulatory judgment, which results in interpretation analysis, evaluation, and inference, as well as explanation of the evidential, conceptual, methodological, criteriological, or contextual consideration upon which that judgment is based. (Facione, 2010 p. 22)

This definition incorporates the following cognitive skills: interpretation, analysis, evaluation, inference, explanation, and self-regulation. The use of these skills is necessary to address problems in decision making about client care, consider alternative actions, and make decisions about what to do. However, one must have more than just the cognitive skills to engage in critical thinking, one must also be disposed to use them. Facione and Facione (1992) also described the elements that increase a person's disposition to think critically. These include:

- Inquisitiveness—a measure of intellectual curiosity and desire for learning
- Systematicity—use of an orderly, focused, and diligent process in the inquiry stage
- Analyticity—use of reason and evidence to research problems
- Truth seeking—honesty and objectivity with findings even if they do not support one's own beliefs
- Open-mindedness—tolerance of divergent views
- Critical thinking self-confidence—trust in one's own reasoning powers
- Cognitive maturity—recognition that some problems have more than one option

Older definitions of critical thinking have been in use in nursing practice also. Watson and Glaser (1964) interpret critical thinking as an attitude of inquiry that includes recognition of the existence of a problem, knowledge to analyze the accuracy and logic of the supporting data, and skill in applying this attitude and knowledge.

Ennis (1985) describes critical thinking as "reflective and reasonable thinking that is focused on deciding what to do or believe" (p. 45). The correct assessment of statements and formulation of hypotheses, questions, alternatives, and plans of action are necessary skills for appropriate decision making.

Kurfuss (1988) defines critical thinking as an "investigation whose purpose is to explore a situation, phenomenon, question, or problem, arrive at a hypothesis or conclusion about it that integrates all available information and that can therefore be convincingly justified" (p. 2).

All of these definitions have similarities. All include identification of a problem that requires a level of inquisitiveness. The problem then needs to be analyzed using pertinent information that has been collected. A decision about how to manage the problem (or develop a hypothesis) using the best evidence available is then made and carried out. Finally, the response to the action decided on must be evaluated. Throughout this process the nurse must be open to new information and be aware of personal biases that could interfere with interpretation of the situation. These are all reflected in the nursing process by which students have been taught to deliver nursing care.

REFLECTION ON PRACTICE

A component of critical thinking is that of reflection. Schon suggests that reflection is a self-conversation analyzing a situation and evaluating the outcomes of the actions taken. He compares it to the thoughts of a quarterback, who on Monday thinks about the decisions and actions he took during the game on Sunday and determines what worked, what didn't work, why, and what he would change to improve his game for the next week. This reflective process has three stages: conscious reflection, criticism, and action (Schon, 1991).

Pesut and Herman (1999) consider the reflection component of critical thinking. They describe three aspects of reflection: content or thinking about *what* you are thinking; process, or thinking about *how* you are thinking; and premise, or thinking about *why* you are thinking what you are thinking.

Intuition plays a key role in reflection. Intuition is an attitude exhibited by the suspension of judgment and the openness to "knowing" the patient with a degree of predictability (Jackson, Ignatavicuis, & Case, 2006). Knowing the patient comes from obtaining the patient's story and understanding both its content and its context. Intuition comes from knowledge of the patient, knowledge from experience, and a connection to similar circumstances, and knowledge of previous evidence. Benner considers intuition a process of clinical forethought and key to the development of the expert practitioner (Benner, Hooper-Kyriakedis, & Stannard, 1999).

Atkins and Murphy (1993) identify two types of reflection: reflection in action and reflection on action. In nursing, these occur as reflection in practice and reflection on practice. Reflection in practice takes place during practice and reflection on practice takes place following the action, similar to the Monday quarterback. During practice, the student thinks about what is being done and why it is done based on past knowledge and experience. After practice, the student reflects on the outcomes achieved including if they met the desired goals. If the goals are not met, the student must think about what could have been done differently reflecting on new knowledge and new options.

EVIDENCE-BASED PRACTICE (EBP)

EBP—that which is based on research rather than tradition—has been recommended by the Institute of Medicine in the United States to form the basis of practice for all health care professionals. Using evidence-based research to drive practice is suggested to both improve the quality of health care as well as contain costs. In Sweden, such practice for nurses is mandated by law (Johansson, Fogelberg-Dahm, & Wadensten, 2010). While the use of EBP is mandated, actual practice often falls short of this goal. In studying EBP-related practices of head nurses in a university teaching hospital, they reported that a significant barrier to using EBP was the lack of time during the work day to find and read research articles needed for such practice. This concern has been widely reported by others as well (Staffileno & Carlson, 2009).

Sackett, Strauss, Richardson, Rosenberg, and Haynes (2000) define EBP for nursing as practice that utilizes available evidence to make decisions about the care of individuals using information from research, clinical experience, client concerns, and preferences. Skills required to do this are those described in the critical thinking section of this study. Nurses must first ask compelling questions related to practice—in other words have an inquiring mind. Then they must be able to critically appraise the evidence and think about ways to apply it in practice (Melnyk & Fineout-Overhold, 2005). At all times, the individual client's capabilities and preferences must be evaluated. Even with the move to incorporate EBP into health care, one must keep in mind that a best practice may not always be relevant to a particular individual. For example, best practice states that a person following a total hip replacement surgery should ambulate and participate in physical therapy on the first postoperative day. However, if the person has experienced severe fluid shifts following the surgery and his blood pressure is unstable, such ambulation could result in harm. Thus, teaching nursing students to use EBP is more than learning how to find best practice as reported in research literature; they must also learn to consider individual client differences and how to apply the best practice guidelines to the individual.

Moch, Cronje, and Branson (2010) have done an extensive review of the literature on the best pedagogy to teach nursing students to develop skill in EBP. Time to apply evidence-based research in the practice setting to individual clients was deemed very important. Moch and Cronje (2010) have developed discussion groups consisting of nursing students and staff nurses to research and apply EBP to particular problems that have arisen in the clinical setting. For example, one of the issues was the management of end of life concerns among a cultural group, the Hmong, who had moved into the area. Through group discussion of relevant literature, new practice patterns were developed to achieve better outcomes for this group.

Thus, to promote nursing student expertise in EBP, several steps need to be followed. The student must be guided into asking relevant questions. These are referred to as the "PICOT Questions" (Cannon & Boswell, 2011). Factors to be included are:

- Who is the patient population (P)
- What intervention is needed (I)
- Condition (C)
- Outcome desired (O)
- Timeframe needed (T)

After the question is formulated, the nurse must search for the best evidence using appropriate resources such as the Cumulative Index for Nursing and Allied Health Care Literature, Medline, or the Cochrane Library. The literature retrieved must be evaluated for its validity and relevance to the particular situation under study. Findings then must be applied to the plan of care for the client. "EBP must be contextualized by the nurse in particular clinical settings and particular patient–nurse relationship" (Benner & Leonard, 2005, p. 181). Evaluation of the outcome is the final step of the process.

CLINICAL REASONING

Another element of expert nursing is development of clinical reasoning or as it is sometimes called "clinical decision making." Clinical reasoning, according to Pesut and Herman (1999), is "... reflective, concurrent, creative and critical thinking...that nurses use to frame, juxtapose, and test the match between a client's present state and desired outcome state" (p. 92). Benner (1984) and Tanner (2000) have long pointed out that expert nurses rely on intuition as an important part of clinical reasoning rather than a step wise process to come to a decision. In fact, they often cannot outline the steps they used in coming to a clinical decision. However, students need a model to develop clinical reasoning. They must learn to organize their thinking in a meaningful way.

Reflection in and on practice is one method that can be used to assist nursing students to think more like a nurse. It helps them develop their metacognitive skills, that is, to think about their own thinking and learning (Angelo & Cross, 1993, p. 4). This metacognition entails knowing what one knows and doesn't know, predicting outcomes, planning ahead, efficiently using resources, monitoring one's ability to solve problems, and to learn. Reflection, or learning how to think and learn, can help students become more intentional, self-aware, purposeful, and motivated in their learning (Huber & Hutchison, 2005, p. 119).

Part of reflection and *if-then* thinking is reframing, which is the process of thinking of alternatives, or looking at the facts from a different perspective. Once the nurse has assessed a clinical situation in one frame, the same situation can be reflected from another frame. This can be done within a theoretical model, a process model (such as Gordon's Functional Health patterns, 2002), different predetermined outcomes (such as Nursing Outcomes Classification, Moorhead, Johnson, & Maas, 2004), or from a systems approach. In addition, the nurse can intervene with a client in need of nursing care from within the framework of nursing models.

Reframing is a two-step process. Step one is to identify one's own filters, attitudes, prejudices, views of the world, and how they influence our data collection and analysis. Step two is acknowledging these filters and then asking the question: how would this situation be different if I thought about it differently? (Jackson, Ignatavicuis, & Case, 2006, p. 51). Framing and reframing is a very difficult concept for nursing students to master. The findings of Kautz, Kuiper, Pesut, Knight-Brown, and Daneker (2005) indicate that describing patterns within a frame and making decisions based on these frames requires repeated experiences. The student is being asked to self-monitor, self-observe, self-judge, self-react, and then structure the environment for problem solving. This type of thinking is not automatic (Kautz et al., 2005). The role of faculty is to facilitate this reflection, reframing, and deep thinking.

Murray and Atkinson (2000) suggest that at the novice level, students want to be told the "right answer." They are very uncomfortable with ambiguity. As they progress through the nursing program, the faculty intent is that they move to the competent level. Here, they are able to grapple with the fact that the right answer will depend on the circumstances. They realize that there are several solutions to any issue and they must explore each to determine which may be best. Faculty struggle for ways of developing the thinking skills of students to help them achieve this level of competency. Literature supports the need for developing teaching strategies that promote clinical reasoning in student nurses.

THE VALUE OF CLINICAL REASONING AND CRITICAL THINKING THEORIES IN THE AIM

The purpose of a nursing model is to provide a framework for practice. The purpose of theory is to explain how that practice can be carried out. Therefore, the more knowledge the practitioner has about nursing theories, the more the theories can be used to enhance nursing practice. The novice nurse has few skills in assessing, planning, and evaluating nursing care because of limited knowledge about nursing theory. However, the novice nurse can still use the framework of the AIM as a means of organizing data collection, negotiating values, and organizing a joint plan of care. By learning clinical reasoning skills through study and practice, the novice nurse can move in the direction of becoming an expert nurse. The novice nurse gathers data about the biological, psychosocial, and spiritual subsystems and then the focus of the situation that will assist in identifying the main concern of the patient or of the nurse. The novice nurse can then follow the steps of the AIM in the situational environment to bring about resolution of the main concern. The resolution of the main concern is determined by rescoring on SSOC. If no resolution of the concern has occurred, the desired and actual outcomes can be compared by determining possible gaps between them. The student nurse then begins the process of gathering additional data about what the patient knows and values, and the resources and behaviors the patient has available to resolve the main concern and uses the process of the AIM to work toward resolution of the main concern.

When the nurse adds theories such as the ones presented in this chapter about clinical reasoning, critical thinking, and skills in using EBP to his/her knowledge base, the AIM can be used with greater efficiency. In fact, the steps of the AIM process do not need to be spelled out because the expert nurse can move quickly to an understanding of the situation and can assist the patient to resolve the main concern. The greater the repertoire of nursing theories and knowledge about clinical situations the nurse has, the less the processes of the model are needed to bring about resolution of the main concern.

CONCLUSION

Learning to think like a nurse is a necessary part of nursing education. The skills discussed here, use of EBP, critical thinking, and clinical reasoning form the basis for such growth. These skills will help the nursing student move from rule-based care using predetermined care plans to independent, individualized care that honors the input of the client. With the nurse and client working together to determine goals for the nursing care provided, the client's sense of coherence can be enhanced.

REFERENCES

Angelo, T., & Cross, K. (1993). *Classroom assessment techniques* (2nd ed.). San Francisco, CA: Jossey-Bass.

Atkins, S., & Murphy, K. (1993). Reflection: A review of the literature. *Journal of Advanced Nursing, 18*, 1188–1192.

Benner, P. (1984). *From novice to expert: Excellence and power in clinical nursing practice*. Menlo Park, CA: Addison-Wesley.

Benner, P., Hooper-Kyriakedis, P., & Stannard, D. (1999). *Clinical wisdom and interventions in critical care*. Philadelphia, PA: W.B. Saunders.

Benner, P., & Leonard, V. (2005). Patient concerns, choices, and clinical judgment in evidenced-based practice. In B. Melnyk & E. Fineout-Overhold, *Evidence-based practice in nursing & healthcare: A guide to best practice* (pp. 163–181). Philadelphia, PA: Lippincott.

Benner, P., Sutphen, M., Leonard, V., & Day, L. (2010). *Educating nurses: A call for radical transformation*. San Francisco, CA: Jossey-Bass.

Bevis, E., & Watson, J. (1989). *Toward a caring curriculum: A new pedagogy for nursing*. New York, NY: National League for Nursing.

Cannon, S., & Boswell, C. (2011). Application of evidence-based nursing practice with research. In C. Boswell & S. Cannon (Eds.), *Introduction to nursing research: Incorporating EBP* (2nd ed.). Retrieved 5/10/2010 from www.jbpub.com/samples/0763740403/40403

Ennis, R. (1985). A logical basis for measuring critical thinking. *Educational Leadership, 43*, 44–48.

Facione, N., & Facione, P. (1992). *The California critical thinking dispositions inventory*. Millbrae, CA: California Academic Press.

Facione, P. (2010). *Critical thinking: What it is and why it counts*. Retrieved 4/1/2010 from www.insight assessment.com

Gagne, R. (1980). Learnable aspects of problem solving. *Educational Psychologist, 15*(2), 84–92.

Gagne, R. (1984). Learning outcomes and their effects: Useful categories of human performance. *American Psychologist, 37*, 377–385.

Gagne, R. (1985). *The conditions of learning* (4th ed.). New York, NY: Holt, Rinehart, & Winston.

Gordon, M. (2002). *Manual of nursing diagnostics* (10th ed.). Philadelphia, PA: Mosby.

Huber, M., & Hutchings, P. (2005). *The advancement of learning: Building the teaching commons*. San Francisco, CA: Jossey-Bass.

Jackson, M., Ignatavicuis, I., & Case, B. (2006). *Conversations in critical thinking and clinical judgment*. Sudbury, MA: Jones & Bartlett.

Johansson, B., Fogelberg-Dahm, M., & Wadensten, B. (2010). Evidence-based practice: The importance of education and leadership. *Journal of Nursing Management, 18*, 70–77.

Kautz, D., Kuiper, R., Pesut, D., Knight-Brown, P., & Daneker, D. (2005). Promoting clinical reasoning in undergraduate nursing students: Application and evaluation of the outcome present state test (OPT) model of clinical reasoning. *International Journal of Nursing Education Scholarship, 2*(1), 1–19.

Kurfuss, J. (1988). *Critical thinking: Theory, research, practice, and possibilities (ASHE-ERI Higher Education Report No 2)*. Washington, DC: Association for the Study of Higher Education.

Melnyk, B., & Fineout-Overhold, E. (2005). *Evidence-based practice in nursing & healthcare: A guide to best practice*. Philadelphia, PA: Lippincott.

Moch, S., & Cronje, R. (2010). Empowering grassroots evidence-based practice: A curricular model to foster undergraduate student-enabled practice change. *Journal of Professional Nursing, 26*(1), 14–22.

Moch, S., Cronje, R., & Branson, J. (2010). Undergraduate nursing evidence-based practice education: Envisioning the role of students. *Journal of Professional Nursing, 26*(1), 5–13.

Moorhead, S., Johnson, M., & Maas, M. (2004). *Nursing outcomes classification* (3rd ed.). Philadelphia, PA: Mosby.

Murray, M., & Atkinson, L. (2000). *Understanding the nursing process in a changing environment* (6th ed.). New York, NY: McGraw-Hill.

Pesut, D., & Herman, J. (1999). *Clinical reasoning: The art and science of critical and creative thinking*. Albany, NY: Delmar.

Sackett, D., Strauss, S., Richardson, W., Rosenberg, W., & Haynes, R. (2000). *Evidence-based medicine: How to practice and teach EBM*. London, UK: Churchill-Livingstone.

Schon, D. (1991). *The reflective practitioner* (2nd ed.). San Francisco, CA: Jossey-Bass.

Staffileno, B., & Carlson, E. (2009). Providing direct care nurses research and evidence-based practice information: An essential component of nursing leadership. *Journal of Nursing Management, 18,* 84–89.

Tanner, C. (2000). Critical thinking: Beyond the nursing process. *Journal of Nursing Education, 39*(8), 338–330.

Tanner, C. (2009). The case for cases: A pedagogy doe developing habits of thought. *Journal of Nursing Education, 48*(6), 299–300.

Watson, G., & Glaser, E. (1964). *Watson-Glaser critical thinking appraisal manual*. San Antonio, TX: Psychological Corporation.

9

The Artinian Intersystem Model in Nursing School Education

Pamela H. Cone, Barbara M. Artinian, and Katharine S. West

The Artinian Intersystem Model (AIM) is eminently suited to nursing education because of its focus on the two systems, teacher and student, and how they negotiate effective learning.

Students come to us with intrasystems consisting of their existing knowledge and understanding of life and health care, their personal values and meanings, and their resultant behaviors, and we as teachers, having our own *intrasystem* elements, must reach our students in ways that are meaningful and sense making to them, thus engaging in intersystem negotiation. According to nurse educator Helen Gordon (2010), we live and teach in an era where "we have a whole new kind of learner filling the chairs of our classrooms, learners that call for us to engage them in the process of their learning" (p. 77).

While many nursing schools have chosen not to use a theoretical framework or model for nursing education, others have applied various models or theories as their framework, a practice that has recently been highly encouraged by our nursing education accrediting bodies such as the National League of Nursing (NLN) and the Council for Collegiate Nursing Education. In the Southern California area, very few nursing schools use a nursing model. Some examples of those that use a model include California State University at Northridge, which has chosen Orlando's Self-Care Nursing Model for its program, and University of California at Irvine, which has chosen Jean Watson's Model of Caring for both their medical center and the academic nursing program. California State University at San Bernardino uses the AIM, though it is less emphasized now than it was previously. This lack of a theoretical framework in nursing programs in general raises a concern about the scholarly level of nursing education. The editors of a 2004 issue of the *Teaching Professor* wrote in response to the question of whether or not teachers are engaging in the scholarship of teaching that this lack is a "pervasive issue" in collegiate education (p. 4).

For over 20 years, the Azusa Pacific University School of Nursing (APU-SON) has used and continues to use the AIM to help bachelor of science in nursing (BSN) students understand the theoretical underpinnings of nursing science and practice (Artinian, 1991). It is used throughout the curriculum to develop critical thinking and create nursing care plans. Its use keeps the element of spiritual care foundational to the core of the curricula. In addition to its use in undergraduate education, the graduate nursing program presents the AIM as one of the nursing models for advanced practice nurses to explore and select for their nursing practice. The AIM is often chosen by MSN students for their comprehensive examinations because of its practicality, its congruence with a university that has a focus on spirituality, and its applicability to all types of nursing practice.

In this chapter, the congruence of the AIM with the nursing philosophy of APU-SON is addressed. In addition, the principles of Ernest Boyer (1996) are highlighted in this discussion. Two formats for recording intersystem interactions are introduced: the block form developed for three levels of undergraduate students and a narrative outline for seniors and graduate students. Student case studies illustrating the progression of how students learn to use the AIM are presented at the freshman, junior, and senior levels at APU-SON. Finally, the use of the model at the graduate level is discussed, and a lesson plan is presented that describes how the AIM was introduced to graduate students. A creative method of introducing students to the concept of *model* is described. The chapter closes with examples of student philosophies of nursing.

PHILOSOPHY OF APU

As a Christian institution, APU presents students with a Statement of Faith, a Mission Statement, a Statement of Essence, the Four Cornerstones, and a "God First" Motto. These elements are foundational to the university and provide a clear presentation of our Christian worldview. According to Azusa Pacific University (2010a), "Azusa Pacific University is an evangelical Christian community of disciples and scholars who seek to advance the work of God in the world through academic excellence in liberal arts and professional programs of higher education that encourage students to develop a Christian perspective of truth and life" (APU Mission Statement, para 2).

The APU-SON philosophy (2010b), which is congruent with the university philosophy, states that "Consistent with the mission and purpose of the university, the SON is a Christian community of discipleship, scholarship, and practice. Its purpose is to advance the work of God in the world through nursing education, collaborative projects, church and community service that encourages those affiliated with the SON (whether faculty, staff, student, graduate, or colleague) to grow in faith and in the exercise of their gifts for service to God and humanity" (APU-SON Mission Statement, para 1).

In the Undergraduate Program, nursing students are encouraged to read a number of nursing philosophies and to develop their own philosophy, which they place in their Nursing Portfolio. Over the course of their nursing education, they revisit their personal nursing philosophy and revise it as personal and professional growth occurs. The overall goal of the Undergraduate Program (2010c) is to produce a graduate nurse who "integrates faith and ethics as a skilled and knowledgeable practitioner, accountable professional, health care educator, and advocate and coordinator of care" (Program Competencies, para 1). This is done in part using the AIM.

The Graduate Program also has a mission statement and philosophy that is congruent with both the university and the SON mission statements. As with undergraduate education, all graduate education is based on the foundation of a Christian Worldview. The goal of this program is to prepare nurses for advanced practice that is culturally competent, clinically excellent, and theoretically sound and to prepare nurse leaders in various clinical specialties. Graduate nursing education is mutually negotiated and planned by the student and a faculty advisor, another evidence of the congruence of the AIM and APU-SON.

The overall goal at the APU-SON is to provide excellence in all of its nursing education programs. To that end, faculty members are encouraged to pursue personal and professional growth, to stay current with the nursing literature, and to implement the highest quality of teaching that is possible. As nurse educators, we have found that Boyer's principles of education are sound and his priorities for learning are beneficial to curriculum planning.

BOYER'S PRIORITIES FOR QUALITY SCHOOLS

In his 1996 work, *5 Priorities for Quality Schools*, scholar and educator Ernest L. Boyer discussed the basic elements that need to be present for quality education to occur. These include a "sense of community," the "centrality of language," a "curriculum with coherence," a "climate for creative learning," and a "climate that affirms the building of character for every student" (p. 4). Passamore (2008) reminds us that Boyer encouraged educators to be "building connections in learning by organizing the disciplines differently to integrate subject matter...[presenting] the human commonalities which include life cycle, symbols and aesthetic response" (p. 46). With these in mind, contemporary nursing educators must work at both the science and the art of nursing education. The following discussion of APU undergraduate nursing education will use Boyer's five components of education to demonstrate the use and efficacy of the AIM in nursing education. Graduate nursing education addresses many of the nursing models, but the AIM is exemplified by two student philosophies.

Sense of Community

Mutuality, a concept congruent with the AIM, is an important part of education, and it is strongly emphasized at APU. Connectedness and community, mutual respect, and an interactive relationship between teachers and students all foster a sense of community. In fact, community is one of the Four Cornerstones (Christ, Community, Scholarship, and Service) of APU's vision and mission as a university (APU Web site, 2010). Class sizes are kept below 50 in the SON, and clinical groups usually have 10 students per clinical instructor. Negotiation of assignments is an accepted practice, and students are encouraged to work together with instructors to make changes that will enhance their learning experiences. Yair (2008), in his discussion of the Scholarship of Teaching, points out the "centrality of the student-teacher relationship" (p. 447) in effective learning situations. When teachers build a sense of community in the classroom or the clinical setting, mutual negotiation, a key element of the AIM, occurs more readily, and learning is enhanced.

Centrality of Language

Students develop a language of nursing and of the AIM to record their nursing care plans. Artinian uses the theory of the *sense of coherence* (SOC; Antonovsky, 1987) to evaluate the patient situation by learning about the patient's knowledge, value, and behaviors related to a main concern. This is an example of the importance of the centrality of language. By developing a measure to assess the patient response to a nursing intervention, nurses are able to make sense of and quantify subjective information. Using the *situational sense of coherence* (SSOC) measurement scale and reporting their findings on their Case Study Data Forms enable students to develop a nursing care plan that has measurable goals that are mutually negotiated. This is particularly important in their early years as novice nursing students. They become more adept at the use of the AIM to guide their nursing processes with each semester and clinical rotation.

Curriculum With Coherence

As mentioned previously, the AIM is used as the guide for all of the Case Study Data Forms over the 4-year program. Even students in the RN to BSN degree completion program at APU-SON are introduced to the model. In their introductory course, they are excited to see how the use of the AIM provides a focused direction and thus enhances their care plans. By the time students are in their Critical Care rotation as seniors, they are able to work through the various elements of the AIM in their heads and develop a nursing care plan quickly and efficiently. Students learn to distinguish when to develop a nurse-organized plan of care (physical care only) versus a mutual plan of care with input from the patient or family based on their ability to participate in the planning of care.

The use of the Case Study Data Form across all levels has provided continuity and coherence to student formation in critical thinking and the development of effective care plans for their patients. In addition, the AIM's three-part view of person, with biological, psychosocial, and spiritual subsystems (Artinian, 1991), is both congruent with the Christian heritage and focus of APU (body, soul, and spirit) and the holistic approach of nursing that addresses all aspects of the person.

Climate for Creative Learning

One of the positive aspects about the AIM is its versatility and congruence with creativity. Gordon (2010) mentions that it is particularly important with our current generation of students to facilitate learning by being "engaging and creative while infusing content with relevance anchored in the student's thinking" (p. 77). Relevance and meaningfulness are highly prized by our current students; they often resist assignments that, from their perspective, lack these qualities. By introducing the Intersystem Model (Artinian, 1991), students connect these qualities to patient care. Using the Assessment Guide as shown in Table 9.1, an expanded form of the original table (see Table 3.1), students explore their own as well as the patient's knowledge, values, and behaviors as they relate to the main concern. They then score the patient in each area of SSOC (*comprehensibility, meaningfulness,* and *manageability*). The student nurse identifies goals to increase SSOC and assesses the ability of the patient and nurse to work together to resolve the main concern. This is an effective tool for learning and practice. Students are encouraged to find creative ways, including multimedia and visuals (Gordon, 2010), to meet the identified goal. Mutuality, a concept very important to this generation of students, is stressed.

Climate That Affirms the Building of Character for Every Student

APU is a private Christian institution of higher education that promotes a rich learning environment for students. Excellence in teaching is stressed, and the use of scholarly experiences that enhance transformational learning is encouraged. Yair (2008) described his findings in a qualitative study that explored key learning experiences in higher education that were transformational in nature. Yair identified the following three themes: (1) the centrality of personalized student–teacher relations, (2) the identification and integrity of the faculty providing students with role models to emulate, and (3) excellence in the skills of teaching (p. 447). These themes have rekindled interest in the academic community in pursuing the art, science, and profession of teaching.

The focus on mutuality in the Intersystem Model (Conger, 1997) makes connection between student and teacher more meaningful. This lays the groundwork for the experience of transformational learning to occur. In addition, the use of the AIM for nursing care plans provides a theoretically based model for student practice. Finally, the progressive use throughout the program of the AIM-based Case Study Data Forms allows for consistency among professors and helps them become more proficient in teaching. As nurse educators, APU-SON faculty strive to implement Boyer's elements of excellence in pedagogy. Our goal is to provide quality nursing education, and using the AIM helps us to reach that goal.

ADOPTION OF THE AIM AT APU

The AIM is the result of the work of many years of study, exploration, and revision. Before coming to teach at APU, Artinian developed the Intersystem Model, based on Kuhn's 1974 work, *The Logic of Social Systems*. At APU, she was an educator during the refinement and subsequent publication of the initial Intersystem Model (1991). Before the adoption of the Intersystem Model by the faculty at the SON, the APU-SON used the Nursing Process Systems Model developed by Brown (1981) for curriculum development. Modifications made in the mid-1980s included combining the two models and adding the work of Antonovsky (1987) with his SOC to describe health. At that time, "the name of the model was changed to the Intersystem Model to reflect the interactional process that takes place between patient and nurse in using the nursing process to develop a plan of care" (Artinian, 1991, p. 196). Recently, graduate nursing students began to identify the Intersystem Model with Artinian and call it the AIM, just as they identify the Roy Adaptation Model with Roy. In a classroom discussion with graduate students trying to understand the heart of the Intersystem Model, I (Cone) explained, "the aim of the AIM is a mutually negotiated plan of care." AIM has now become the new name of the model to reflect the additions made to the earlier models.

In the early 1990s, the APU-SON chose to use the Intersystem Model (1991) as a theoretical framework for undergraduate nursing education. This entailed using the definition of person to drive the gathering and reporting of patient information and the model itself as the guide for the Case Study Data Form used from the freshmen through the senior year. Faculty members worked together to develop the block form used in undergraduate student case studies. Over time, the form was leveled according to year in the nursing program so that beginning students focused on more general data gathering and use of the model, moving on to a more complex application over time in a novice to expert nursing student format (Benner, 1982). In graduate education, students were introduced to the AIM by Dr. Artinian herself. As the originator, Dr. Artinian clarified the elements of the model and its various uses in advanced nursing practice.

UNDERGRADUATE NURSING EDUCATION AT APU

The 4-year nursing program at APU-SON is one of a small percentage of nursing schools that introduces clinical practice into the first year of college. Artinian (1997a) writes that the AIM can "be used by the novice practitioner as well as by the expert because the complexity of the model derives from the knowledge base of the user, not from the structure of the model" (p. 16). At APU-SON, students begin their clinical experiences with a lecture in their Foundations of Nursing course on the Nursing Process. This is followed by a detailed lecture on the use of the AIM to develop a plan of care that is mutually negotiated. Then students are given the 1991 Artinian article to read and are shown how the AIM focuses on the measurement of the patient's comprehensibility (knowledge/understanding), meaningfulness (value/meaning), and manageability (behaviors/actions) related to the main concern. Student understanding of mutuality is enhanced as nursing students study the intrasystems of the patient and of the nurse (see Table 9.1). Assessing the biological, psychosocial, and spiritual

TABLE 9.1 Assessment Guide for the Biological, Psychosocial, and Spiritual Subsystems

PATIENT INTRASYSTEM	NURSE INTRASYSTEM
Biological subsystems	*Biological subsystems*
1. What does the patient know about the physical subsystems related to the presenting problem?	1. Does the nurse have knowledge about the presenting problem? What data are derived from the physical assessment of the patient/client? How does this compare to norms? What further information does the nurse need to complete the knowledge base?
2. What attitudes and values does the patient/client have about physical subsystems related to the present problem?	2. What attitudes and values does the nurse have about physical subsystems related to the presenting problem?
3. What behaviors does the patient/client manifest or what technical skills does s/he possess relative to presenting problem?	3. What behaviors does the nurse manifest that may affect the interrelation, i.e., fatigue, shyness, technical skills?
Psychosocial subsystems	*Psychosocial subsystems*
1. What does the patient/client know about treatment, prognosis, or resources available for management of the presenting problem?	1. How much information does the nurse have about cultural, developmental or role characteristics of the patient/client or about family or community resources?
2. What attitudes and values does the patient/client have that may motivate a plan of care?	2. What biases does the nurse have that may affect the plan of care?
3. What coping strategies or role relationships does the patient/client have that will assist in carrying out the care?	3. What supportive role relationships does the nurse have that will facilitate the providing of care for others?
Spiritual subsystems	*Spiritual subsystems*
1. What spiritual beliefs does the client/patient have that may influence presenting problem?	1. What spiritual beliefs does the nurse have that may affect presenting problem of patient/client?
2. What attitudes or values does the patient/client have that provide strength to face presenting problem?	2. What attitudes or values does the nurse have that provide strength to enable offers of assistance to patient/client?
3. Does the patient/client have religious practices that may be disrupted by presenting problem or that may interfere with the plan of care?	3. Are there any practices the nurse would not be able to do because of spiritual values?

Source: Artinian (2011). Adapted from Artinian (1997).

subsystems gives them knowledge about the patient and nurse that allows them to identify the main concern. For many students, it is the first time they have explored their understanding and personal values regarding patient care. Thus, the questions used in the assessment process are important for student growth. Because students have only a rudimentary understanding of theory, they think concretely at this stage, gather data, and report on their patient assessments accordingly.

With further experience, students learn how to use the Case Study Data Form based on the AIM and are instructed in the mutual negotiation of a care plan. They begin to apply critical thinking to the conceptual elements of the AIM. The use of the Case Study Data Form helps students to clarify the patient's main concern and to identify nursing diagnoses related to the concern in each of the subsystems. An evaluation form for faculty to use to evaluate the student understanding has been developed. The key assessment factors leading to development of the Care Plan are scored according to a rubric to assess the student's level of achievement (see Table 9.2). This table has been enhanced for this chapter based on the Case Study Care Plan Rubric for the undergraduate course, Foundations of Professional Nursing.

Although students identify only one main concern and implement a mutual plan of care to resolve it, students are expected to be aware of other potential concerns and to develop nursing diagnoses in each of the subsystems that relate to the main concern. These concerns are listed as nursing diagnoses that could become a new main concern of either the patient or nurse when the first concern is resolved. These diagnoses are analogous to the concept used in business project management as "parking lot" items (Brenner, 2007). When an idea occurs that is not pertinent to the current focus of the project, but may be important someday soon, it is "parked" so it will be remembered for consideration at a later time. For nursing students, the greater their theoretical knowledge and awareness of the complexity of patient subsystems, the more diagnoses students can "park" as potential problems that may be advanced to the priority main concern at a later time. Over the 4 years of study, students develop a facility with AIM-based nursing care plans. In addition, students are shown how to attain excellence in writing and reporting as they prepare their care plans using the scoring rubric for a guide.

Case Study Vignettes

Following are three case study vignettes from my students at different levels in the APU-SON program. With my help, in each case, nursing students

TABLE 9.2 Rubric for Assessing Achievement in Undergraduate Care Plans

CRITERIA	LEVEL OF ACHEIVEMENT		
	EXEMPLARY	PROFICIENT	UNSATISFACTORY
Physical or biological subsystem	<ul><li>Physical assessment 100% complete</li><li>Good description of assessment</li></ul>	<ul><li>80% of physical assessment data completed</li><li>Vital signs and pain assessment data complete with BSA and BMI</li></ul>	<ul><li>Less than 80% of physical assessment data completed</li><li>Answers brief and not informative.</li></ul>
Psychosocial subsystem	<ul><li>Identifies developmental stage</li><li>States cultural influence/health beliefs and values</li><li>Describes family challenges and/or strengths</li></ul>	Completes at least 3 concepts in this subsystem	Incomplete assessment of individual and/or family
Spiritual subsystem	All concepts of the subsystem addressed	Identify spiritual strengths and needs of patient	No spiritual concerns are identified
Nursing diagnosis	<ul><li>Comprehensive list of patient care needs</li><li>Prioritize pt care needs</li><li>Five diagnoses presented</li></ul>	<ul><li>Identify patient needs f or the day</li><li>Uses NANDA diagnoses</li><li>Minimum of three nursing diagnoses are prioritized</li></ul>	<ul><li>Diagnoses not in NANDA format</li><li>Key patient needs not identified</li><li>Nursing diagnosis not prioritized.</li></ul>

Care Plan		
■ Comprehensive list of assessment factors ■ All 5 columns of the care plan accurately completed with good evidence-based support for interventions ■ Care Plan is mutually negotiated	■ Complete first 4 columns of the care plan ■ Use NANDA for all diagnoses ■ Continuity between goals & interventions ■ Patient goals are measurable & realistic for that day of care ■ Scientifically bases rationale for interventions	■ Incomplete or inaccurate data and Care Plan ■ Key assessment factors used to determine diagnosis not provided ■ Goals unrealistic or not measurable ■ Rationale for interventions not evidence-based

Key assessment factors leading to development of the Care Plan for resolving the Main Concern

Main Concern

Nursing Diagnosis:
_____ Related to _____ Manifested by
Mutually negotiated ____ Yes ____ No

Planning (Goals)	Intervention (Implementation)	Rationale for intervention	Evaluation
One Short-Term goal: patient-oriented, measurable, and specific One Long-Term goal	Two nursing interventions provided per goal	Scientific rationale for each intervention	Evaluation of accomplishment of each goal

Source: Cone (2011). Adapted from the APU-SON Fundamentals of Nursing course.

identified the main concern of their patients and worked toward its resolution. These scenarios give a brief description of each case study. Sample care plans can be found in the online adjunct manual.

Case Study 9.1

Freshmen Case Study

Nursing students in their first year have a beginning understanding of the nursing process when they are introduced to the Intersystem Model (1991). They acknowledge the importance of mutual negotiation, but they often focus on what the nurse feels is best for the patient. One care plan was developed for an elderly man who was in the hospital to have a hip replacement. The patient was angry and unwilling to cooperate with the student nurse. The nurse was anxious about the patient's body alignment and pain level but was unable to negotiate a mutual care plan due to the patient's angry attitude. After reassessing the situation with her instructor, the student was able to focus on the patient's main concern, which was that the Christian-based hospital had Christmas decorations in patient rooms that offended her patient, who was Jewish. The student apologized for this insensitivity on the part of health care providers and removed all of the decorations, offering to find some that celebrated his religious holiday. The patient immediately calmed down. Once this main concern was resolved, the patient was willing to negotiate with the student another a plan of care to address his physical concerns.

Case Study 9.2

Junior Case Study

At the junior level, students progress from individual care plans to family care plans. At first, students find it difficult to use appropriate terminology for family diagnoses, but over time, they become adept at identifying concerns in all three subsystems of the family. In this case study, the family was struggling to deal with four small children at home during the hospitalization of 2-year-old Kimberly who was burned by hot porridge in a pot knocked off the stove. The entire family was concerned about her pain and her healing, but their family routine was completely disrupted by the mother's need to stay with Kimberly at the hospital. The student was very creative in developing a mutual plan of care that involved the extended family support system to address the logistical needs of this young family in order to meet Kimberly's individual needs. Her health progressed rapidly after this concern was resolved.

Case Study 9.3

Senior Case Study

Community health is taught at the senior level at APU. Students learn to care for groups of people. In negotiating a plan of care for homeless people with diabetes, students working with the APU-SON Nurse Practitioner Clinic for the Homeless performed a needs assessment by surveys of the people they were serving. They identified that accessibility of health care services was the main concern of the diabetic patients. The students then researched possible sites where homeless people could be served and posted a list at the homeless shelter. This list was also distributed at the Nurse Practitioner Clinic for the Homeless so that those who needed such help could find out where to get their blood sugar tested and where to get supplies for their particular needs. While this did not entirely solve the main concern of access to health care services, it did give homeless clients information about facilities that could meet some of their diabetic needs.

GRADUATE NURSING EDUCATION AT APU

When students enter the graduate program at APU-SON, they bring with them a variety of experiences in their use of nursing models. Some students are negative about the use of models because they were required as undergraduate students to use a particular model as adopted by their previous school to guide the curriculum. Others feel that models are irrelevant to practice because they do not see how they can be helpful in a hospital setting to provide care to patients. Still others have had successful experiences in the use of models and want to learn more about them. When Dr. Artinian taught the course that introduced nursing models to the students, her goal was to change their global orientation to the use of models so that they would understand the use of models (*comprehensibility*), see them as useful for their practice (*meaningfulness*), and be able to incorporate them into their practice in a manageable way (*manageability*).

Graduate education at APU-SON has a broad approach to the use of nursing theories and models. Students are introduced to several models, including the AIM, and are encouraged to explore in detail one theorist and model. Many continue to choose the AIM because of its simplicity, its focus on mutuality, and its congruence with a faith-based approach to nursing. There is a strong connection between nursing philosophy, theory, and models; therefore, the philosophy of the APU-SON is addressed as part of this discussion on the use of the AIM for graduate nursing education.

Through the curriculum review process, the theory course that current graduate nursing students take at APU-SON has changed somewhat over the last few years. However, I (Cone) continue to use the methods that Artinian put in place in her years as the theory professor in the graduate department. I also use in my current teaching the diagram of the model revised in 2009 that introduced color-coding for each section (see Figure 1.7). Students report that the colors make it easier to follow the process and learn how to use it effectively in writing care plans. Teaching graduate students about models by using the AIM as an example is a process enjoyed by both students and faculty.

LESSON PLAN FOR TEACHING THE AIM TO GRADUATE STUDENTS

Lesson plans are modified each semester to keep up with new health care information and changes in the curriculum. Educators use many methods to introduce theoretical foundations for nursing practice. These differ according to course and professor. The AIM lends itself to flexibility in this ever-changing teaching environment. The "Research and Theory in Advanced Practice Nursing" course at APU-SON introduces all nursing models using lesson plans developed for the presentation of each model. Table 9.3 shows Artinian's lesson plan introducing the AIM to graduate students when she taught this course.

The concepts from the SOC (Antonovsky, 1987) help students understand how a theoretically based model can be useful in their advanced nursing practice. Knowing and understanding the use of models (*comprehensibility*), valuing their use in practice (*meaningfulness*), and using them effectively (*manageability*) develops over time as students move from their early theory course toward their comprehensive examinations.

TABLE 9.3 Artinian's Lesson Plan for Introducing Models and Theories to Graduate Nursing Students

1. Discuss student experiences in providing nursing care	▪ Ask students to write an essay on "What is important to me when I provide nursing care?" ▪ Analyze essays to identify areas of importance for nursing.		
2. Differentiate between the concepts of models and theories using examples that correspond to each other		**Model**	**Theory**
		Represents the structure of a concept or an object	*Explains the "How?" or "Why?" of a phenomenon*
		A model airplane	Aerodynamic Theory
		Epidemiological model (Agent–Host–Environment) (Clark, 2008)	Germ Theory
		Critical Incident Stress Debriefing (CISD) model (Davis, 2006)	Selye's Stress Theory
		Artinian Intersystem Model	SSOC Theory of Recovery (Artinian, 1997b; Hill, 1949)
3. a. Introduce the use of models in practice b. Present selected models for study, including the AIM	▪ Discuss problems students encounter when attempting to apply a model in practice. ▪ Discuss how to select an extant model that is congruent with personal philosophy.		

4. Acquaint students with the concepts of AIM	▪ Give AIM diagram to orient students to process of using AIM
	▪ Give narrative outline care form
	▪ Present the concepts of AIM
	▪ Give examples of successful use of the model
	▪ Examine forms for writing care plans
	   ☐ Block care plan template
	   ☐ Community health care plan template
	   ☐ Standard care plan template
	   ☐ Narrative care plan template		

5. Discuss examples of care plans written in varying formats	▪ Truncated care plan ▪ Full text care plan ▪ Annotated care plan ▪ Referenced care plan ▪ Group care plan ▪ Care plans based on Grounded Theory research (See online adjunct manual for examples.)		

Source: Artinian (2011). Adapted from the APU-SON Graduate Nursing Syllabus.

Comprehensibility

During the first three weeks of Artinian's original theory course, the emphasis was on clarifying the distinction between a model and a theory. The simplest way to differentiate between these concepts is to see a model as a framework or representation of an actual thing and a theory as an explanation of a phenomenon that allows predictions to be made. By understanding the separate use of each, it is possible to understand how they are integrated to form an actual nursing model. For example, in the Intersystem Model (1997), the Kuhn Model (1974) is used to describe the interaction between the patient and nurse in a helping situation that involves communicating information, negotiating values, and carrying out a mutual plan of care. In addition, the theory of SOC (Antonovsky, 1987) has been adapted to measure the effectiveness of the interaction between the nurse and patient by scoring on the SSOC. When this distinction between a model and theory is understood, students are able to increase the usefulness of models by bringing to them their theoretical understanding of many theories. During this time in the course, no mention of specific models was made, but students were encouraged to begin thinking theoretically.

Meaningfulness

To help students realize that models are useful in practice, students were asked, during the first three weeks of the course, to write their philosophy of nursing, answering the question "What is important to you when you provide nursing care to patients?". Their beginning attempts to express in words what they actually tried to do in providing care were often sketchy, but as students read aloud their early thoughts and discussed them in class, their reflections were clarified and they were able to define what was important for them. Analysis of these papers provided clues to suggest what extant nursing model might be compatible with their practice.

Manageability

Although students were required to follow the total process outlined in a nursing model when writing a care plan for the models they selected, it was made clear, that in actual nursing practice, it is not possible to write an in-depth care plan for each patient and each situation. Rather, the learning of the process of a model provides a framework for mentally assessing each patient situation, so that all of the important aspects of care are considered. In Chapter 1, a truncated form of an AIM care plan is presented that can be used to document the main structure of the model, and in Chapter 12, an example is given for converting the process of the model into SOAPIE charting (see online adjunct manual for detailed Care Plans and SOAPIE notes). A care plan developed from Cone's (1997) doctoral research is used to illustrate the use of the AIM to teach graduate nursing students (see Chapter 16).

ANOTHER APPROACH TO INTRODUCING MODELS

When introducing undergraduate students to the practical aspects of using models at another university, I (West) have found it helpful to explain models using examples from students' daily life. The best example I have found, and one with which everyone is familiar, is that of getting places using street maps as a portable "model" of real towns and geographic spaces. We also discuss the evolution of how different cultures give directions to places, comparing oral tradition societies where directions must be memorized to cultures where the acquisition of written literacy and technology inspired maps as models of neighborhoods. In oral or very rural societies, directions consist of instructions noting key landmarks such as "walk along the river's edge" or "next to the cornfield." Where footpaths, roads, and structures become more abundant, directions become more sophisticated, to "turn left at the second lane after the old oak tree" or "third house past the fire station." With the spread of literacy and writing, drawings and depictions of the river, the cornfield, and the fire station could be represented on portable material that could be easily carried for reference along the way. These pocket maps are not the "real thing" but rather an approximate representation of real features in the landscape. Societies find maps useful precisely because they model the world and can be used to navigate and referred to as needed. Maps, or models of real geography, allow one to not have to memorize directions for details along the way, as an oral tradition would require.

Models can guide rerouting to accommodate changes in plans or determine alternative routes as the journey progresses in case of unforeseen circumstances, unexpected barriers, or even serendipitous opportunities. As GPS technology is acquired by the average citizen, people intuitively understand the need to input My Location and Destination in order to secure directions via such vendors as Google Maps or MapQuest. Neither would a mountain climber begin the assent of a mountain without first establishing a Base Camp and assessing the route to the Summit. It is an easy transition for students to use nursing models to describe the nurse–patient relationship, serve to guide assessment, and plan a route through the health care experience to their goals together when they have a familiar example of how models are "maps."

In a like manner, the AIM provides nurses and clients a way to establish a baseline location together and mutually agree on a plan to guide them to their destination, or outcome(s). With the AIM, mutuality is the norm, and the SSOC allows quantification of the start and the finish, to observe and measure change. As the care plan is implemented and unexpected events occur, the AIM provides a reference to restrategize the route, just as looking at a city map allows rerouting in case of a road closure or other event. This teaching approach to the use of models in nursing is readily grasped by students at all experience levels, whether or not they have used nursing models before. Completing and actually using the care plan then becomes more than an academic exercise; the care plan becomes a useful tool to refer to and revise as needed, to achieve the mutual resolution of the main concern.

SAMPLE PHILOSOPHIES OF NURSING

Currently, the APU-SON Graduate Program has a course that introduces models and theories to advanced practice nursing students. In that course, students explore a number of models, including the AIM, and are shown how to apply them to nursing practice. At one time, Dr Artinian taught that course.

The following two essays were written by students at the beginning of Artinian's graduate theory course to identify what they considered to be of importance in their nursing practice. The students discussed and analyzed their essays to identify the major themes. Throughout the course, as the many nursing models were discussed and the main focus of each model was identified, the students would match their personal themes with those of each model. Ultimately, they selected one of those models that was most congruent with their personal style of practice. This chosen model was then analyzed in depth, and a care plan was developed using the format of that model. These two essays identify congruence between the student's personal philosophies of nursing and the AIM.

Philosophy of Nursing 9.1

Philosophy of Nursing and the Intersystem Model (1997) Approach to Nursing[1]

Sarah Templeton, MSN, RN

My philosophy of nursing centers around three dimensions. These dimensions include caring, competency, and instilling hope and confidence in patients. I believe that all of these aspects encompass what matters most when caring for a patient.

I believe that caring is vital to my practice as a nurse. My motivation for caring comes from my belief that patients are valuable because they are uniquely made in the image of God. Therefore, each patient will have his/her own unique set of thoughts, beliefs, and reactions toward illness. Recognizing that each patient is an individual and understanding his/her point of view are essential to the expression of care. All hopes of following a treatment plan are lost if patients feel their needs and values are not considered. Part of caring includes giving my patients any further explanation regarding their diagnosis as well as treatment options. It is important to me to have patients make well-informed decisions. I will always tell my patients what I believe is the best option for treatment; however, I respect the right to self-determination and believe that ultimately the decision is up to them. Caring for my patients also involves being confident that their needs are met. I maintain open dialogue with them during my care for them and encourage feedback from them. It is my belief that patients respond positively to a nurse who genuinely cares for them.

I believe that patients have a right to competent nursing care. During the time any patient is under my care, I realize that he/she is dependent on my knowledge and skills at a time when he/she often most vulnerable. I am motivated to provide excellent care and strive toward becoming an expert because I care. Competency is vital to establishing a relationship with a patient. Patients will begin to trust me when they can see that I am knowledgeable and that I have their interests in mind. Likewise, I believe that maintaining my integrity is part of building this trust with patients. I am committed to honesty

(Continued)

---

[1] Used with permission from Sarah Templeton, MSN, RN.

in all aspects of my care even if this means admitting an error in care. I do not believe that I can be truly competent if I am not morally accountable for my actions to my patients, my peers, and to God. One of the most important aspects of becoming competent is the continual process of learning. I believe that outside of education, one of the best tools for learning is the very patient I care for. As I begin a relationship with a patient, I want to learn what his/her perspectives are, what his/her values are, and what his/her subjective complaints are regarding his/her illness. If I am a student of my patient, we can begin to formulate a plan of care that embodies the things that are most important to him/her. It is important for me to have a patient do what is best even in my absence. Therefore, as I include the patient input in the plan of care, the patient will be more likely to follow through with it.

As a nurse, I believe that instilling hope and confidence in my patients is essential in promoting self-care. I am interested in assisting patients to meet their goals by providing them with the resources and care they need to do so. When people feel in charge, they also feel hopeful and therefore have a sense that they can do what is required to maintain health, conserve health, or return to health. When I work with a patient, I give them options and help make goals that they feel are attainable. With this in mind, I realize that I may need to provide resources to help them be successful. This may mean medicating them for pain so that they can ambulate or it may mean praying with them when they are overcome with frustration. In addition, I believe that confidence is created when I explain how the goals we agree on will increase their own autonomy as they move closer to self-care. Finally, I believe that educating my patients on how to care for themselves in my absence is part of building confidence. I believe that if I am not teaching my patients, I may be holding them back and keeping them from accomplishing what they are capable of doing. Sharing what I know with patients is so important for me because this is one of the very reasons they are seeking me out. Part of confidence is removing the fear that many patients have because they simply do not understand what is happening to their bodies. As a nurse, I believe it is my duty to help alleviate this fear through education.

Congruency of My Philosophy With the [Artinian] Intersystem Model

My philosophy of nursing is most congruent with the Intersystem Model. The following is a description of the concepts that can be found in both. The first section of my philosophy focuses on the idea of caring. The ideas I listed within this section match with many of the core ideas found in the Intersystem Model. For example, both require that the nurse and client work together to negotiate mutually agreed upon goals between the nurse and the patient. Likewise, the essence of both is a sense of collaborative planning between the nurse and the patient. In order for this to be successful, both require that the nurse understands the life situation of the patient (Artinian, 1997a). Both systems recognize the need for patient input in his/her plan of care in order for it to be meaningful to the patient and for him/her to follow it. My philosophy states that the nurse is motivated to include the patient in decision making because the nurse cares and because the nurse wants the patient to continue to work on goals even outside of the nurse's immediate presence in his/her care. Likewise, the Intersystem Model borrows from the theory of caring by Benner and states that the impetus behind the desire of the nurse to understand the client's perspective and honor the client values in planning care is caring. As defined by Benner and Wrubel (1989), caring means that person, events, projects, and thing matter to people. Caring as a word for being connected and having things matter works well because it fuses thought, feeling, and action (p. 1).

The next section of my philosophy focuses on the importance of the nurse being competent in his/her care of the patient. It seems that there is also congruency with Intersystem Model with this concept as well. Both the philosophy and the model recognize the importance of building trust with the patient. The assertion is that the nurse bears the responsibility for initiating and developing his sense of trust. Both agree that trust is developed as the patient realizes that the nurse who is caring for him/her is both competent and interested in knowing what he/she values. The Intersystem Model asserts that patients feel confidence in their nurses when the nurse competently attends to their needs. Likewise, my philosophy states that nurses should "be a student of their patients" so that he/she can better incorporate the patient's values into the plan of care and instill within the patient the idea that the nurse is tracking with what is most important to him/her. This aids in the development of trust between the two systems because nursing actions are guided by how the nurse perceives the world of the patient. To foster this type of trust, both my philosophy and the model indicate that the nurse must provide expert care through technical proficiency and explain what is happening and provide reassurance. If the patient is not confident in the nurse's skills and abilities, then trust is lost. This may also affect the ability for connection between the two intrasystems. This means that the ability to collaborate and in this way help the patient move toward wellness is stifled.

Finally, my nursing philosophy states that instilling hope and confidence in the patient is essential to providing nursing care. Though not explicitly stated, it seems that the Intersystem Model expresses ideas about assisting the patient to move toward wellness that are similar to my ideas within my philosophy. Both agree that assisting patients to use their coping mechanisms is essential in achieving wellness. For example, by providing patients a means for pain control, the patient is better able to use his/her resources to complete the tasks needed to be done and successfully adapt to the situation. This is what I mean when I state in my philosophy that nurses play a large role in providing patients with the resources they need to be successful in their care. Education seems to be one of the primary ways that both my philosophy and the model use to help patients learn about various coping strategies. Both the model and my philosophy focus on the fact that the nurse must keep in mind the patient's individuality. If the nurse is attempting to provide the patient with coping strategies, then the nurse must know exactly how one patient's needs differ from that of another patient. This is the key to not only developing mutual care planning for your patients but also to making the entire model work properly. There is no set care plan for every patient. Each intrasystem (patient) is unique. Therefore, to make the model work, the nurse must understand this. It seems that this idea is congruent with my entire nursing philosophy. Therefore, I conclude that the Intersystem Model is the appropriate model for my personal philosophy of nursing. It tells me how I do nursing.

In summary, I believe that this model makes significant contributions to health care. It reflects a holistic approach to patient care. It encompasses all of the domains of a person as it includes also a spiritual component. In addition, this model provides patients with choice and "say" in their care. It fosters a partnership between patients and the health care system. This is perhaps the most significant contribution because patients are more likely to follow through with care that they have agreed to. This is essential in obtaining better patient outcomes and more patients achieving wellness. Therefore, the overall utility of this model is recognized and seen as valuable in providing care to patients of all kinds.

> *Philosophy of Nursing 9.2*

My Philosophy of Nursing[2]
Mary Hull MSN, RN

When I look back at the two out of four years of my nursing career that I have been a labor and delivery nurse, I wonder: What is important for me to be as a nurse? What are the desires that I have for myself as well as for every day of caring for the mothers and babies? What are my daily goals? The answers came to me clearly and I will express them as well as I am able to.

My philosophy is encompassed in the following three factors. The first is to strive to develop an effective nurse–patient relationship so that the mother will work with me toward the outcome of having a safe delivery. My hope for the mother is that she will have adequate knowledge regarding her individual plan of care beginning from the time of admission. My role at this point is to discuss the reason for her admission that can range from admission for an induction, cesarean section, an emergency situation, or for observation and to answer questions regarding the plan of care.

The second factor is to make it certain that the patient is able to feel that her specific plan of care is significant although challenging. I believe that the patient should take part in every decision. This can be done by listening to the views of the patient including stories regarding her past labor and delivery experiences. It is also done when the nurse and physician offer their explanations and opinions and thoughts so that the patient has adequate information to understand her plan of care. When she understands the reasoning behind the nurse/physician suggested plan of care, she is in a position to participate in the decision of a selecting a plan to improve her care.

The third factor is for the patient to be able to view the complete plan of care as one that she will be able to control with the help of the nurse and physician. This can be done by encouraging the patient to freely express her preferences and by discussing alternatives to her decisions if they are necessary.

These three factors demonstrate the importance of the nurse and patient working together as a team, although they are two

(Continued)

---

[2] Used with permission from Mary Hull, MSN, RN.

individuals with differing opinions, knowledge, and values. By working together, a true relationship between the nurse and patient can develop that is characterized by communication, negotiation, and hopefully, patient satisfaction.

Congruency Between My Philosophy of Nursing and the [Artinian] Intersystem Model

The main goal of my philosophy of nursing is to strive to develop a nurse–patient relationship that fosters working together toward the same goal: a safe delivery. The goal of the Intersystem Model is to foster mutual goal setting so that the nurse and patient work toward an agreed upon goal that moves the patient the patient to a successful outcome.

The first factor in my philosophy of nursing is for the client to have adequate knowledge regarding the individual plan of care. This equates to the concept of comprehensibility that describes the level of knowledge of the client in relation to what he or she needs to do about the situation. The second factor is for the patient to be able to feel that her plan of care is significant although challenging. This equates to the concept of meaningfulness. This is in relation to motivation the patient has and how much effort the patient is willing to put into resolving the concern. The third factor is for the patient to feel that the plan of care is one that she can control with the help of the nurse. This equates to the concept of manageability in relation to resources available to manage the particular concern.

In summary, the value of using the Intersystem Model is that is allows the nurse to see patients as whole persons responding to the contextual settings in which they are placed. The movement of health care into community settings with a focus on families and communities as well as individuals is a new challenge to nursing and this model can serve as a structure for implementing this change. The Intersystem Model lends itself to all aspects of current nursing education and also to future developments in education. It is dynamic and flexible, and it provides a rational, concrete, and organized manner for approaching nursing practice.

CONCLUSION

Nursing education is a good venue for the use of the AIM. The AIM can be used in many ways to meet patient, family, and community needs. In addition, various teaching pedagogies can be used to introduce and explain the AIM to students at all levels of nursing education. The examples provided in this chapter are only a sampling of the many uses of the AIM in nursing education. Boyer's elements of excellence in teaching pedagogy were used to demonstrate the quality of our nursing education at the APU-SON and the use of the AIM in nursing education. It is our view that the AIM assists us in reaching our goal for educational excellence in our programs. It is our hope that nursing faculty at other institutions will use some of the strategies and examples in their own programs and classrooms (see Appendix and online adjunct manual for blank forms and templates). We encourage the use of the AIM as a model to guide curriculum planning, course development, and lesson plan formulation for all levels of nursing education.

REFERENCES

Antonovsky, A. (1987). *Unraveling the mystery of health: How people manage stress and stay well*. San Francisco, CA: Jossey-Bass.

Artinian, B. (1991). The development of the Intersystem Model. *Journal of Advanced Nursing, 16*(2), 194–205.

Artinian, B. M. (1997a). Overview of the Intersystem Model. In B. M. Artinian & M. Conger, *The Intersystem Model: From theory to practice* (pp. 1–17). Thousand Oaks, CA: Sage Publications.

Artinian, B. M. (1997b). Situational sense of coherence. In B. M. Artinian & M. Conger, *The Intersystem Model: From theory to practice* (pp. 18–26). Thousand Oaks, CA: Sage Publications.

Artinian, B. M., & Conger, M. (1997). *The Intersystem Model: From theory to practice*. Thousand Oaks, CA: Sage Publications.

Azusa Pacific University. (2010a). *About APU*. Retrieved from http://www.apu.edu/about/mission/

Azusa Pacific University. (2010b). *About the School of Nursing*. Retrieved from http://www.apu.edu/nursing/about/

Azusa Pacific University. (2010c). *Undergraduate nursing*. Retrieved from http://www.apu.edu/nursing/undergraduate/

Benner, P. (1982, March). From novice to expert: The Dreyfus model of skill acquisition. *American Journal of Nursing, 82*, 402–407.

Benner, P., & Wrubel, J. (1989). *The primacy of caring*. Menlo Park, CA: Addison-Wesley.

Boyer, E. L. (1996). 5 priorities for quality schools. *Education Digest, 62*(1), 4–8.

Brenner, R. (2007, September 12). Using the parking lot. *Point Lookout*. Retrieved from https://www.chacocanyon.com/pointlookout/070912.shtml

Brown, S. J. (1981). The nursing process systems model. *Journal of Nursing Education, 20*, 36–40.

Clark, M. J. D. (2008). *Community health nursing: Advocacy for population health* (5th ed.). Upper Saddle River, NJ: Pearson Education, Inc.

Cone, P. (1997). Connecting: A basic social process of spiritual care giving. In B. M. Artinian & M. Conger, *The Intersystem Model: From theory to practice* (pp. 270-288). Thousand Oaks, CA: Sage Publications.

Conger, M. (1997). Fostering mutuality in clinical practice. In B. M. Artinian & M. Conger, *The Intersystem Model: From theory to practice* (pp. 226-243), Thousand Oaks, CA: Sage Publications.

Davis, J. A. (2006). *Providing Critical Incident Stress Debriefing (CISD) to individuals and communities*. American Academy of Experts in Traumatic Stress. Retrieved from http://www.aaets.org/article54.htm

Editors. (2004). Are faculty doing the scholarship of teaching? *Teaching Professor, 18*(7), 6-11.

Gordon, H. (2010). Faculty matters. *Nursing Education Perspectives, 31*(2), 76-78.

Hill, R. (1949). *Families under stress*. New York, NY: Harper & Row.

Kuhn, A. (1974). *The logic of social systems: A unified, deductive, system-based approach to social science*. San Francisco, CA: Jossey-Bass.

Passamore, K. (2008). Human commonalities and art. *School Art, 108*(1), 46-47.

Yair, G. (2008). Can we administer the scholarship of teaching? Lessons from outstanding professors in higher education. *Higher Education, 55*(4), 447-459.

10

AN EMERGING NURSING PROGRAM IN A DEVELOPING COUNTRY

Darlene E. McCown and Barbara M. Artinian

A PROGRAM TO PREPARE professional nurses at the baccalaureate and graduate levels is being developed under the direction of Dr. Darlene McCown, Director of Nursing, for the nursing program at Hope Africa University (HAU) in Burundi, Central Africa. The program is developed based on the salutogenic model of Antonovsky (1987) and the Intersystem Model (Artinian & Conger, 1997). Although the students are the survivors of a brutal tribal/political war, they demonstrate a strong sense of coherence (SOC). In spite of the fact that their environment has not been predictable or well structured, they exhibit an amazing sense of perseverance and confidence in the future and life. The nursing students at HAU see the goal of the BSN degree as worth the investment of work and see it as a challenge worth pursuing. These students look to the future with great expectations for service to others and a better life for themselves.

BACKGROUND OF THE PROGRAM

HAU is a Free Methodist institution under the leadership of the African Free Methodist Church. It is assisted by an organization in the United States called "Friends of Hope Africa University." The university is located in Bujumbura, the capital city of Burundi, in Central Africa. The mission of the university is to "transform students for the development of character and for service through academic and professional programs that glorify God and serve mankind."

Burundi is a small landlocked, resource-poor country comparable in size to the state of Maryland. It is bordered by the Democratic Republic of Congo on the west, Rwanda on the north, and Tanzania on the east and south. Burundi is recovering from 12 years of civil war between Hutu and Tutsi factions and now has an elected president since 2005. It is one of the poorest countries in Africa ranking 174th out of 182 countries in the world according to the United

Nations' Human Development Index (HDI; United Nations Development Programme, 2009). The total population of Burundi is 9,511,330 with only 10% of the total population living in urban areas. Nearly half the population is children under 14 years of age (46.3%). The median age of the population is 16.8 years. Adults 65 and over represent only 2.5% of the population (Central Intelligence Agency, n.d.).

The United Nations Development Programme (UNDP) looks beyond the GNP to evaluate the well-being of a country using the HDI. The HDI measures the potential to live a long and healthy life, being educated, and having a decent standard of living. For citizens of Burundi, life expectancy at birth is 50.1 years, the adult literacy rate is 59.3%, and the GDP per capita is $362US (UNDP, 2009). The majority of the labor force (93.6%) is employed in the growing of coffee and tea, accounting for 35% of the GDP (Central Intelligence Agency, n.d.). The Human Poverty Index (HPI-I) for Burundi shows that a third of the people suffer severe deprivation with a 33.7% probability of not surviving to age 40. A decent standard of living is further measured on the HPI-I by the unweighted average of people not using an improved water source (29% in Burundi) and underweight children under age 5 (39% of Burundi's children). The infant mortality ranks Burundi at 192 of 224 nations globally with 64.86 deaths per 1,000 births. Only one in two children go to school, and approximately one in 15 adults has HIV/AIDS (Central Intelligence Agency, n.d.). Prematurity, malnutrition, infectious diseases, accidents and trauma, postpartum infections, HIV, TB, diabetes, malaria, sexually transmitted diseases, depression, and alcoholism are among the common health problems faced by children and the nation. Treatment for complicated conditions such as neurological, birth defects, cancer, and chronic disabling conditions is generally nonexistent. Burundi is predominantly Christian, with Catholicism the major Christian affiliation and Free Methodist the major Protestant affiliation.

Currently, there are 44 district hospitals with one medical doctor for 34,744 persons and one nurse for 35,000 persons. Burundi is a country with less than 200 doctors. Many nurses are currently lay-persons prepared on the job or prepared at the high school level of nurses' aides or practical nurses. Medical doctors are poorly trained and lack experience with current medical procedures and equipment. There is a lack of equipped facilities and trained human resources in all aspects of the health care sector. Existing health infrastructures are outdated and damaged by war and lack of resources and leadership and are unable to provide minimal required basic services.

It is into these challenging circumstances that HAU was founded with a commitment to facing African realities and finding African solutions for Africa's problems. The concept of HAU was born out of the Central East Africa

Free Methodist Church in the 1980s. HAU is an associate member of the Association of Free Methodist Educational Institutions that include Roberts Wesleyan College in Rochester, New York.

DEVELOPMENT OF HAU

In February 2000, the school opened with 27 students in Nairobi, Kenya. In 2003, HAU was relocated to Bujumbura, Burundi. The university was granted governmental approval for its academic programs. In 2004, all these initial university programs were accredited by the Burundi Minister of Education, and the first 37 students graduated. Construction of the Bujumbura campus progressed and by 2006 enrollment topped 700 students. By 2007, enrollment doubled and by 2010 reached 3,165 students in both graduate and undergraduate programs.

The Burundi Minister of Education accredited the Schools of Medicine, Nursing, and Physiotherapy in 2009. The first classes graduated in January of 2010. It must be noted that a significant number of HAU students have been orphaned by the civil war and lack family and financial support. The university bears a financial burden in providing higher education for a population with extremely limited financial resources. This is especially true for programs such as nursing and medicine that demand scientific equipment, clinical training, laboratories, and professional oversight.

THE NURSING PROGRAM

The Nursing Program at HAU was established in 2005. The first class graduated in January of 2010. This program was developed to meet the need for professional nursing in a developing country that has a substandard medical system and lacks the basics of good health care. Prior to the graduation of the first nursing class, there were no nurses prepared at the baccalaureate level in the country. The baccalaureate program is a 4-year program. Currently, there are about 250 nursing and medical students enrolled with equal numbers in each program.

Early in their studies, students are introduced to the basic nursing process and documentation using the SOAP process. For the first graduating class, the instructors were primarily medical faculty. Resources for the students are very limited but they are improving. In the past, the students did not have textbooks.

They were taught by lecture and recitation, note taking, and memorization. This is changing. The nursing program has been able to obtain 37 copies of basic physical assessment and diagnosis texts by various authors. Each student now has the use of the textbook for the course on physical assessment. Since the students never had access to any books or learned how to find information for themselves, they were taught how to use the table of contents and indices. The students also had difficulty manipulating medical equipment because they lacked manual dexterity that comes from experience using toys as children.

The School of Nursing has developed a philosophy of nursing that is consistent with the principles of the Intersystem Model (1997). The School of Nursing philosophy states:

> Nursing is a caring profession. It is a professional discipline based on the social, biological, natural, and medical sciences. Nurses assist individuals, families, and communities to prevent and recover from illnesses, restore disabilities, or to achieve a peaceful death. Hope Africa University Department of Nursing views women, men, and children as persons of value with physical, spiritual, social, and environmental attributes. Nursing at Hope Africa University continues in the tradition of Florence Nightingale (1893), the founder of nursing.
>
> Nurses are independent and collegial members of the health care team. Nursing is viewed as a process that requires assessment, diagnosis, planning for interventions, and evaluation. Nursing care incorporates specific nursing therapeutics such as comfort measures, health teaching, and emotional support. The skills required for professional nursing care include critical thinking, problem solving, manual dexterity, leadership and team-work, administration, effective communication, accountability, and compassion.
>
> Hope Africa University faculty members believe that nursing requires a baccalaureate level education. Research and scientific inquiry are valued components of the curriculum. Nursing at Hope Africa University is founded on Christian principles of service, confidentiality, truthfulness, faithfulness, and compassion for those in need. (D. McCown, personal memo, 2005)

The medical program is staffed by up to five African doctors onsite and additional medical doctors from abroad who volunteer their academic and clinical services. The nursing faculty has three US-educated registered nurses with masters and doctoral degrees and two African nurses who are the directors of a regional hospital and a high-functioning clinic. Lecturers from the medical school also provide instruction in the nursing program. Teams of volunteer faculty from the United States in both medicine and nursing are scheduled on a regular basis throughout the year. Screening of volunteer applicants is facilitated through the Friends of Hope Africa University executive committee. Preparations are underway to prepare the first four nursing graduates for faculty positions and for service in the Hope Africa University Community Health Center due to be opened in December 2010. These new graduates have been hired by Hope Africa Community Hospital in Kibuye under the direction of the full-time medical staff with the expectation that they will become faculty in the nursing program. Dr. Darleen McCown will launch the masters program in Nursing in 2011.

The Masters Program in Nursing

McCown (2010, March 17) developed the proposal for the Hope Africa University Masters of Nursing Science Program (Table 10.1). This masters program curriculum represents the first step toward preparing the first six nursing graduates for faculty positions and for administrative positions at the Hope Africa University Community Health Center.

As undergraduates, the students were introduced to SOC Theory (Antonovsky, 1987) and the Intersystem Model (Artinian & Conger, 1997).

TABLE 10.1 Hope Africa University Masters of Nursing Science Program

HAU MSN CURRICULUM

Prerequisites	
Baccalaureate in Nursing or a closely related field of study	
Registered/legally licensed nurse in Burundi or other cooperative countries	
One year of clinical nursing practice or equivalent experience	
Advanced entry credit	5 credits
Nursing major courses	
Studies in Nursing Theory, Practice, and Research	6 credits
Teaching Methods and Curriculum Preparation	3 credits
Nursing Education Practicum Experience	3 credits
Advanced Nursing Skills	5 credits
Advanced Applied Pharmacology	5 credits
Required Courses in Nursing Major	27 credits
Electives: Must be at the 300–400 level	
Business Management Course	3 credits
Education or Social Work Course	3 credits
Premedicine (Medical Psychology recommended)	10 credits
Required Elective Courses	16 credits
Master's Project	7 credits
TOTAL REQUIRED CREDITS	**50 credits**

TABLE 10.2 Modules in the Graduate Course, "Readings in Nursing Theory, Practice, and Research"

Nursing Theories

Theories to be studied have been selected from the book, *The Intersystem Model: Integrating Theory and Practice* (Artinian & Conger, 1997). They include:
- Developmental theories (Chapter 3)
- Psychosocial theories (Chapter 6)
- Theories affecting the spiritual experience (Chapter 7)
- Family theories (Chapter 8)
- Learning theories (Chapter 12)

Nursing Models

Various topics about nursing models will be presented. Discussion of the use and value of nursing models will be based on chapters from the book, *The Intersystem Model: Integrating Theory and Practice* (1997), including:
- Overview of the Intersystem Model (Chapter 1)
- Situational sense of coherence (Chapter 2)
- Context of involvement (Chapter 4)

Nursing Research

Standard topics in nursing research have been selected for study by the students in this program and include the following:
- Types of quantitative research and reliability and validity
- Qualitative research: Grounded theory
- Methods of data collection
- Critical analysis of nursing studies
- Evidence-based practice

Rationale

The Intersystem Model (1997) is useful for application in practice in a Christian nursing program because the Intersystem Model:
- provides a systematic way to assess the patient and provide care
- places the spiritual subsystem at the core of the person
- respects the dignity of the patient by making the patient part of the decision-making process
- explores the developmental environment of the patient
- identifies the main concern of the patient or nurse
- explores what the patient knows about the main concern, what the patient wants to do, and the resources patient has to resolve the main concern
- scores patient on Situational Sense of Coherence (SSOC)
- evaluates the success of the intervention by rescoring on SSOC

Source: B. Artinian (2011).

At the graduate level, students will apply SOC theory to patient situations by using the Intersystem Model (1997) in their clinical practice. To use the model effectively, the knowledge base of the graduate student must include understanding theories developed by nurses and others, the value and use of nursing models in practice, critical thinking, clinical diagnostic skills, ability to assess the impact of cultural environment on development, and evaluation of research studies. The purpose of the course "Readings in Nursing Theory, Practice, and Research" is to provide a knowledge base in theory and research. A description of the modules in the course is given in Table 10.2.

Future of the Program

HAU has been requested by the government of Burundi to develop a health clinic to serve their geographical sector of the capital city. As new facilities are added to the HAU campus, additional clinical sites will be available to the students. The developing Community Health Center will be staffed by medical and nursing faculty; recent graduates and current students will have clinical rotations there as part of their nursing and medical education. Construction of the clinic has begun, and changes have already been made in the design to significantly enlarge each of the clinic wings including the pediatric and maternity areas to accommodate the ever-increasing population. In addition, a station for giving pediatric immunizations, a covered outdoor patio patient waiting area, as well as conference and office space for medical and nursing students and faculty have been added. Funding for equipping the clinic has been generated from grants and gifts from generous individuals were committed to Hope Africa University. Ongoing support for the clinic will be funded by the Burundi government that pays for maternity and pediatric care for children under the age of 5 and by fees for service from patients. The completion of the building is scheduled for December 17, 2010. It is expected that students and patients will begin using the clinic by January 2011.

The development of Hope Africa University Schools of Nursing and Medicine, including the establishment of a Community Health Clinic, is a major achievement brought together by the cooperative work of African leadership and assistance from interested participants in the United States and Canada. This venture reflects the success of cross-cultural cooperation and a high level of leadership, trust, and vision.

REFERENCES

Antonovsky, A. (1987). *Unraveling the mysteries of health: How people manage stress and stay well.* San Francisco, CA: Jossey-Bass.
Artinian, B., & Conger, M. (1997). *The Intersystem Model: Integrating theory and practice.* Thousand Oaks, CA: Sage Publications.

Central Intelligence Agency (CIA). (n.d.). *CIA—The World Factbook*. Retrieved from https://www.cia.gov/library/publications/the-world-factbook/geos/by.html

McCown, D. (2010, March 17). [Hope Africa University Masters of Nursing Science Program Proposal Draft 1]. Hope Africa University Archives, Bujumbura, Burundi.

United Nations Development Programme. (2009). *Human development report—Burundi* [Country Fact Sheets]. Retrieved from http://hdrstats.undp.org/en/countries/country_fact_sheets/cty_fs_BDI.html

11

FOSTERING MUTUALITY IN CLINICAL PRACTICE

Margaret M. Conger

Nursing has long espoused joint planning with client and nurse for development of a plan of care (Joint Commission on Accreditation of Healthcare Organizations, 1989). In practice, however, this is not commonly done. Many health professionals operate on the premise that they know best what is good for the client. The values of paternalism and beneficence are strongly held beliefs in much of clinical practice. The use of the Artinian Intersystem Model (AIM) makes it possible for the patient to participate in the planning of care on a more equal basis. The shared decision making that incorporates both the client and nurse values in the development of a plan of care is defined in this chapter as mutuality.

In this chapter, examples are presented in which student nurses have been effective in identifying client value systems and developing nursing interventions based on mutually agreed-on goals. The students cared for these clients during a clinical rotation in an Advanced Nursing Practicum at Northern Arizona University. Each example is explored using the Intersystem Model (1997) as a framework.

The geographical environment in which these situations occur is important. The client population includes a large American Indian population that still retains many traditional values, along with a geriatric population living in retirement types of communities. In addition, the local medical center serves not only the immediate community but also a large population of tourists who develop health problems as they travel in the high altitude in Northern Arizona. This very diverse client population makes this a rich area for nursing students to develop skill in meeting unique client needs.

INTERACTIVE NURSING

A number of authors (Benner & Wrubel, 1989; Gordon, 1987; Orlando, 1972) focus on the importance of an interactive experience between the nurse and the client. Nursing can no longer be "doing for the patient," but rather must involve working with the client to determine mutual goals. Orlando (1961) identifies the need for the nurse to focus on the individuality of the client. From her early work to the present, she has maintained that the nurse–patient interaction is the most important component of nursing care. Her perception of the nursing process is that the nurse responds to an observed client behavior by sharing his or her understanding of the behavior with the client. The nurse and client together identify appropriate actions to resolve the problem identified in the behavior. The nurse does not assume that his or her assessment of the situation is correct unless its validity is explored with the client (Orlando, 1972).

Also, the nurse cannot rely on past experiences to know the correct intervention for a particular client. Two patients who present with the same behavior may require interventions that are quite different. Even hospital protocols cannot serve as appropriate reasons for deciding on the use of a particular intervention. At times, it is the responsibility of the nurse to resolve conflicts between the client's need for help and institutional policies (Orlando, 1972).

Benner and Wrubel (1989) also see the need for the nurse to function as the client advocate. A role of the nurse is often to act as a client advocate to the physician and family. Many times, the physician or family concerns differ from those of the client; in such cases, the need for an advocate for the client is essential.

Gordon (1987) explores the need for mutuality between the nurse and client as the plan of care is being developed. She states that the client must contribute personal perceptions of the problem under consideration and plans for health care practices. The nurse must consider the meaning of the situation to the patient. In this encounter, both the patient and nurse value systems must be considered.

Jones and Brown (1993) state that decisions for determining the nursing care required must be made based on the patient's point of view. The nurse and patient need to negotiate between alternative points of view that incorporate the situational context.

Benner and Wrubel (1989) also look at the nurse–client interaction as the plan of care for the client is developed. They state that "if the plan of care does not incorporate input from the patient, a gulf is created between the nurse and patient" (p. 91). They state that the personal concerns of the client are what determine what is "at stake" for a person in any situation. It is the responsibility of the nurse to interpret the concerns that influence the client's understanding of the illness.

Culture

The client's culture must be taken into account in the process. Even when the culture of the client is different from that of the nurse, some understanding of culture must be attempted. Benner and Wrubel (1989) suggest that, through elements of shared culture, it is possible to develop and understand a culture different from one's own.

Munhall (1993) describes some of the difficulties that are encountered when attempting to see a problem from another's perspective. The nurse needs to spend time communicating with the client, reflecting on what is being said, and then validating his or her understanding of what the client has said. It is hard for the nurse to live out the belief that personal perceptions of the world and of health may not be held by the patient.

Mutuality

Current studies in both the nursing and psychiatric literature emphasize the importance of mutuality in providing client care. Sahlsten, Larsson, Sjostrom, Lindencrona, and Plos (2007) explored with a number of nurses their understanding of the concept of mutuality among the nurse and client. Their findings suggest that when the nurse and client work mutually to plan care, the client's motivation and satisfaction with received care was increased. Mutuality was found to be a precursor to negotiation about planned care. A sense of equal partnership was necessary to the process.

In the psychiatric literature, this concept is also explored. Proctor (2010) suggests that if one works from an ethic of mutuality, the power of the therapist over the client is minimized. If the client feels powerless, his or her distress will be increased. When the client's sense of powerless is reduced, recovery is more likely. This need for mutual interaction is also an important component when working interculturally (Lago, 2010). The therapist needs to understand how dominant cultural values can negatively affect therapy when working with a client of a different cultural background. The value system of both the therapist and the client must be examined in order to provide therapeutically effective care.

TEACHING THE CONCEPT OF MUTUALITY

Discussion of how to teach nursing students the concept of mutuality is important. Because this teaching is more directed to the affective domain as opposed to the cognitive domain of learning, classroom exercises and discussion alone are not sufficient. Continued reinforcement in the clinical area is needed. The AIM is a helpful tool to use with students to encourage incorporation of mutuality into their clinical practice. Artinian and Conger (1997) describe the interaction process that occurs when the model is used. In the developmental environment, the nurse works with the client to seek information about the state of both his or her internal and external environments. When the main concern of the patient or nurse is identified, the nurse will assess the client for situational sense of coherence in the three areas. The first area is how comprehensible the situation is to the client. Does he or she have adequate information to make cognitive sense of the situation? Second, how meaningful is the situation to the client? Does life make sense emotionally? Is the challenge of the situation worth the effort it will take to develop adequate coping skills? Finally, is the situation manageable? Are the resources available adequate for the problem to be managed or does the client has a sense of victimization? It is important to understand the value system the client brings to the situation prior to developing outcome goals. Only when the client's value system is recognized can a mutually acceptable plan of care be developed and carried out.

In the clinical practicum, students assess the situational sense of coherence of their clients as part of the care plan. In doing this assessment, the student is required to think about how the individual client is coping with his or her health status. An outcome of this assessment is the identification of the client value system. Information obtained in this assessment forms the basis for development of a plan of care.

Teaching students to value mutuality in clinical practice is an ongoing lesson. Often in the practice area, students are exposed to examples of health care professionals who fail to consider the values of the client when making clinical decisions. Nursing instructors need to counter such behavior with examples of positive applications of mutuality. This example demonstrates how students can be guided in their practice to consider the values of the client when planning nursing care.

Example

A young Native American man was brought to the hospital following a fall from a cliff. He suffered numerous broken bones and contusions involving his chest area leading to considerable pain, which hindered his breathing. Both his wife and mother were constantly at his bedside. The student caring for the client was concerned about his pain level and its effect on his ability to take deep breaths. However, when offering the client pain medication, he denied that he had any pain.

The nursing student came to the instructor to talk about her frustration with the situation. We talked about cultural values of Native Americans and the need for men to appear strong in front of others especially women. The student was encouraged to explore this possibility with the client. She returned to the client's bedside and encouraged his wife and mother to go to the cafeteria for a break. While the family was gone, she again approached the client about the need for pain medication explaining why it was so important to help him take deep breaths to prevent further lung complications. This time he agreed to take the pain medication.

Using this as a clue to understanding the client's value system, the student then planned a medication management plan that coincided with regular meal times for the family. This allowed her to provide pain medication when the family was not at the bedside. The client's value system of appearing strong in front of his family was preserved, and administration of needed medication allowed him to take deep breaths as needed.

Client Vignettes

Because the clinical setting is the environment in which the nursing student best learns effective nurse–patient interactions, early exposure to differentiating between institutional values and client values is important. As will be seen in several of the vignettes that follow, the institutional environment is often hostile to this concept. An important role the instructor can play is in shielding the student from a hostile environment so that mutuality can be achieved. It is hoped that students exposed to nursing practice in which mutuality is valued will internalize this value. In time, as more nursing students incorporate this value into their practice, changes can be made in the institutional environment as well.

The following vignettes are examples of student interactions with clients in which the client's concerns were identified and the student attempted to include the client in mutual planning. Two of the vignettes focus on the constraints that the environment can bring in preventing a client from reaching a higher state of health. Another focuses on identifying spiritual values held by the client. The last vignette focuses on the challenges that working with a client from the nondominant culture brings.

The amount of time needed for the nurse and client to clarify values can vary from a brief encounter to a more prolonged one. Some of the vignettes occurred in just a matter of minutes. At other times, it may take much longer for the nurse to be able to identify the client's value system. The first student vignette describes the interaction of Amy, a senior nursing student, and B, an elderly client with a chronic health problem of diarrhea.

Case Study 11.1

The Wrong Pill[1]

Amy M. Stilley, BSN, RN

"Guess what, it's time to take another pill. Are you ready?" I asked B, a 76-year-old patient who had been lively and cheerful throughout my shift as a team leader in a rural hospital.
"Oh sure, I'm ready. I'm always ready."
"OK, now what pill is this?" I asked, holding a small white pill.
"I don't know. I can't keep track of them anymore because there are so many different kinds."
"Well, this is Lomotil. Do you know what it is for?"
"It's so I won't get diarrhea."
"Right." I then gave him the pill cup and watched as he swallowed the pill.
"You know, that is the generic brand, huh?"
"It sure is," I replied, thinking that it was good that the hospital saved the patient money by giving generic medication whenever possible. I was caught off guard when B's reaction was not what I expected. His face grew very serious and he said,

> I have tried both kinds, the generic and the brand name. The generic just does not work as well as the brand name. I told my doctor that, but he said the only difference is in the fillers. Well, I don't know, but maybe it has something to do with the fillers; but the generic one does not work as well. You know, I am getting old, and I've had surgery on my stomach a few years ago, and have had diarrhea since then. I can't even go to the bathroom normally with this diarrhea. The brand name makes me normal. The generic kind of takes that away, for I'm always trying to make it to the bathroom.

---

[1] Used with permission from Amy M. Stilley.

I listened and let him know that I understood. I told him that I would try to get for him the brand-name form. I called the pharmacy to explain the situation and found that the brand name was not carried. The pharmacist, however, said that B could bring in his own pills and they would then be supplied to him in place of the generic brand. The doctor would need to write an order to cover this exchange.

I found B's wife and asked her to bring in the medication when she returned to the hospital that afternoon. I also spoke with the doctor and received order for the substitution of the brand name for the generic brand. At this point, I left for a lunch break.

When I returned from lunch, my supervising RN informed me that B was distressed over not having his Lomotil before eating lunch. She said that she tried to explain to him that he had received the medication, but B would not accept her answer. I quickly went to B's room. He looked very worried and had his arms tightly crossed over his chest.

"Hello, Mr. B."

"I don't want to talk about it. You have to do what you have to and that's it."

"What do you mean?" I asked as I sat down next to him.

"I'm old and I don't work like I used to. Some days I don't think living is worth it at all. For the longest time after my stomach surgery, I could not control myself, but the brand name helps. I'm not rich and don't have money to throw around, but I don't mind paying more for those pills. I feel human again when I am on time. Can you understand what I'm saying?"

"Yes, I understand that the brand name works better, and that they make life bearable for you. Mr. B, you have every right to feel the way you do. It must be very difficult for you right now. I know you got the generic brand of Lomotil before lunch today and that you believe that this brand does not help you as much as the name brand. As soon as your wife brings in the prescription bottle, you will be able to begin taking the name brand. Will your wife be here before four thirty?"

"Oh yes, by three o'clock."

"Great, then your next pill at five should be the name brand."

"Thanks for understanding. You're the only one who would listen."

On returning to B's room 15 minutes later, I found him fast asleep.

Analysis

In this vignette, Amy took time to explore B's value system. She learned that B believed that the brand-name form of Lomotil gave him more control over his diarrhea than did the generic brand. She also learned that the use of the brand-name product made him feel that his life was worth living and was worth the extra amount of money that it cost. Amy also had to evaluate her value system of believing that it was good to save money through use of a generic form of a drug.

Amy's interventions focused on the client's value system rather than the values of the institution. She took B's concern seriously, giving validity to his situation. By working with the pharmacy, doctors, and the client's wife, she was able to bypass an institutional restraint and provide the desired pill. She kept B informed of the negotiations needed to achieve the joint goal. Finally, Amy was able to evaluate the effect of her interventions when she went back to check on B and found him able to rest. This was far different from the very anxious person she had seen earlier.

In evaluating this situation in terms of B's situational sense of coherence, the area of comprehensibility was high—B knew all about his reaction to both the generic and the brand-name form of Lomotil. He found meaning for his life in the control of the diarrhea that the brand name gave him. His ability to manage the situation, however, was at risk. He was fighting against an institutional environment that had a very different value system—namely, that the generic form of drug was most cost-effective. Only as this value system was seen from the client's perspective could this problem be resolved.

Case Study 11.2

The Twelve-Hour Journey[2]
Vince Martinez, MS, RN

I participated in a unique clinical experience during my senior year as a nursing student at Northern Arizona University. I was assigned to care for Mike, a 40-year-old Caucasian male diagnosed with histiocytic lymphoma of 2 years' duration. He had been treated at a well-respected cancer institute with aggressive therapy, but his body did not respond, and he was told that his condition was terminal.

---

[2] Used with permission from Vince Martinez.

Mike and his family eventually accepted that he would only live 4 to 5 months and that only palliative treatment was recommended.

Mike lived with his wife, Dana, and his 12-year-old stepson in New Hampshire. He also has two grown daughters who are married and have young children of their own. The family mutually decided to travel to the Western states in a motor home so that they could spend some quality time together. Mike was given a thorough physical exam by his doctor and cleared for this trip.

The first week of the trip went without incident. The family made positive gains toward their goal of quality time. Mike began to feel slightly ill with the onset of diarrhea toward the end of the second week. His family hoped it was just stress related to the traveling, but his condition rapidly deteriorated. He developed a fever, generalized edema, blood-tinged stools, and uncontrolled epistaxis. The family had no option but to stop at the nearest hospital.

Mike was admitted to the Intermediate Care Unit through the Emergency Department, diagnosed with pancytopenia. His initial platelet count was 3,000 and only increased to 9,000 following infusion of 30 units of platelets. He also received several units of packed red blood cells. He developed more gastrointestinal bleeding, oral thrush, gross lymphedema, generalized petechiae, severe muscle weakness, severe body pain, and a deeply bruised upper soft palate.

Mike was presented with the option of having multiple invasive diagnostic procedures to fully understand his current crisis. He realized that these procedures would not alter the course of his disease process and that he would eventually die. Mike subsequently refused all of the procedures.

When I started my first day with Mike, I asked the staff nurse what the plan for Mike would be. He answered, "He's going to die here. He's too sick to travel." The physician had spoken candidly to Mike and his family and had suggested that he would probably not live more than 48 hours with the degree of bleeding he was experiencing.

Mike was placed in a reverse isolation room, given liberal pain medication, and soft diet as he could tolerate it, and no further invasive procedures. The reality of impending death left Mike and his family with many sudden concerns and decisions. Mike spoke openly of his desire to die at his peaceful farm home in the presence of his family. At first, this did not seem to be a possibility for him. As the day went on, I noted that Mike was becoming increasingly depressed. He and his family expressed frustration and anger over

(Continued)

the difficult situation. His insurance would not cover the cost of a medevac flight home, although it would pay for the equal cost of the invasive procedures and hospitalization.

Mike decided to leave the hospital, even though it meant attempting to drive home in the motor home and dying somewhere along the highway. The stark reality of this decision finally prompted the hospital staff to work with him to develop an alternate plan. The social service worker was able to find a low-cost commercial transport that would get him home in about 12 hours. Mike would fly in a first-class section of the plane with his wife and a sister, who was a nurse, accompanying him. The family would drive him to Phoenix in the motor home and help him on to the flight. Another family member would meet him in Boston and drive him directly to his home. He would theoretically be in his own bed within 12 hours of being discharged from the hospital. The remainder of the family would drive the motor home back to New Hampshire.

The plan immediately hit many stumbling blocks. Airline personnel denied Mike the ticket when they realized how sick he was. They reluctantly agreed to reinstate the tickets when assured that a nurse would be accompanying him on the flight. The family also realized that all but Mike's wife and sister would be traveling about 4 days and would probably not see Mike alive again after they said goodbye at the airport.

Preparation for this journey was begun. Mike would be given an infusion of both platelets and packed red cells just prior to transport. He was also given PO pain medication and an antiemetic. We made every effort to accommodate the family needs. The reverse isolation guidelines were adhered to by all hospital personnel, but the family members were not required to wear masks, gowns, and gloves. There was always a family member with him at his bedside.

I noticed that the family was evidencing increased stress during the waiting period. I worked with Mike's sister to help her plan for the flight. We put together a kit of supplies to help manage any emergency that might arise. We talked through all of the potential problems and decided on a plan of action for each. The time for his discharge had to be delayed owing to the onset of a new GI hemorrhage. The physician was very pessimistic about the outcome of this transport because of the new bleeding. He said "He'll probably be dead well before he gets home." He did, however, order more platelets to be given. No platelets were available here and we had to wait for some to be flown up from Phoenix.

Mike left the hospital at five o'clock in the afternoon to begin the 12-hour journey. I woke up at five o'clock the next morning and wondered if Mike had actually made it home to die in his bed with his family at his side. I never found out the ending to this story, but what truly matters most is that Mike was allowed to work at realizing his goal of dying at home. His dignity in the dying process was preserved.

Analysis

In this vignette, Vince was able to look beyond the institutional value of Mike's need for intensive medical care to the greater need for Mike to control his own dying process. He determined to become engaged with Mike as a person and care for his personal values rather than the institutional value system. He was able to see that quality of life for Mike meant taking a big risk—the journey home.

His interventions changed from a cure model to a care model. He was able to assist the family to spend quality time with Mike both while in the hospital and again in undertaking a risky journey. He was able to make it possible for the entire family to set out on the biggest risk they would probably ever have to take. In doing so, however, they were able to satisfy their need to provide Mike with a quality death. In evaluating this situation in terms of the situational sense of coherence of Mike and his family, their level of comprehensibility was high. They knew about his disease and its ultimate consequence. The area in which they needed assistance was in the manageability of the situation. They had to work against institutional values of both the hospital and the airline to take Mike home. The positive support that Vince was able to give them in preparing for this journey gave them the confidence that it could be done. Once given the emotional support they needed, they were able to work with Mike to achieve his most cherished goal. Not once did Vince suggest to them that their initial plan for the journey to the West had been foolish and now they were paying the consequence.

Case Study 11.3

A Missed Identity[3]
Margaret Bond, MS, RN

When I first met Robert in a nursing home, he was slumped in his wheelchair and looked at me with sad, melancholic eyes. Tethered to his room by his oxygen tubing, the furthest Robert could venture was into the hallway, just past his room, where he sat quietly in his wheelchair, watching as the nursing home staff hurried about. Robert had been placed in the nursing home for 4 months prior, following an episode of congestive heart failure that had left him too weak to ambulate more than a few steps.

During my assessment of Robert, he told me that, although the nursing home record identified his occupation as a retired masonry contractor, he was also a Christian minister, which he considered his "true" profession. He described his current health as "I'm an invalid, I can't do anything I want to do. That depresses me." Robert was a Hopi Indian. He expressed dissatisfaction with having to eat "white man's food" and longed for his traditional foods. When I asked him what I could do to make his life more comfortable, he responded by saying that he wanted to go outside to walk. He also said, "I like to read the Bible, but my eyes are so bad that I can't."

Based on my assessment data, I determined that a major problem for Robert was spiritual distress related to his inability to practice his own faith as he desired because of his immobility and decreased visual acuity. One of my plans was to obtain a larger print Bible that he could read without any visual aid. I also planned to work with the physician and Robert's wife to provide him with the traditional food he desired.

Obtaining a large-print Bible proved to be a great challenge. Each agency I called cited a lack of resources and referred me to another agency. Finally, in desperation, I contacted a friend who worked in a local religious thrift shop and pleaded my case. My friend located a large-print Bible and had it delivered to my home "at no charge." I was thrilled!

The following Tuesday I took the Bible to Robert and explained that it had been donated anonymously. He asked me to read a passage to him, and then, he read a passage to me. He again asked

---

[3] Used with permission from Margaret Bond.

me to read to him, as the effort seemed too great for him to read aloud. Afterward, we sat quietly while the afternoon sun warmed the room. He seemed to be at peace. Promising to return the following Friday, I left the Bible with Robert.

When I returned on Friday, I found Robert's room empty, his bed stripped. I found the charge nurse and questioned her. "Robert died in his sleep last night." My friend had quietly slipped away. His last days were spent sharing readings from his new Bible with his wife and eating traditional foods she had prepared for him. Robert had reconnected with his spiritual side.

Analysis

In Margaret's assessment data collection process, she found what any nurse could have seen had they stopped to look at Robert. He was the picture of social isolation resulting from his immobility and dependence on the oxygen generated from the compressor in his room. She went a step farther, however, and discovered the unexpected—a Hopi Indian who was a Christian minister. Robert made it very clear to her that he considered his role as a minister to be the important part of his life's work. Robert was also depressed about his inability to do anything he wanted to do. He could not walk outside, and he had to eat the wrong kind of food.

Margaret was able to meet his spiritual need by procuring the large-print Bible for him. She was also able to meet his desire for his traditional food. She tried to get a portable oxygen system but was not successful in working through the bureaucracy for that. The simple intervention of providing for his spiritual need, however, had a life-altering effect on him. Even though he had the Bible only for a few days, it provided him with a peaceful death.

Robert's situational sense of coherence at the time Margaret first met him was very low. He had no ability to manage his life to accomplish even his simple desires related to spiritual practices, traditional food, and ability to go outside. He seemed to have no ability to know how to even begin to procure these things he desired. His motivation was also low, probably as the result of 4 months of living in the nursing home where no one seemed to know or care anything about his desires.

The intervention Margaret used was simple yet very effective. Often, it does not take a great deal of energy to help a client satisfy his spiritual needs. A simple act of caring enough to find out what is important to the client proved to be sufficient.

Case Study 11.4

Who Decides[4]

Elena Kirschner, BSN, RN

The provision of nursing care that is congruent with perceived client desires can be an extreme challenge. This was my experience in caring for an 89-year-old Navajo grandfather and traditional medicine man. The client had been transferred from a small hospital on the reservation for surgical repair of a yet unset fractured hip. Once admitted to the Intermediate Care Unit, he was given a long list of medical diagnoses: fractured hip, end-stage renal disease, hypercalcemia, anemia, ruptured tympanic membranes, sepsis, and malnutrition. The associated high-technology interventions for each medical diagnosis were immediately initiated.

It was apparent to me, as a nursing student, that the value system of the hospital unit and its staff, rather than the client's wishes were guiding the course of care for this patient. The primary medical goal was stabilization of the patient for surgery. This remained the goal for several days after it was clear that the patient was experiencing multisystem failure and was unlikely to survive his hospital stay.

To achieve this stabilization, the client's nutritional status needed improvement; therefore, an attempt was made to place a central line for the delivery of total parenteral nutrition. The client fought this procedure, and the attempt was unsuccessful. He was left with gross ecchymoses from shoulder to groin. Even though the first attempt at placement of the central line was extremely difficult for the client, the staff nurse, while obtaining a telephone consent from the family for a second attempt, described the procedure as "strictly routine." This attitude is an example of the institutional value system that persisted despite the nonverbal objections of the client.

Lack of a common language and client deafness made verbal communication impossible. Thus, nursing assessments had to be based on careful observation of the client's responses to interventions. A good understanding of the cultural context of the situation was also helpful. It was my observation that the client strongly objected to invasive procedures, especially those requiring movement. He objected by using hand movements motioning away

---

[4] Used with permission from Elena Kirschner.

the staff. He also used facial grimacing, loud and disapproving speech, and agitation. As more and more procedures were performed, the client's disapproval became less overt. He began to withdraw into a semiconscious state. Objective findings such as an increased blood pressure, tachypnea, tachycardia, and diaphoresis during procedures suggested a pain response.

For me, the client's withdrawal indicated that the situation (continuous invasive procedures) was becoming intolerable to him. I identified the nursing diagnosis of pain and social isolation and began interventions related to them. My nursing interventions included regard for the client's need for contact. Regular hand holding and gentle touching were instituted. I made contact with a Navajo translator, and daily social contacts with a Navajo speaker were arranged. I also advocated for a pain management protocol. I eventually was able to get the attending physician to prescribe the pain medication needed.

The client's response indicated that these interventions were well received. He seemed to regain a sense of control when his admonitions affected staff behavior (his complaints resulted in removal of painful stimuli). He was greatly calmed by touch and reached out for a hand when offered. He was able to rest more easily and endure procedures when given the pain medication on a regular basis. The client's interest and attention increased when he was spoken to in his own language. The Navajo translator was able to verify my understanding of the cultural response to the high technology on the part of this traditional medicine man. She indicated that the cultural value was a harmony with nature and that high-technology interventions that prolong suffering were probably in conflict with the client's belief system.

The medical prognosis for this client was extremely poor. As his nurse and advocate, I felt that his nonverbal communication efforts should be heeded and he be allowed a comfortable and dignified dying process. However, this was not the institutional value system and invasive procedures continued. These included placement of the central line, TPN administration, daily hemodialysis, IV antibiotic therapy, invasive suctioning, and a host of miscellaneous procedures.

I attempted to provide nursing care that honored the client's desires. I was only partially successful in this goal. My status as a nursing student was prohibitive to effecting a change in the existing mindset. Therefore, comfort care was unfortunately provided, so to speak, between the cracks. Today, as a staff nurse, I use the frustration of this situation to remind me to base my nursing practice on the needs of the client and not the institutional setting.

Analysis

Elena used data sources for assessments that were in accord with the client situation. Because of the language barrier and the deafness of the client, she focused on the nonverbal clues given. She also used her understanding of Navajo culture to predict the response of an elderly medicine man to the high-technology environment of the modern hospital. Her understanding of the culture was further validated by using the resources of a Navajo translator.

Although Elena's interventions were not successful in preventing further painful interventions for this client, she was able to reduce his discomfort by providing for pain needs and giving emotional support through touch. Perhaps the most important outcome of this interaction was the learning provided to the student. Elena has pointed out how this experience has affected her practice as a nurse. She now is in a position in which she can have a greater effect on the institutional practices and has been able to better advocate for clients to prevent the use of high-technology approaches that are inconsistent with the client's belief system.

The Navajo medicine man's situational sense of coherence at the time Elena cared for him was extremely low. His ability to have any control or management of the situation was not present. He was not consulted about his wishes regarding any of the medical treatments. His knowledge level also was low. He had had little prior contact with the high-tech hospital and had no family members present to intervene for him. His motivation to participate in the therapies presented was low. During the time Elena cared for this client, she was able to begin to give him a minor control over the situation. Some of the hospital staff also began to respond to his nonverbal messages and not insist on performing painful procedures that he did not want. After several days of this kind of negotiation, the client was moved out of an intensive care environment and was allowed to die peacefully.

CONCLUSION

The interventions presented in this chapter were guided by the student's evaluation of issues of profound importance to each of the clients. In each case, the concepts outlined by Orlando (1972) were employed. It was necessary to clarify with the client what his or her true needs were. Even in the case of Elena working with the Navajo grandfather who was unable to communicate in English, the client's value system was identified through observing his body language. His response to comfort measures was seen as approval of the interventions. As the uniqueness of each of these clients was validated, and as the plan of care was altered to include the value system of each, the deepest needs of the clients were met and each increased in situational sense of coherence. This occurred despite that in three of the five vignettes, the client's final outcome was death.

Each of the interventions was focused at the deepest level of the person's being. The nurse made no attempt to try to bring the client into conformity with the institutional values present. It would not have been appropriate for the nurse to try to alter the client's value system. Instead, he or she worked to bring the institutional value system into accord with that of the client. In this way, the client advocate role was expressed and the nurse was able to meet the identified need.

According to Orlando's (1972) conceptual framework, if the client's need has not been clarified, then the nurse has done nothing. In each of these vignettes, the student was able to identify and meet the client's most fundamental needs by moving beyond the ordinary practice of nursing care. A truly individualized plan of care in which the client and nurse were mutually active in the goal-setting process was accomplished. These vignettes demonstrate that mutuality is possible in today's health care environment.

REFERENCES

Artinian, B., & Conger, M. (1997). *The Intersystem Model: Integrating theory and practice.* Thousand Oaks, CA: Sage Publications.
Benner, P., & Wrubel, J. (1989). *The primacy of caring.* Menlo Park, CA: Addison-Wesley.
Gordon, M. (1987). The nurse as a thinking practitioner. In K. Hannah, M. Reimer, W. C. Mills, & S. Letourneau (Eds.), *Clinical judgement and decision making: The future with nursing diagnosis.* New York, NY: John Wiley.
Joint Commission on Accreditation of Healthcare Organizations. (1989). *Nursing standards task force: Revision process.* Chicago, IL: Author.
Jones, S. A., & Brown, L. N. (1993). Alternative views on defining critical thinking through the nursing process. *Holistic Nurse Practitioner, 7,* 71–75.
Lago, C. (2010). On developing our empathic capacities to work inter-culturally and inter-ethnically: Attempting a map for personal and professional development. *Psychotherapy & Politics International, 8,* 73–85.
Munhall, P. (1993). "Unknowing": Toward another pattern of knowing in nursing. *Nursing Outlook, 41,* 125–128.
Orlando, I. J. (1961). *The dynamic nurse-patient relationship: Function, process, and principles.* New York, NY: G.P. Putnam.

Orlando, I. J. (1972). *The discipline and teaching of nursing process.* New York, NY: G.P. Putnam.

Proctor, G. (2010). Boundaries or mutuality in therapy: Is therapy mutually really possible or is therapy doomed from the start? *Psychotherapy & Politics International, 8,* 44–58.

Sahlsten, M., Larsson, I., Sjostrom, B., Lindencrona, C., & Plos, K. (2007). Patient participation in nursing care: Towards a concept clarification from a nurse perspective. *Journal of Clinical Nursing, 16,* 630–637.

PART

IV

THE ARTINIAN INTERSYSTEM MODEL IN PRACTICE

Barbara M. Artinian

IN THIS SECTION, selected examples are given to illustrate various ways the Artinian Intersystem Model (AIM) has been used in individual clinical practice and with interdisciplinary teams. In Chapter 12, Erdmann-Nell gives an example of its use by individual nurses in an outpatient setting with patients seeking cosmetic procedures. The use of SOAPIE charting is introduced. Chapter 13 explores how the AIM was used by Conger to develop a system for delegating nursing assignments for hospital personnel at various levels of licensure, including a nursing assessment decision grid.

The model has also been used by clinical nurse specialists who have developed programs to coordinate the efforts of interdisciplinary teams that provide care for special groups of patients. An ongoing example of the use of the model with an interdisciplinary team is given in Chapter 14. This program is designed for patients with heart failure with the purpose of reducing hospital readmissions. A nurse coordinator works with all the team members to bring about very successful outcomes for the patients. The role of the patient care coordinator is described showing the relationship between the recommendations of Taylor (1997) for developing a salutogenic program (see Chapter 2, Situational Sense of Coherence: The Salutogenic Model) and the actual operation of the program.

The final example is that of a nursing home that is based on the AIM. A model for "resident-centered care" is described in Chapter 15. The program at the Ararat Nursing Facility is described using actual admission, evaluation, and teaching materials. Reference is made to the many awards for excellence the facility has received. The congruence of the program with the recommendations Taylor made for the development of a salutogenic program is given. The abstract for a research study using the methodology of grounded theory titled "Family Making" is included.

Since the AIM closely follows the ideology of Glaserian Grounded Theory, the purpose of Chapter 16 is to illustrate how research findings can be implemented in practice. Selected research studies as reported in the book *Glaserian Grounded Theory in Nursing Research: Trusting Emergence* (Artinian, Giske, & Cone, 2009) provide the basis for care plans in this book. A summary of the care plan for each study is preceded by an abstract of the associated theory with its conceptual map. These specific patient situations are presented from original data. The full corresponding care plan is available in the online adjunct manual.

REFERENCES

Artinian, B., Giske, T., & Cone, P. (2009). *Glaserian grounded theory in nursing research: Trusting emergence.* New York, NY: Springer Publishing.

Taylor, D. (1997). *The implications of sense of coherence for the early treatment of people who have had a traumatic spinal cord injury.* Unpublished doctoral dissertation, University of Wollongong: Wollongong, Australia.

12

Advanced Practice Nursing in an Ambulatory Setting

Christine Erdmann-Nell

Clients who seek cosmetic or plastic surgery services differ from patients in an acute setting in that they are usually not sick and that they are seeking care on an elective basis to improve their quality of life. This does not mean that their problems are insignificant or that their problems do not greatly influence their ability to carry out the normal activities of daily life. In many cases, the patients have experienced the problem for a number of years and have finally reached the point where they have decided that something must be done. These patients are seeking care on an elective basis and often enter the clinical setting with firm ideas about the type of care they want and want to be active participants in the decision-making process. Therefore, a nursing model that allows for negotiation of values and developing a joint plan of care is needed.

Nurses who work in an outpatient dermatology clinic or a plastic surgeon's office practice on a more independent basis than compared to nurses in a hospital setting and are not subjected to the rules and regulations of a large institution. This offers advantages and disadvantages. The advantage is that they are free to implement their own style of practice. Many nurses who work in cosmetic nursing fail to use a nursing model to guide their practice because they are only familiar with nursing models in which the nurse is responsible for creating the plan of care and the patient is expected to comply with the nurse-created plan of care. Advanced practice nurses know that in a cosmetic practice, the patient's views must be the focus of care. The purpose of this chapter is to describe how the Artinian Intersystem Model (AIM) has been used to focus on the negotiation of values between patient and nurse and to develop a mutual plan of care that enhances the sense of coherence (SOC) of the client.

The AIM provides a systematic approach to resolving the main concern of the patient. An assessment of the biological, psychological, and spiritual subsystems of the patient as well as the stated reason for the visit allows the nurse to identify the main concern of the patient. Both the patient and nurse are seen as having their own knowledge about the concern and their value systems regarding it. The first step of the process pertains to knowledge: what does the patient know regarding the problem, and what does the nurse know regarding it? The second step pertains to attitudes and values: what are the patient's values, and what are the nurse's values? The third step deals with behaviors: what does the patient want in regard to a plan of care, and what does the nurse want? An analysis of this information sets the stage for intersystem interaction in which information is communicated, values are negotiated, and a joint plan of care is developed. If the nurse and patient are not able to come to an agreement on the plan of care, they must renegotiate until they arrive at a plan of care that is agreed upon by both parties.

Although patients receiving cosmetic procedures are not facing life-threatening situations, they still experience a period of disorganization during the time of treatment. It is during this period of time that the nurse has the opportunity to make it possible for patients to participate in the planning of care to enhance their situational sense of coherence (SSOC) and allow them to achieve a higher level of SOC than they had prior to the treatment.

SELF-ESTEEM RELATED TO SKIN DISEASE AND COSMETIC PROCEDURES

The encumbrance of skin disease is a multifaceted condition that involves social, psychological, and financial consequences for clients as well as for their families. Even though most chronic skin disorders are not immediately life threatening, they do cause a substantial burden on health status and quality of life (Basra & Shahrukh, 2009). The adolescent who feels self-conscious about his/her appearance will often be absent from school, work, or social functions. This lack of social interaction adds to feelings of isolation and depression. One study found that acne clients reported levels of emotional, psychological, and social problems as vast as those reported by clients with arthritis, back pain, diabetes, epilepsy, asthma, or chronic disabling asthma (Kellet & Gawkrodger, 1999). Another study conducted with adolescents found a strong correlation between body image and appearance-related burden level. Clients increased bodily satisfaction levels and decreased appearance-related burdens following cosmetic surgery. Psychological, social, and physical burdens associated with appearance satisfaction improved significantly in both corrective and reconstructive adolescent clients (Simis, Hovius, de Beaufort, Verhulst, Koot, & The Adolescence Plastic Surgical Research Group, 2002).

Self-esteem refers to the extent to which people value or accept themselves for what and who they are. It also refers to the amount of satisfaction or dissatisfaction individuals have with themselves (Baumeister, 2001). This reflects one's evaluation of self-worth. The literature review shows a strong, direct correlation between cosmetic surgery and self-esteem levels. Cosmetic nurses should be especially aware of how their clients' self-esteem and body image is affected by cosmetic procedures. Nurses need to respect and value clients for whom they are and for what they are experiencing throughout this sensitive period in their lives (Figueroa, 2003).

USE OF THE AIM IN COSMETIC NURSING PRACTICE

Cosmetic procedures have a direct effect on increased SOC because the client has increased self-esteem resulting in a better outlook on life. These individuals who have undergone cosmetic procedures and/or dermatological medical treatment for a skin condition feel more comfortable entering into new situations and social encounters because they experience increased self-esteem. Several examples illustrating the interaction between the nurse and client follow.

The first example of how SOC can be enhanced with cosmetic procedures is the use of BOTOX. Not only does BOTOX relieve forehead wrinkles but it can also eliminate migraine headaches. There are different theories as to why BOTOX works on migraine headaches, but the most popular theory is that BOTOX eliminates muscle tension, which can be a primary cause of migraines. Some clients who suffered from debilitating migraines and used several ineffective medications found BOTOX improved their headaches. These clients enhanced their SOC by looking better and feeling better.

The AIM can also be used in understanding the client's attitude toward the acceptability of different types of medications and procedures. There are some clients who are uncomfortable with the idea of any type of oral medication for the treatment of their condition; whereas, there are other clients who would be dissatisfied with their care if they did not receive a prescription for at least one oral medication for their ailment. In addition, there are clients who are very interested in the idea of laser treatment, but refuse to use any sort of prescription topical and/or oral medication or vice versa. Sometimes it is difficult for the nurse to understand why a client accepts one treatment modality over another. However, one must refrain from making judgment on another's choices. The nurse must accept the client's values for what they are and continue with the negotiation process in order to achieve an appropriate joint plan of care.

One client who came in to see me for the treatment of moderate acne vulgaris illustrates the positive outcome that can result when the nurse and patient agree on a mutual plan of care. The client indicated that she did not want to be treated with antibiotics. As her nurse practitioner, I knew that this patient needed antibiotics to treat the inflammatory lesions effectively. With further conversation, I realized that it was the idea of oral rather than topical antibiotics that concerned the patient. Although I would have preferred to prescribe oral antibiotics on a short-term basis for this client, I knew she would not take the oral antibiotic. To do so would violate her values, she would lose trust in my ability to treat her within her comfort level, and I would become frustrated with her noncompliance. Therefore, I offered her treatment with topical antibiotics instead. She agreed she would prefer that treatment plan and would fill the prescription. We were able to agree on a mutual plan of care that satisfied both parties.

Another example was a client who came to see me for the treatment of wrinkles and a number of severe acne scars. She expressed fear of anything being injected into her skin such as dermal fillers or BOTOX. However, she was extremely interested in laser treatment for skin rejuvenation. Upon further questioning and clarification, it turned out that the client had misconceptions and had heard rumors about injectables. I felt the best possible treatment outcome would be realized with a combination of dermal fillers, BOTOX, and a series of Smoothbeam laser treatments. After thorough education regarding the truth and safety of these injectables as well as dispelling any associated myths, the client stated she would like to start with laser treatments. She would think about the future possibility of adding other injectable treatments. Since the laser stimulates collagen production, I knew it would help her condition, even though better results could be obtained with laser plus injectables. Together, we decided to begin with laser treatments and see how she looked at the end of her series of treatments. Perhaps, she and I would both be content with the results of laser alone. Later, she could reconsider the addition of injectables if she wanted a better cosmetic outcome. We were both satisfied with this plan of action. In this scenario, the nurse and client understood each others' knowledge and values. They then negotiated an agreeable joint plan of care to resolve the main concern of the client.

A final example describes the interaction between the nurse and a patient who wanted removal of facial hair on her chin but did not want to wait for the best procedure. By providing information about the procedure, the advanced practice nurse was able to negotiate a solution acceptable to both patient and

TABLE 12.1 The SOAPIE Note

S:	Complaint of hairs to chin for 10 years. Wants to get laser hair removal. Currently tweezes hair daily. Has not tried shaving or laser hair removal. Has wedding to attend in 1 week.
O:	Face-dark course hair to chin, tanned skin
A:	Hirsutism
P:	Schedule laser hair removal session in 1 month.
I:	Educated regarding need to wait 1 month prior to laser hair removal treatment due to recent tweezing and current suntan. Refrain from tweezing or waxing hair; shave instead. Refrain from sun exposure prior to laser treatment.
E:	Client verbalized understanding regarding need to wait until her tan fades and for more hair growth prior to laser treatment. Client agreed to shave hair prior to laser treatment and understands that shaving will not stimulate hair growth.

nurse. This interaction has been published (Erdmann, 2003) and a description of how the negotiation was carried out is presented in the full care plan available in the online adjunct manual.

SOAPIE CHARTING

I believe the best way to document the use of the AIM is through a SOAPIE progress note (Using SOAP, 1999.) The S stands for *subjective findings*, O for *objective findings*, A for *assessment*, P for *plan of care*, I for *intervention*, and E for *evaluation*. It is the most widely used form of charting in cosmetic settings and provides effective documentation of AIM interactions.

Within the subjective or S portion of the SOAPIE note, the provider can make note of the developmental environment as well as the intrasystem analysis of the patient. The organization of behaviors and nursing goals are documented in the plan or P of the SOAPIE note. The SOAPIE note shown in Table 12.1 is based on an actual patient care plan.

CONCLUSION

There has been an extremely positive response from clients as well as from other health care professionals to the introduction of the AIM within the cosmetic dermatology field. Clients are thrilled that their voices are being heard and that we professionals value their opinions. There is a sense of control among clients about taking a more active role in the decision-making process. Increased compliance among clients is one of the most exciting rewards of utilizing this approach.

Health care professionals who saw my *Dermatology Nursing* article on utilizing the AIM in a cosmetic setting (Erdmann, 2003) emailed me that they agreed that the use of this model is highly effective for cosmetic dermatology. Another dermatology nurse practitioner told me that she finds this to be the only model that makes sense for use within her specialty.

Since cosmetic procedures are not based on medical necessity but are based on clients' desires, clients will only accept the treatments they choose. All clients are healthy and able to take an active role in their treatment process. This is why I believe the AIM is the best model to use in cosmetic nursing. Nurse and clients negotiate values and interventions.

REFERENCES

Artinian, B. M. (1997). Overview of the intersystem model. In B. Artinian & M. Conger (Eds.), *The intersystem model: Integrating theory and practice* (pp. 1–17). Thousand Oaks, CA: Sage Publications.

Basra, M. K. A., & Shahrukh, M. (2009). Burden of skin diseases. *Expert Review of Pharmacoeconomics & Outcomes Research, 9*(3), 271–283.

Baumeister, R.F. (2001, April). Violent pride. *Scientific American, 284*(4), 96–102.

Erdmann, C. (2003). The value of the intersystem model for cosmetic nursing practice. *Dermatology Nursing, 15*(4), 335–338.

Figueroa, C. (2003). Self-esteem and cosmetic surgery: Is there a relationship between the two? *Plastic Surgical Nursing, 23*(1), 21–24.

Kellet, S. C., & Gawkrodger, D. J. (1999). The psychological and emotional impact of acne: The effect of treatment with isotretinoin. *British Journal of Dermatology, 140*, 273–282.

Simis, K., Hovius, S., de Beaufort, I., Verhulst, F., Koot, H., & The Adolescence Plastic Surgical Research Group. (2002). After plastic surgery: Adolescent-reported appearance ratings and appearance-related burdens in patients and general population groups. *Plastic & Reconstructive Surgery, 109*(1), 9–17.

Using SOAP, SOAPIE, and SOAPIER formats. (1999, September). *Nursing, 29*(9), 75. Retrieved September 1, 2010, from ProQuest Health and Medical Complete. (Document ID: 44463116).

13

DELEGATION DECISION MAKING

Margaret M. Conger

DELEGATION DECISION MAKING in health care becomes more important as the demand for health care services increases during a nursing shortage. As people age, there is an increased demand for health care services because of the numerous health concerns of the elderly. Also, as health care reform is accomplished, there will be many more persons able to seek health care. One approach to meet the increased demand is to have registered nurses (RNs) play a larger role in managing chronic health problems. However, while the need for professional nurses is increasing, their numbers are decreasing. Rosseter (2010), with the American Association of Colleges of Nursing, reports that "the U.S. nursing shortage is projected to grow to 260,000 registered nurses by 2025. A shortage of this magnitude would be twice as large as any nursing shortage experienced in this country since the mid-1960s" (Current and Projected Shortage Indicators, para 3). It is expected that some of the need for nursing services will thus be filled by increasing the number of assistive personnel (AP). These include persons trained at a lower level than the RN such as licensed practical nurses, nursing assistants, and nurse technicians.

The use of APs to assist RNs in delivery of client care increases the responsibility of the RN. In addition to direct client care, the RN must also oversee care given by the AP. Data collected by the AP must be interpreted and decisions made from it. To use these APs effectively, RNs need to learn to make delegation decisions so that health care can be administered in a safe and effective manner (Boucher, 1998). Unfortunately, many nursing programs do not include teaching about safe delegation decisions (Parsons, 2004).

DEFINITION OF DELEGATION

What is delegation? While there are many definitions, one that is commonly used throughout management literature is that delegation is the act of assigning to another person responsibility for a task or project that would normally be the responsibility of the first person. While the wisdom of doing this may be questioned by some, there are many advantages to be gained by learning to be an effective delegator. Aside from the efficiency that should occur if the delegation is done properly, the person who is given the delegated task will have the opportunity to grow in ability and to develop a greater sense of participation in the project. But many supervisors are hesitant to delegate some of their workload to others for fear that the job may not be done correctly or some just fear that sharing with others will in some way diminish themselves. Parsons (2004) confirmed these same issues among nurses when asked about barriers they had experienced when working with an AP. The fear of taking responsibility for the work of others was expressed. However, effective delegation can lead to improved productivity and an enhanced sense of team work. Thus, it is well worth while for any person working in the health care setting to develop skill in the art of delegation.

LEARNING EFFECTIVE DELEGATION DECISION MAKING

As nurses work in team environments that incorporate a variety of levels of health care workers, delegation decisions become more common. Several states have incorporated into their State Board of Nursing practices, guidelines for effective delegation. Massachusetts has developed a guide that includes an algorithm on when and how to delegate nursing care to an assistive person (2002). The Iowa Board of Nursing has a Delegation Decision-making Grid that includes elements to consider when making a delegation decision (2003). It provides a framework for assessing the needs of the client, the skills of the AP, and potential harm in delegating an activity.

These tools are similar to the Nursing Assessment Decision Grid (NADG) developed by Conger (1993, 1994). This tool has been used as a teaching device for RNs to learn safe delegation decision making (Conger, 1999; Parsons, 1997, 2004). Such teaching is needed because many RNs reported a lack of knowledge about delegation (Hansten & Washburn, 1996; Parsons, 1997). Parsons (2004) reported that in her study nurses agreed that there needs to be an accepted standardized baseline for knowledge about delegation. She concluded that delegation decision making must be a part of every RN nursing program. It also must become part of staff development programs for RNs who did not have this type of education in their basic nursing program.

MODEL FOR LEARNING DELEGATION SKILLS—NURSING ASSESSMENT DECISION GRID

The NADG shown in Table 13.1 is a tool developed for teaching RNs to identify those aspects of nursing care that they must retain and those aspects that can be safely delegated to a lesser skilled nurse (Conger, 1993, 1994). Its design is such that it leads the learner through a number of steps to analyze a client situation and then make a decision about the nursing needs of that client. These steps have been developed using the Intersystem Model (Artinian, 1991) as the conceptual framework.

The NADG requires the learner to go through a four-step process that is shown in Table 13.1. In the first step, the learner lists the tasks that he or she identifies as needed for client care. These tasks are pieces of assigned work that could result from a physician order such as administration of a medication or treatment, a nursing order such as the need to turn a client frequently, or unit policies such as frequency of vital sign assessment.

The second step is to consider each of the biological, psychosocial, and spiritual subsystems as described in the initial Intersystem Model (Artinian, 1991) and carried forward to the current Artinian Intersystem Model to identify the Main Concern that a client may be experiencing. For ease in the use of the NADG in the clinical setting, the spiritual subsystem assessment was grouped with the psychosocial subsystem assessment.

The third step is to evaluate the client's adaptation to his or her situation using the construct of situational sense of coherence (SSOC). This construct was adapted from Antonovsky (1987) and incorporated into the Intersystem Model (Artinian, 1991). The elements in the SSOC are a sense of comprehension or knowledge needed to understand the main concern, the ability to manage the main concern, and the motivation and meaningfulness to be involved in resolving the main concern. Because the goal of nursing is to assist a client to move toward the health end of a wellness–illness continuum, attention to the client's adaptation to a given situation is important. As the client's SSOC improves, movement toward health can be seen. It is this third step in the grid that sets this tool apart from other delegation models previously mentioned. It moves the nurse beyond just identifying tasks related to the client's health condition and puts importance on how the client is responding to the situation. Boucher (1998) stresses the need for the nurse to focus on client responses to care, not just completing tasks as ordered. Using the SSOC framework, the RN can learn to do just this.

The fourth step is to make a delegation decision based on the data collected in the first three steps. Having objective data about both the client and the care provider gives a solid foundation for the delegation decision.

TABLE 13.1 The Nursing Assessment Decision Grid: A Model for Learning Delegation Skills

DELEGATION DECISION-MAKING ASSESSMENT PHASE

Step 1. List all required nursing tasks and rate them according to institutional policy and skill level of AP

    1 AP can do independently
    2 AP needs to be taught
    3 RN must do

Step 2. Identify health problems in client subsystems and rate on the rapidity of change

Biological
  Regulatory (neurological, endocrine, immune)
  Circulatory–respiratory
  Musculoskeletal
  Gastrointestinal
  Renal
  Reproductive

    1 Stabilized
    2 Moderate change
    3 Rapidly changing

Psychosocial/spiritual
  Anxiety
  Family process
  Fear
  Grieving
  Hopelessness
  Spiritual distress

Step 3. Evaluate situational sense of coherence and rate each aspect

Knowledge of patient
    1 Has adequate knowledge
    2 Needs some instruction-review
    3 Needs intense instruction

Manageability of problem by patient
    1 Able to manage problem
    2 Needs minimal assistance with problem
    3 Needs extensive assistance

Meaningfulness to patient or nurse (motivation for action)
    1 Problem resolution unimportant
    2 Problem resolution moderately important; moderate willingness to resolve problem
    3 Problem resolution highly important and worth the effort

Step 4. Make the delegation decision

Criteria for decision:
  AP can do all aspects of care rated 1
  AP must be taught to manage all aspects of care rated 2
  RN must retain all tasks rated 3

Source: Conger (2011). Adapted from Conger, M. (1993). Delegation decision making: Development of a teaching strategy. *Journal of Nursing Staff Development, 9*(3), 131–135.

USE OF THE NURSING ASSESSMENT DECISION GRID

The NADG consists of a set of rules or guidelines that the nurse uses in the client assessment process. In the classroom setting, in which the nurse is learning to make delegation decisions, the NADG is used in conjunction with client vignettes developed by Conger (1994). In the clinical setting, it is applied to actual client situations.

In the first step of the process, the nurse identifies tasks needed for client care using principles outlined by a number of authors (Manthey, 1989; Neumann, 1989; Poteet, 1984; Rabinow, 1982). Many nursing tasks fall into the category of mandatory practice because their source is physician orders or institutional policies. Other tasks are mandated by professional practice through nursing orders. Identification of client problems is more complex.

In the second step, the client's personal subsystems are assessed. The conceptual framework for problem analysis in the NADG is derived from the Intersystem Model (1991) construct of *person* as having biological, psychosocial, and spiritual subsystems. In the Intersystem Model (1991), *spiritual* is used as the descriptor of the inner center of the person (Emblen, 1997) and is made up of one's beliefs, values, and religious practices. Moving outward from the center is the psychosocial system. The subsystems in the psychosocial dimension include the cognitive, affective, and interactional behaviors of the person. The biological subsystem corporately maintains all the physiological functions needed for life and consists of the following: (a) regulatory, which includes the neurological, endocrine, and immune; (b) circulatory and respiratory; (c) musculoskeletal; (d) gastrointestinal; (e) renal; and (f) reproductive.

In the third step, the client's knowledge base, values, and the ability to manage personal care needs are assessed. Both the client's knowledge base about the problem and his/her ability to manage the situation are evaluated. A third element is also vital to this assessment. What is the meaning of the problem to the client? Is he/she motivated to address the problem? Both positive and negative factors that affect the client's SSOC are analyzed. This information is vital for development of a mutual plan of care.

Scoring Strategies

Both the tasks that are required for client care and nursing problems identified through a review of the client's biological, psychosocial, and spiritual subsystems are analyzed using a three-point rating scale found in the NADG. Scoring of nursing tasks is based on education and demonstrated competence of the staff member, licensing laws, and institutional policy relative to nursing practice. Those tasks restricted to RNs by law such as the administration of intravenous medications are always rated as 3. Those tasks that an AP can do according to institutional policy are rated as either 2 or 1. If the AP has not yet demonstrated competence in the task, it would be appropriate to provide teaching, thus giving the task a rating of 2. If the AP has already demonstrated proficiency in the task, it can be rated as 1 and safely delegated.

The scoring on client problems is more complex. Rapidity of change in a client problem is one parameter that can be used in determining if the care can be delegated to an assistive person. If the client is experiencing a rapid decline in a problem such as deterioration in respiratory function, then close assessment by a professional is needed and a score of 3 would be assigned. If the client's problem is a stable condition, such as a client with a chronic respiratory pattern, less assessment is needed. This client's care could be safely delegated to an assistive person and scored as 1. In contrast, for a client with a problem that is gradually deteriorating, the RN could give guidance to the assistive person to observe for specific parameters and thus delegate the care. This situation would be scored as 2.

The scoring on the SSOC follows the general guidelines established by Artinian (1991). The RN should first assess the client's motivation to participate in care (meaningfulness). If the client shows a high degree of motivation (rated as 3), the RN needs to retain care of this person because a great deal of emphasis will be placed on client and family teaching. These responsibilities have been determined to be within the scope of nursing practice in terms of ethics (American Nurses Association, 2001) and law (California Nursing Practice Act, 2003). If the client is not motivated to participate in personal care, a rating of 1 is given and the care can be delegated to an assistive person. A rating of 2 is used if the level of motivation to be involved in the problem is moderate. The decision to delegate the care of this person can be based on the total demands of the day's assignment. However, if the main concern is viewed as important by the nurse, a rating of 3 can be given even though the patient shows no motivation to act. The role of the nurse is teaching and negotiating values so that the patient may view resolving the concern as worth the effort.

The knowledge and manageability needs of the client are determined in a similar manner. A knowledge need that is new to the client should be rated 3 because it requires the skill of the RN to assess the learning needs and develop the teaching program. If the client simply needs reinforcement of prior learning, a rating of 1 would be appropriate. An example of this would be a person who has been following a salt-restricted diet for a period of time.

Reinforcement of knowledge about the salt-restricted diet can be safely delegated to the assistive person. If the person needs moderate teaching about the diet, the problem is rated as 2 and the delegation decision is again made based on the demands of the day's assignment. When the client is well aware of diet restrictions but continues to select inappropriate food, a 3 would be given because the RN is needed to assess what attitudes contribute to this continued noncompliant behavior.

The scoring for the client's ability to manage health needs would be similar. A client with a problem that will require considerable assistance for management, such as with a new colostomy, requires the intervention of the RN and is scored 3. A client with a lesser problem, such as assisted ambulation with crutches, could be handled by the assistive person and scored 2. A problem that the client is able to manage independently or needs only minimal assistance would be scored as 1.

Following scoring of the nursing tasks required, client issues, and the client SSOC, delegation decisions are made. All areas rated as 1 can be safely delegated to the AP. Items rated 2 require that the AP be educated about the issue before it can be safely delegated. All items rated 3 must be retained by the RN. Following these principles, the RN and AP can jointly care for clients to provide a safe environment for care.

An example from practice gives guidance about scoring client assessment using the NADG. An 18-year-old male was admitted to the hospital with out of control diabetes. His history showed that this was the fourth such admission for this problem within the year. At this time, problems in his biological systems that were important were related to dehydration, electrolyte imbalance, and elevated blood glucose levels. All of these issues were rated 2 because they were fairly stable at this time. However, the psychological issues were of concern to the nurse and rated 3. Thus scoring on the SSOC became very important when determining that his care should be retained by the RN.

When approached about the idea of scheduling a conference with the dietician about food choices, he became very angry and refused the offer. He said he was tired of being restricted in what he could and could not do in his life because of his disease. Rather than deciding to delegate his care to an assistive person, the RN chose to retain his care and explore the problem further even though he demonstrated little interest in working on the problem. Later that morning the RN started a conversation about what he wanted for his life. His response was that he was angry about spending so much time in the hospital. The suggestion was made that if he learned to find ways to control his blood sugar, he would have fewer uncontrolled diabetic episodes. The next morning, the young man asked if he could meet with the dietician and explore how better to manage his diabetes. The role of the RN at this point was to meet with the dietician to explain the situation and jointly help the young man plan strategies for better diabetes control. Even though at the initial encounter with this client, the RN could have been tempted to delegate his care to an assistive person, she wisely chose to retain it. The knowledge and concern that prompted the RN to explore ways to enhance his motivation for a changed life style demonstrate professional responsibility.

Teaching Delegation Skills

As stated earlier, many nurses report they are unsure of how to make delegation decisions (Parsons, 2004). In the clinical setting, the nurse needs to be able to rapidly identify the critical elements of care required for a client and make appropriate delegation decisions. Educational programs utilizing the NADG are intended to achieve this outcome.

The effectiveness of the NADG in improving delegation decision making has been tested in the classroom setting (Conger, 1999; Parsons, 2004), where the teaching–learning environment was based on the 4MAT® system as developed by McCarthy (1980). The 4MAT® system is a model depicting four quadrants of learning styles and instructional techniques (Figure 13.1). This system has been further developed and studied by McCarthy and McCarthy (2006) and Nicoll-Senft and Seider (2009). Using this teaching strategy, differences in individual learning styles are recognized, and instructional techniques encourage

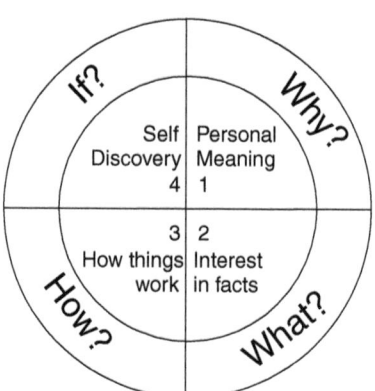

FIGURE 13.1 The 4MAT system.
Source: M. Conger (2011). Adapted from *4MAT System*. [Art]. Retrieved September 15, 2010, from About Learning: Official site of Bernice McCarthy's 4MAT System: http://www.aboutlearning.com/what-is-4mat/what-is-4mat

all participants to be engaged in the process. The inclusion of learning activities to meet the needs of all participants is especially important in a classroom setting in which the instructor is unfamiliar with the learning styles of individual participants. While each person has a preferred style of learning, it is important to experience all four quadrants of the learning cycle. The learner moves from experiencing a new situation to reflecting on it, then uses the new information, and finally integrates the experience into active practice. This cycle must be completed for learning to occur (McCarthy & McCarthy, 2006). Learners were categorized into four styles by the nature of the question they ask of a learning experience (McCarthy, 1981; McCarthy & McCarthy, 2006).

The Type 1 learner is interested in the personal meaning of the lesson. The preferred method for learning is through the use of sensing and feeling. This learner is described as the person who asks the question: "Why?" When working with this type of learner, a clear objective for the lesson must be established early or the learner will "tune out" what is happening and not participate in the activity.

The Type 2 learner is characterized by an interest in facts. The question asked by this type of learner is: "What?" This learner needs to be able to integrate new concepts into an organized system to deal with them effectively.

The Type 3 learner is characterized by an interest in how things work, asking the question: "How?" This type of learner works best by actively trying out a new idea to find out how it works. This process allows the person a means of becoming actively involved in the learning experience.

The Type 4 learner is characterized by an interest in self-discovery. This type of learner frequently asks the question: "If?" The individual wants to expand on the learning and extend it to new situations (McCarthy, 1981; McCarthy & McCarthy, 2006).

Classroom activities are designed to incorporate each of these styles of learning so that the effectiveness of the NADG will not be biased by a classroom environment not conducive to some of the participants' learning style. In teaching the use of the NADG, the classroom session begins with a discussion of why delegation is important, thus engaging Type 1 learners. Then, the "rules" of the NADG are presented answering the "What?" question. The students are guided through the steps of the process to Step 3, when client vignettes are presented depicting actual clinical situations. The participants are then led through an exercise using the vignette in which the nursing tasks and client problems are identified and delegation decisions about which aspects of care need to be retained by the RN and which aspects can be delegated to the assistive person. Experimenting with the "rules" of the NADG is vital to the learning process. Finally, the discussion leads to thinking about how delegation decision making affects both the client and the nursing staff. This step completes the 4MAT® cycle and reinforces the learning process.

This teaching strategy, using the NADG applied to client vignettes, is based on the theoretical constructs advocated by Benner (1984) in assisting nurses to move from novice to expert practice. Benner suggests an effective learning strategy for novices is the use of vignettes with a set of "rules" to guide the learner in a decision-making process. She also suggests that repeated use of a problem-solving approach will lead to skill acquisition that can be transferred to the clinical setting.

Outcome Assessment of the NADG

Testing of the NADG in institutional settings has been reported by Conger (1999) and Parsons (2004). The RNs participating in the learning experienced significant improvement in delegation decision making based on scores

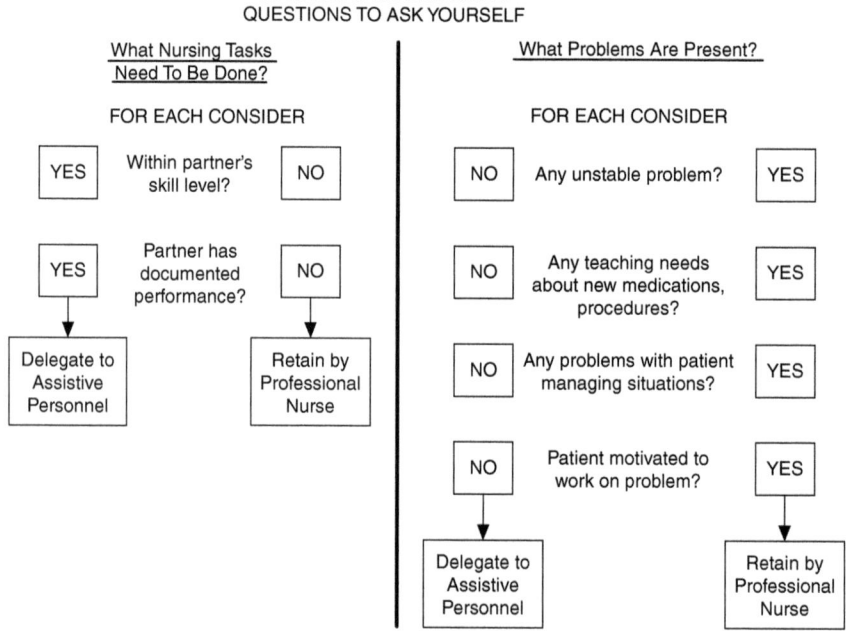

FIGURE 13.2 Delegation Decision Algorithm.
Copyright © 2011 M. Conger.

comparing pretest and posttest results. One of the gratifying outcomes of this study was that when participants were divided into high- and low-performing groups based on pretest results, the low-performing group demonstrated a statistically significant gain on posttest results compared with the high-performing group. This finding suggests that a rule-based educational activity can improve the delegation decision-making ability of nurses shown to be novices in this area (Conger, 1999).

Follow-Up Activities

As the nurse moves from the classroom setting to the clinical area, the principles of the NADG need to be reinforced. The chart shown in Figure 13.2 was developed by the author to provide such reinforcement. The principles of the NADG are used to think about the client situation and the appropriateness of delegation to the assistive personnel. Pocket-sized cards were distributed to the nurse attendees at the training sessions for a ready reminder of the classroom learning.

CONCLUSION

As partnership models of nursing delivery systems increase, teaching strategies to prepare nurses for this environment are vital. A critical element of any partnership delivery system is the ability of the RN to make safe and cost-effective decisions about the utilization of all the various levels of nurses being introduced into the workforce. It is suggested that use of the NADG is one approach to this need.

Theoretical models were used in the development of this theory-based approach to practice. The decision process for analyzing nursing tasks was developed from a variety of sources in the nursing literature. The decision process for analyzing client problems was developed using the Intersystem Model (Artinian, 1991). The teaching strategy used is based on the "novice to expert" concept developed by Benner (1984) and the 4MAT® system (McCarthy, 1981; McCarthy & McCarthy, 2006).

Nursing partnerships between RNs and various levels of nurses are on the rise. Nursing administrators need to carefully consider the professional implications of such practice. The use of the NADG provides a means for the RN to retain the professional role of client assessment in directing the activities of nonprofessional nursing assistants. Because this tool is grounded in theoretical concepts, it provides a means for transferring theory into clinical practice.

REFERENCES

4MAT System. [Art]. Retrieved September 15, 2010, from About Learning: the Official site of Bernice McCarthy's 4MAT System: http://www.aboutlearning.com/what-is-4mat/what-is-4mat

American Nurses Association. (2001). *Code of ethics for nurses with interpretive statements.* Kansas City, MO: Author.

Antonovsky, A. (1987). *Unraveling the mystery of health: How people manage stress and stay well.* San Francisco, CA: Jossey-Bass.

Artinian, B. (1991). The development of the Intersystem Model. *Journal of Advanced Nursing, 16*(2), 194–205.

Benner, P. (1984). *From novice to expert.* Menlo Park, CA: Addison-Wesley.

Boucher, M. (1998). Delegation alert. *American Journal of Nursing, 98*(2), 26–32.

Nursing Practice Act. (2003). *Business and Professions Code of California.* Chapter 6, Article 2, § 2725–2742.

Conger, M. (1993). Delegation decision making: Development of a teaching strategy. *Journal of Nursing Staff Development, 9*(3), 131–135.

Conger, M. (1994). The nursing assessment decision grid: Tool for delegation decision. *Journal of Continuing Education in Nursing, 25*(1), 21–27.

Conger, M. (1999). Evaluation of an educational strategy for teaching delegation decision making to nursing students. *Journal of Nursing Education, 38*(9), 419–422.

Emblen, J. (1997). Theoretical foundations for the spiritual subsystem. In B. Artinian & M. Conger (Eds.), *The Intersystem Model: Integrating theory and practice.* Thousand Oaks, CA: Sage Publications.

Hansten, R., & Washburn, M. (1996). Why don't nurses delegate? *Journal of Nursing Administration, 26*(12), 24–28.

Iowa Board of Nursing. (2003). Delegation decision-making grid. *Nursing Newsletter, 22*(2), 3.

Manthey, M. (1989). The role of the LPN or the problem of two levels. *Nursing Management, 20,* 26–28.

Massachusetts Nurses Association. (2002). *Accepting, rejecting and delegating a work assignment: A guide for nurses.* [Brochure]. Canton, MA: Author.

McCarthy, B. (1980). *The 4MAT system.* Barrington, IL: Excel.

McCarthy, B., & McCarthy, D. (2006). *Teaching around the 4MAT cycle.* Thousand Oaks, CA: Sage Publications.

Nicoll-Senft, J. M., & Seider, S. N. (2009). Assessing the impact of the 4MAT teaching model across multiple disciplines in higher education. *College Teaching, 58*(1), 19–27.

Parsons, L. (1997). Delegation decision making: Evaluation of a teaching strategy. *Journal of Nursing Administration, 27*(2), 47–52.

Parsons, L. (2004). Delegation decision-making by registered nurses who provide direct care for patients with spinal cord impairment. *SCI Nursing, 21*(1), 20–28.

Neumann, T. A. (1989). A nurse's guide to fail-safe delegating. *Nursing, 19*(9), 63–64.

Poteet, G. W. (1984). Delegation strategies: A must for nurse executives. *Journal of Nursing Administration, 14*(9), 18–21.

Rabinow, J. (1982). Delegating safely within the law. *Nursing Life, 2*(5), 48–49.

Rosseter, R. (2010). *Nursing shortage fact sheet.* American Association of Colleges of Nursing. Retrieved from http://www.aacn.nche.edu/media/factsheets/nursingshortage.htm

14

Care Management of Heart Failure Patients in the Outpatient Setting

Laurie Carson and Louise Della Bella

Congestive heart failure (CHF) is one of the most common diagnoses for patients discharged from Saddleback Memorial Medical Center (SMMC). SMMC is a 325-bed not-for-profit hospital, with tertiary level cardiac services, that serves a large retirement community as well as other groups. More than 520 patients with CHF are admitted every year. Many of these patients are readmitted following discharge, and most readmissions are accompanied by a decreased quality of life and reduced functional status. Between 2006 and 2007, SMMC had 500–600 CHF discharges and 11% of these were readmitted for heart failure.

THE HEART FAILURE MANAGEMENT PROGRAM AT SMMC

A heart failure outreach patient program (HFOPP) was developed to address this problem. The initial planning began in 2005. The process began by securing funding from a foundation grant so that HFOPP services could be provided to patients at no cost. A grant was awarded in 2007 to begin the program and a nurse coordinator was hired. Between 2007 and 2009, a multidisciplinary advisory committee met every month to provide direction and oversee the program. The advanced practice nurse who had been hired to be the nurse coordinator chaired this committee. The departments represented were rehabilitation, home health, marketing, professional development, care management, social services, senior community social service, nutrition, and cardiac services. In 2009, the Continuum of Care Partnership Council replaced the multidisciplinary committee to assume the role of Advisory Committee. The Saddleback Foundation provided a second year of funding from 2009 to 2010.

The goals of the program were to decrease preventable readmissions for any cause, improve physical functioning, and to improve quality of life. The objectives were to provide individualized educational and counseling efforts to increase compliance with medical directives, to promote positive health behaviors, and to aid in the development of self-care skills. An additional objective was to link the inpatient services with the medical doctor's office and outpatient services to enhance continuity and integration of care and to provide smooth transitions from inpatient services into increased accessibility and utilization of outpatient services.

Hospitalized patients who were at high risk for readmission were informed about the program and enrolled. The majority of patients were frail, of advanced age, had multiple comorbidities, and had limitations that impacted psychosocial and physical functions. Utilizing the hospital electronic medical record, all pertinent clinical information was compiled before discharge and an outpatient plan of care was created that would be implemented upon discharge.

The specific interventions of the HFOPP were (1) to visit the patients while they were hospitalized, (2) to collaborate with the inpatient care manager to ensure appropriate patient referrals and to communicate for effective continuity of care, (3) to ensure that the bedside nurses used the hospital stay to teach the patient self-care skills, (4) to work with the primary care physicians to ensure rapid follow up for appointments and full transfer of data, and (5) to provide home visits, phone calls, and other interpersonal follow up. The responsibilities of the advanced practice nurse coordinator were to provide collaboration, communication, and integration of all patient services and to make possible long-term follow up and referrals that took into consideration all significant problems including the social/psychological issues for these patients. She did this by providing personal contact and support through phone calls and community visits. Through these contacts, the nurse developed and maintained a supportive connection with the patients, tracked signs and symptoms of fluid volume overload, and monitored deterioration of the condition of the patient. The nurse also provided reminders of classes the patients needed to attend and tracked the next MD appointment and helped the patient prepare for it. The nurse reviewed instructions with the patients and provided counsel as needed. The nurse also made referrals for treatment when early recognition of patient problems was noticed in order to prevent unnecessary admissions or emergency room visits.

VALIDATION OF TAYLOR'S RECOMMENDATIONS FOR A SALUTOGENIC PROGRAM IN HEART FAILURE MANAGEMENT

The advanced practice nurse uses the Artinian Intersystem Model (AIM) to plan her interventions. The AIM is a salutogenic model that enhances health care in a positive way. She views each patient as a unique individual with biological, psychosocial, and spiritual needs. She focuses on mutual decision making and the development of a joint plan of care with both the nurse and patient being active participants in this process. In reviewing the 15 recommendations for a salutogenic rehabilitation program developed by Taylor (1997) in his dissertation research, the advanced practice nurse realized that she had implemented Taylor's recommendations in the development and implementation of the HFOPP. The full text of Taylor's recommendations is given in Chapter 2. Taylor's recommendations as implemented in the HFOPP are discussed below.

Recommendation 1

Use the salutogenic model. A one-page goal sheet and a teaching packet were developed to meet the patients' requests for needing all the information about heart failure management on one page. This page contains every basic and essential point for the development of self-care maintenance and management of heart failure at home. On the first day of hospitalization for heart failure, patients are given this goal sheet as their self-directing guide to achieve their goals for successful self-care. Throughout the hospitalization, multidisciplinary staff such as nutrition, rehabilitation, and nursing, all work with the patients and families to assist them with their goals. Patients are encouraged to use the goal sheet for making notes. The staff members use a salutogenic approach by asking the patients and families, "Which of these goals have you already attained?" and "Have you identified an area you need help with?" They also provide an opportunity for patients to practice the self-care practices they will use at home. This replaces the pathogenic model that would say, "You have a disease and listen to me, I will tell you what to do. Do you understand? Repeat back what I have said."

There is a check box next to each goal to be marked off when patients feel that they understand the goal and can verbally state it or demonstrate it. By doing this, patients can advocate for their specific needs and goals and are able to retain what they are already doing that works for them. They can also develop processes that fit their needs and preferences. In the home setting, nurses are trained for this ongoing coaching approach to helping the patient achieve successful self-care. Patients are at the center of the process, and all others partner with them as they move from needing intense assistance into greater independence. The patients themselves decide what level of assistance they need and this can change if greater needs arise. The patients and nurse work together to decide what level of assistance is needed.

Recommendation 2

Use a systems approach. In a systems approach, there is a synthesis of parts into the whole and a focus on interpersonal and environmental interactions. Patients want their separate care services integrated and not fragmented. By taking into account their values, skill level, knowledge, and psychosocial and spiritual needs, and by making connections among them, nurses can help them to move forward. As they integrate all parts of their lives into an organized whole, they are able to increase their sense of coherence (SOC). Through various communication and collaboration processes, this understanding of the patient and family is carried into every patient encounter. For example, Mr. H did not want to take his water pill immediately before a social event and so we worked together to devise a schedule so that he would wake up very early to take the pill well before the event. Other patients have found that a blood pressure medication makes them sleepy and so a plan was made to take the medication in the evening before going to bed rather than in the morning. This information is communicated to the treatment team by having the patient share the medication record with them. In addition, end of life care is offered according to patient preference. Patients are offered the choice between comfort care rather than medical care, the patient signs the appropriate directive, and this is given to all providers.

Recommendation 3

Focus on problem prevention. Problems can be prevented when there is a transfer of an accurate history of the patient to all providers. Surveillance levels that track progress, trends, and change in status are all intended to prevent problems. Using appropriate surveillance technology helps the treatment team to focus resources when needs arise thus reducing unnecessary calls or visits and saving time for the most needy, unstable patients. These unstable patients are the ones who are frequently readmitted to the hospital and who especially need to have individualized care to coordinate the activities of all team members. The nurse coordinator sets alerts for monitored readings that fall outside of acceptable ranges. When an alert occurs, teaching and coaching are reinforced in a timely manner before the problem becomes significant. For example, if there is a significant increase in weight, the nurse is notified and the patient is coached on what to say to the medical doctor and what to ask for. As the nurse helps the patient to follow the instructions given by the medical doctor, the nurse helps the patient to safely implement the new program. In this process, the nurse provides help only if needed and the patient implements the program independently when able.

When patients progress to lower levels of care, information about their status is monitored by the health information center. Patients are encouraged to keep a list of questions and are given guidance on how to talk to the medical doctor using their own outpatient record. Patients are also provided guidance for negotiating caregiver help. If the patient needs to move into an assisted living home to meet self-identified needs for higher assistance, placement specialist referrals are made. If the need is for rehabilitation programs, locations are given and information about what transportation is available as well as the type of classes and support groups that are available. The focus is on problem prevention and improved levels of quality of life.

Recommendation 4

Assume that the behavior of the patient is a normal consequence of the illness event. Studies show that up to 48% of heart failure patients have significant clinical depressive symptoms, which increase mortality and readmissions two-fold (Song, Lennie, & Moser, 2009). A large proportion of patients have anxiety as well. Many patients are angry, are grieving, or have various levels of denial. Some feel hopeless and helpless following a hospitalization for heart failure. Many experience increasing disability and frailty, and therefore, vulnerability. They feel that they are a burden and that they are powerless over aging and disease progression.

When these behaviors are seen by the nurse to be part of the illness experience rather than as medical problems, treatment can be directed at restoring the self-confidence and well being of the person. By connecting with the patients often and long enough and making targeted home visits on a frequent basis, patients often can help themselves without the need for medications for depression and anxiety. We gather the right people around them for dialogue and support and assist them in commenting on some of these feelings and reactions. We encourage them to realize that they are normal and that they can recover. We encourage them to plan ways to regain control and self-direct their health care. We encourage them to get help they can afford and to reconnect with loved ones, engage in social activities, and get out and be active again. We get them started in practical ways and put them in touch with the best providers. We build hope as we point out progress that has taken place in small increments and explain the recovery process and what they can realistically expect.

Recommendation 5

Use a care manager to coordinate all services. It is the responsibility of the coordinator to provide care through communication and collaboration across all outpatient services and programs. Additionally, the activities of all those involved in the patient's care, including family members, physicians and office staff, caregivers, pharmacists, home health providers, physical/occupational therapists, exercise programs, caregiver agencies, wound care specialists, cardiac rehabilitation therapists, the diabetes clinic, and providers of durable medical equipment are coordinated. The coordinator also refers patients and family members to palliative and hospice care and assists in the transition. This helps to reduce unnecessary and inadequate inpatient care for end of life care and symptom control.

Recommendation 6

Be sure that the patient is an active participant in planning for health interventions. One way to be sure that the patient can be an active participant in the planning of his or her own care is to translate any needed information regarding the disease and treatment process from medical terminology into language that can be understood according to the educational and the cognitive level of the patient. We explain, "You have heart 'remodeling' that results in salt sensitivity" rather than "You have heart failure and need to eat less salt." Prior experience and knowledge and level of self-care also influence how the patient can participate in the process. Because each heart failure patient has unique features and highly tailored treatments, participation for each patient is different. Patients are able to participate at various levels of involvement according to their individual preferences. Classes are provided to educate heart failure patients on the disease process and on medication, diet, and exercise and necessary lifestyle changes so that they have the knowledge to optimally manage their condition. Barriers to learning and adopting lifestyle changes are identified, explored, and overcome as the patient becomes a more active participant in managing care.

Recommendation 7

Aim to strengthen SSOC in the treatment process. Upon meeting the patient and family, we begin our assessment of all aspects of the situational sense of coherence (SSOC), the stressors unique to the patient and family, the resources available, and their willingness to incorporate changes into their personal daily lives. Whether the diagnosis is new or chronic, each person copes according to prior experiences with illness and medical care. We introduce the idea that they have within themselves and their surrounding care team, resources for improving their adaptation to life, but they may be underutilized or over utilized. We present a balancing approach that offers this concept: You have within yourself the power to manage this situation well and succeed in your goals. You know what you must access in your environment and can do it. We capture their intense desire to remain out of the hospital and join them in that goal. We present tools and lifestyle changes that they can choose or create their own ways to achieve that goal while improving quality of life that includes greater physical functioning. We help them overcome barriers by encouraging positive responses so they can increase the SSOC. The first part of SSOC, *comprehensibility*, involves self-care training and practice in self-care activities that are self-directed. The second, *meaningfulness*, requires the nurse to convince the patient that it is worth pursing these behavioral changes and new skills, because they really work and make a difference. We point out how much it is helping, or if they do not make progress, then we propose alternatives. The final part, *manageability*, calls for the nurse to encourage the patient to focus on which practices need to continue, what they might consider changing, and new ways of living to achieve success, given this chronic illness. This very elderly cohort has difficulty with understanding the features of living a long time with a chronic illness. All along the continuum, we are prepared to ask again "What is quality of life to you now?" and to build their trust and confidence in themselves and the team to attain it. A good indicator of a stronger SSOC is the improvement in self-care maintenance and management.

Recommendation 8

Identify level of SOC and strengthen it. SOC is the general adaptation level of a person prior to the illness event. The pre-illness SOC is difficult to determine at the first encounter when the patient is experiencing illness. The intersystem assessment is performed to increase SSOC. The goal of the AIM is to assist the patient to reach the former level of SOC, if possible. Therefore, information must be obtained from the patient and family regarding important meanings in the patient's life and the implications of the illness event for those meanings. It is also important to strengthen the patient's manageability of the illness event. Before entry into the program, the patient's team may not have had the time to learn how the patient managed life prior to the illness event. It is often the case that the health care team is not interested in who the patient was in the pre-illness life. However, the contribution of the HFOPP is to come in as a value added quality incentive to encourage the patient to regain his/her former level of SOC with the goal that the HFOPP would become less needed over time. The goal of the program is not to replace any service or to come in as a new service. Most patients in our community have full access to services, but they need help in understanding how to access them and use them effectively.

Recommendation 9

Distribute power so that the patient is fully involved in all decisions. If at all possible, we prefer to have the patient or caregiver or family communicate directly with providers by presenting their self-monitoring data sheets and medication card to be checked for accuracy. In this way, they increase power to accomplish self-directed care management. Only if they are unable to carry

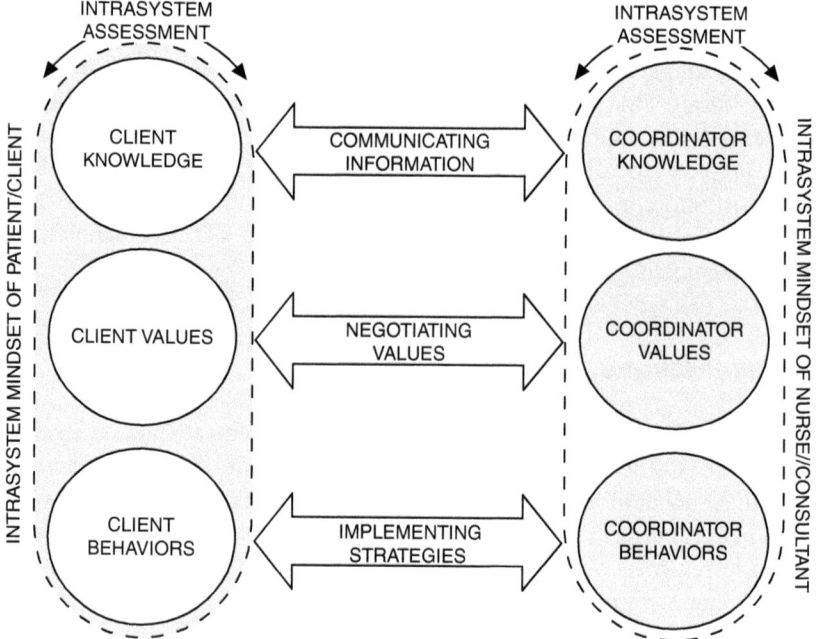

FIGURE 14.1 Home environment: Coordinator makes connection.
Copyright © 2010 B. Artinian.

14. Care Management of Heart Failure Patients in the Outpatient Setting 227

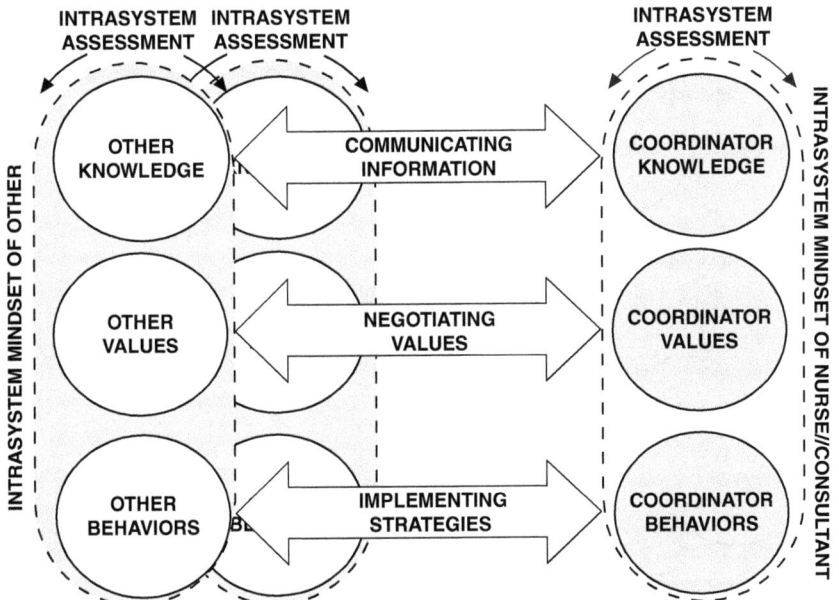

FIGURE 14.2 Coordinator connects to patient family and social network.
Copyright © 2010 B. Artinian.

out this communication do we intervene on their behalf. This is needed early after discharge, but in most patients, the responsibility can be transitioned to them gradually. This is a highly tailored program, highly sensitive to patient preferences and decisions. If it were not so, it would not continue. If patients decide themselves to change something, the change has a greater chance of being maintained over time. Heart failure is a chronic problem and must be continuously managed. This is why motivational interviewing principles and the AIM in practice are so important to them.

An anticipated outcome of the program is to replace the nurse coordinator management with patient self-care management. A series of diagrams have been developed to depict this process.

When a patient returns home after admission for heart failure, the patient is very vulnerable and dependent on the nurse. The first diagram shows the nurse coordinator connecting with the patient in the home environment (see Figure 14.1).

There in the home environment, the coordinator performs an intrasystem assessment of the patient's family and social network to identify available resources and skills and enlists their support (see Figure 14.2).

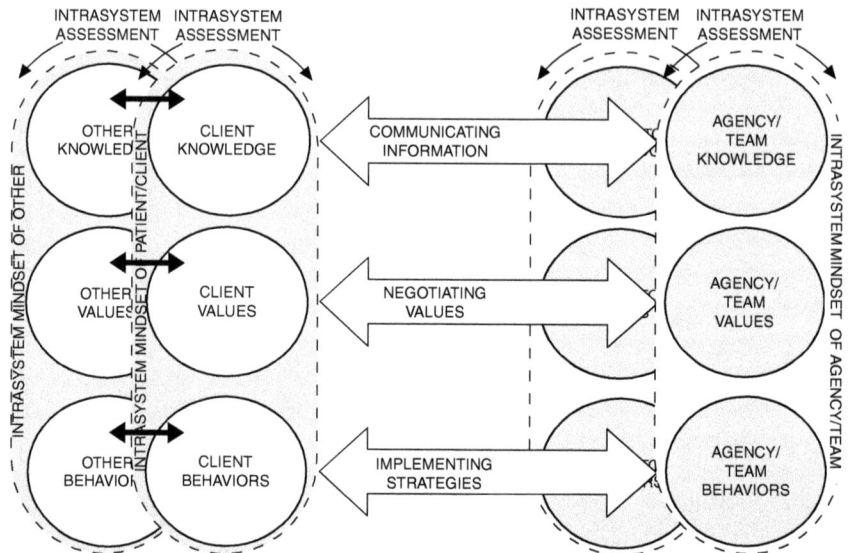

FIGURE 14.3 Coordinator connects to agency.
Copyright © 2010 B. Artinian.

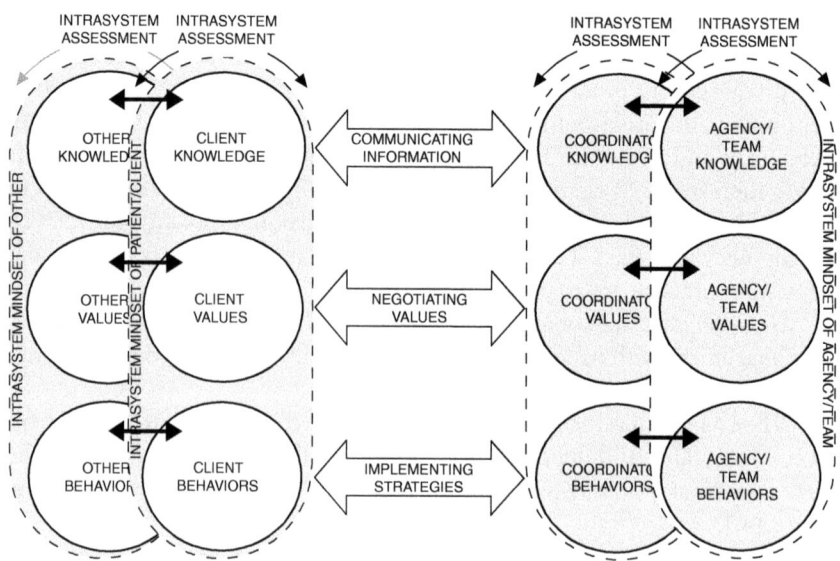

FIGURE 14.4 Coordinator is the connection from agency to patient.
Copyright © 2010 B. Artinian.

After the initial assessment of the patient and family intrasystems, the coordinator has knowledge of her agency's resources and makes referrals as appropriate (see Figure 14.3).

Additional services and resources of the agency needed by the patient, such as lab, outpatient pharmacy, physical therapy, and occupational therapy, are accessed through the coordinator's referrals. In this situation, the values of the agency take precedence over the values of the coordinator (see Figure 14.4).

As the patient increases self-management skills, the patient is better able to communicate directly with the agency and the role of the coordinator lessens (see Figure 14.5).

When the patient is competent in self-care management, the usual model is that the coordinator closes the case and the patient engages directly with the agency and its departments for all further care (see Figure 14.6).

However, in the HFOPP, the coordinator never completely disconnects, but remains available "behind the scenes" ready to reconnect in a prominent role as the patient's condition indicates. The patient knows that the coordinator is available at any time for questions or counseling (see Figure 14.7). The case never completely closes.

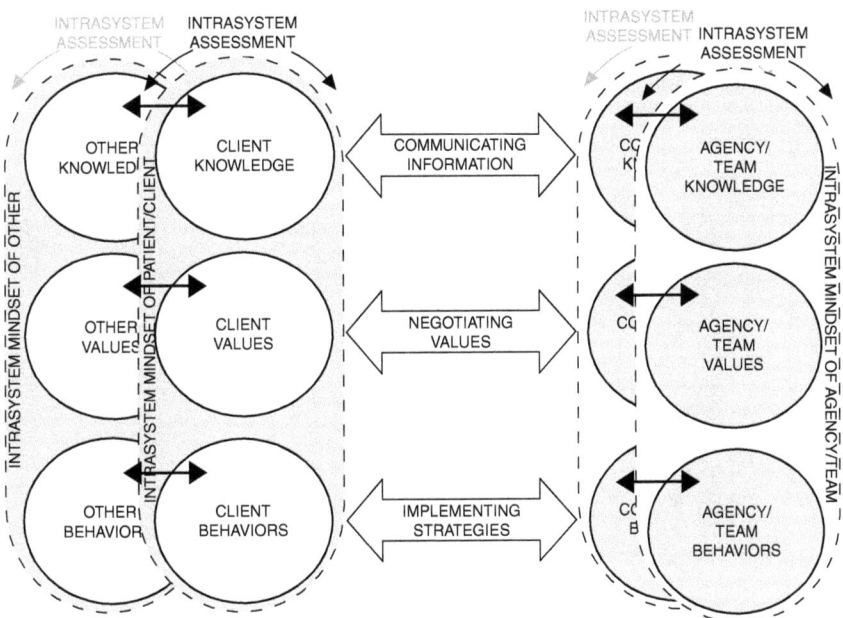

FIGURE 14.5 Coordinator as connector lessens.
Copyright © 2010 B. Artinian.

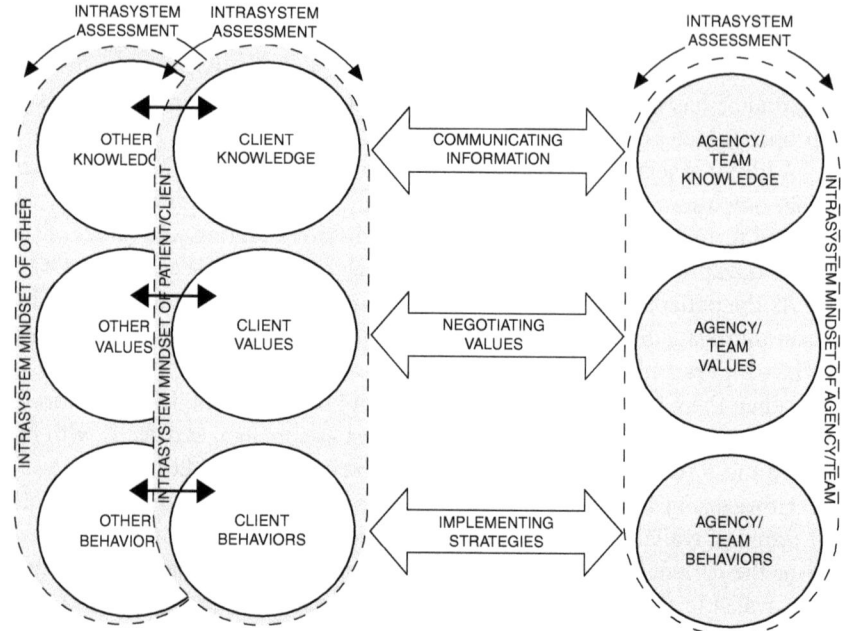

FIGURE 14.6 Does the coordinator disconnect?
Copyright © 2010 B. Artinian.

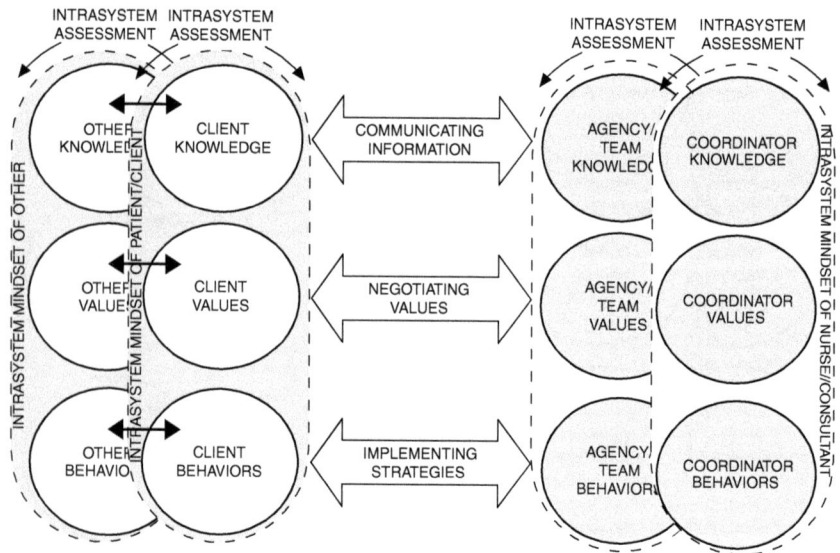

FIGURE 14.7 Coordinator stays connected until needed again.
Copyright © 2010 B. Artinian.

Recommendation 10

Educate patient and staff to reinforce patient's self-care skills. The purpose of the HFOPP is to support newly discharged heart failure patients so that they can learn to manage their care independently. The goals of the HFOPP are to decrease readmissions and to improve physical functioning and quality of life for these patients. Accomplishment of these goals requires the coordinated activities of all members of the health team who come into contact with the patient. The heart failure education program emphasizes reduction of further damage to the heart, identification of symptoms, and treatment of heart failure. This educational program has been developed by the nurse coordinator and is provided to the patients so that they will have the knowledge necessary to understand the ways to monitor their disease and live a more productive life. Because it is important that each care provider gives the same message to the patient, the same information that the patients receive is provided to the health delivery team by the nurse coordinator. This team includes the home health registered nurses (RNs), the case management staff, the emergency and critical care services RNs, the clinical documentation specialists, the SMMC nursing staff, diabetes and chronic illness support groups, and community groups. The coordinator also develops protocols and educates newly hired staff so that they all interact with the patients congruently. The coordinator encourages the active participation of all team members, informing each of them about every aspect of the patient's situation because each heart failure patient has unique features, etiologies, and therefore, needs highly tailored treatment.

Recommendation 11

Obtain feedback about the treatment program. Once a year, we invite our patients to send anonymous suggestions as part of our patient satisfaction survey. The questions on the survey include simple yes or no responses about whether we helped them know more about their condition and whether certain teaching or training sessions and counseling were helpful. We also survey quality of life and physical functioning. The survey is given at the beginning of the program, at 3 months, and every 6 months. Cumulative scores from these surveys are analyzed and they influence changes in the program. We also gather ongoing feedback in an informal way as we analyze responses to the educational materials. This feedback from our patients helps us modify our educational materials so that we can accomplish our goal for them to successfully manage their own care throughout the continuum.

Recommendation 12

Create a long-term relationship with the patient. Our program is intended to develop long-term relationships and the patient determines the nature of the relationship. Patients continue in the program as long as they are able to participate at a minimal level. They can be discharged because of nonparticipation or if they have cognitive dysfunction and there is not adequate caregiver support. Patients are screened carefully for factors that would limit participation prior to being invited to enter the program. Patients remain in the program because of the technology available to monitor their progress coupled with fully integrated disease management programs that are carried out by qualified staff.

Recommendation 13

Integrate acute and rehabilitation phases of treatment. Integrated relationships between the acute care team and the disease management team are the key to success. These teams work hand in hand to educate the patient, prepare the patient for discharge, and start the patient in self-care practices. All the information gathered by the acute care team is made available to the HFOPP team. Extensive excel files are maintained for each patient in an outpatient electronic file with personal notes, encounter notes, and all records of patient symptoms and measurements. These are stored in an organizational memory file. All records are collected, analyzed, and reported. This information directs program change and expansion. Because of the success of the HFOPP at Saddleback Hospital, our corporation, Memorial Health Services, has asked that the program processes be shared with our sister hospitals. We are collaborating now at a systems level to expand these processes to all patients in all corporation hospitals.

Recommendation 14

Design the treatment program to maximize the patient's successful adaptation. If a patient is readmitted to the acute care hospital, we bridge the gap by forwarding any necessary data and insights about the patient learned in the outpatient setting. This information directly influences decisions regarding treatment and admission status, thereby providing a more patient-centered approach to care. For example, a patient was ordered to take a new pain medication at home. She suffered a serious reaction to it and called 911. She did not associate her reaction with the medication and could not remember what the pill was. Therefore, the hospital emergency room notes and subsequent hospital progress notes did not reveal that this was the main issue. The advanced practice nurse communicated the story about the medication and its name to the patient's primary physician. The medication was discontinued and was listed as an allergy on her wallet medication list. We encouraged a short hospitalization since the effects of the medication would wear off after 8 hours and she would no longer be suffering from the effects of the medication. However, because of her frail elderly status and history of heart failure, she was kept longer than was necessary. She was discharged to a skilled nursing facility instead of to her home, and eventually, she went home in the same condition she had been before she took that pill. In another situation, when we had made a graphic chart showing a pattern of weight loss prior to an admission, we sent the information to the acute care team so that they could avoid the iatrogenic problem of inducing low blood pressure and orthostatic changes associated with over diuresis. Our data also show that we are able to reduce unnecessary readmissions and suffering by transferring a patient to hospice care as soon as it is indicated. In this way, we are able to provide the patient an opportunity for a good death.

Because the HFOPP is designed to provide highly personalized care and to develop trust with the patient and the acute care team, there is confidence in the treatment program that comes from a unified team. The coordinator communicates the patient's wishes to the team, thus opening up discussion about the best plan for the patient.

Recommendation 15

Collect data to direct the treatment program and allow for research. We are continuously interviewing our patients at every turn of their lives, when things are up or down as we remain highly connected throughout the continuum of care. We record some of this information in the form of case studies, progress notes, and quality of life surveys. Patients and family members frequently write letters and cards expressing thanks, and these are saved. Therefore, we have both qualitative and quantitative data available for analysis. This information has been analyzed to direct changes in the program. We maintain data sets showing the demographics of the patients, including age, city of residence, and the number of patients actually seen as compared with the potential patients with this diagnosis who were not seen. These demographics identify the numbers in the active caseload, the number eligible but not enrolled in the program, the numbers of patients discharged to a hospice program, the numbers who were discharged from the program for nonparticipation, and the number of patients who expired. We maintain a list of patients who enrolled in the program as well a list of those patients who did not enroll and they could be interviewed for research purposes to compare the two groups. At this time, we do not have the staff to perform this research.

OUTCOMES OF THE PROGRAM

For the period from June to December 2009, it was found that the 57 patients enrolled in the program had a 40% improvement in compliance. Measurement of lifestyle compliance was done by noting if the patient maintained a record of a daily weight and blood pressure reading and pulse, if indicated, by notifying HFOPP of any changes, and by carrying an updated medication list. The expected outcomes for 2009–2010 for 33 participants who were continuously enrolled for 12 months are a 10% reduction in readmission rates for all causes, a 10% improvement in quality of life, and a 10% improvement in functional activity score as measured using standard cardiac rehabilitation assessment tools. In actuality, during the year of 2009, for 33 patients who were continuously enrolled for 12 months, the readmission rate showed a 60% reduction. The cumulative functional percent improvement for the 33 patients showed a 39% improvement using a tool, which measures activities from basic self-care to strenuous sports. For the same group, quality of life improvement was 40% using a second scale that measures positive changes in physical activity, feelings, daily activities, social activities, pain, social support, and perceived improvement.

Program Expansion Needs

Because of the success of the program, there is a plan to expand the program into other areas such as management of diabetes mellitus and chronic obstructive pulmonary disease. To expand the program, there is a need for advanced practice RNs to serve as navigators and coaches for new groups with chronic disease. There is a need for increased health information staff to review remote monitoring records and ensure that appropriate patient follow up is initiated. In the area of technology, there is a need for home remote monitoring devices as for weight, blood pressure, and oxygen saturation measurement. An administrative assistant is needed for statistical data management, to prepare presentations in PowerPoint format, to distribute and score patient satisfaction and quality of life instruments, and to provide support for grant writing. There is also need for research and development. Staff members are needed to assist with identifying grant funding opportunities, proposal writing, and to monitor best practice research.

More work needs to be done to take full advantage of the functionality of the electronic medical record from analysis of heart failure patient data to ready accessibility of multidisciplinary progress notes, thus promoting an individualized, tailored approach to care and avoidance of communication breakdown. It is anticipated that an informatics program will be implemented to combine patient progress notes and outpatient medication lists into the hospital electronic record progress notes.

Heart Failure Outreach Program Opportunities

In the future, the goal will be to increase the number of nurses available to handle caseloads so that all eligible patients in a geographic region can be enrolled. Adding support for a telemanagement team would be useful in accomplishing this goal. There is also a goal for further reduction of readmission rates by identifying and mitigating cofactors such as noncompliance, psychosocial/cognitive factors, inadequate caregiver support, poor dry weight maintenance, and communication and continuity breakdown. Improved telemanagement strategies can be used to identify and develop appropriate telephone outreach for appropriate patients.

CONCLUSION

This chapter has described a program developed at SMMC that is coordinated by an advanced practice nurse. The program is designed to reduce hospital readmissions of heart failure patients. The focus is on education of patients and all team members who provide services to the patient. The goal is to prevent problems before they become severe by identifying physical symptoms and psychosocial problems. The program has been so successful that additional programs are being developed to assist patients with other chronic conditions.

REFERENCES

Song, E. K., Lennie, T. A., & Moser, D. K. (2009). Depressive symptoms increase risk of rehospitalization in heart failure patients with preserved systolic function. *Journal of Clinical Nursing, 18*(3), 1871–1877.

Taylor, D. (1997). *The implications of sense of coherence for the early treatment of people who have had a traumatic spinal cord injury.* Doctoral dissertation: University of Wollongong, Wollongong, Australia.

15

EXCELLENCE IN PRACTICE: A RESIDENT-CENTERED CARE PROGRAM IN A LONG-TERM FACILITY

Margo Y. Babikian, Barbara M. Artinian, and Victoria Winter

THE ARARAT NURSING Facility in Mission Hills, California, has had unprecedented success in the field of elder care. Under the leadership of the Executive Director, the facility has received a number of federal and state awards for excellence in nursing home care, including a zero deficiency evaluation from the California Department of Health Services for the past several years. This nonprofit skilled nursing facility has been providing a special program of compassionate care for seniors since 1995 when the basics of the program were implemented. The program was raised to a higher level in 2005 when the Quality First Covenant was signed. The senior management team made a commitment to practice transformational and transactional leadership that was defined as shared vision and shared governance.

The facility uses a modified form of the Intersystem Model (1997). This nursing model uses an interactional process that takes place between resident and nursing staff in using the model to develop a plan of care. The resident, as a unique individual, is considered to be a whole dynamic entity with biopsychosocial and spiritual needs. The Interdisciplinary Team (IDT) meets systematically with the resident and the resident's family to review the individualized plan of care and validate or develop successful coping strategies of delivery of care. The primary certified nursing assistant (CNA) is an integral part of the IDT. The ombudsman is invited to conduct in-service classes and attend all IDT conferences. There is a collegial professional relationship with the medical staff. The basic principles of the Intersystem Model were fine-tuned to develop a Resident-Centered Care Model. Interlocking and self-directed teams were developed comprising all services. Ultimately, the effect of moving to this new system is evidenced by individualized quality care for the residents.

The innovative Resident-Centered Care Model practiced at the Ararat Nursing Facility reflects a philosophical shift from mass care to individualized services. The organization of the home is based on the Intersystem Model (Artinian, 1997) that focuses on mutual decision-making and the development of a joint plan of care. Residents and caregivers are active participants in this process in collaboration with all staff members of the facility. The paradigm shift seen here is from an authoritarian relationship to a collaborative relationship that supports the resident's individuality as a dynamic entity. The management philosophy of resident-centered care states:

> As leaders, we will be change agents at the Ararat Nursing Home and will practice the fundamental values of employee empowerment, open communication, innovative interventions, compassion, and collaboration with all disciplines.
>
> We will function in a learning organization characterized by flexibility and adaptability to changes benefiting our residents. In this open environment, information will be transformed into a resident-centered standard of practice.
>
> We will be excellence driven, fair, and respectful. Elder talk in all its forms will be discouraged. Our decisions will be based on principles and core values. We will promote cohesive teams, accountability, and positive relationships among residents, families, and staff. We will create an environment where "Being at Home" will be characterized by privacy, autonomy, respect, affection, security, dignity, commonality, and significance.

The Ararat Nursing Facility is a 196-bed not-for-profit, skilled nursing facility with 100% occupancy and a waiting list. The dedicated Board of Trustees supports a progressive environment focused on compassionate care and excellence in services. A modified primary care approach is used and staffing needs are determined by the acuity of the resident population. About 97% of the residents receive aid from MediCal, the California Medicaid program, and the majority of the residents are aged 85 or older. The nursing staff is a culturally diverse team that at this time includes representatives from 13 ethnic backgrounds.

A participatory value-focused management style characterizes the facility. The leadership has taken the initiative to model and then create an environment of trust. This culture of trust is characterized by respect, creativity, teamwork, open environment, employee empowerment and recognition, proactive behavior, celebration, and accountability. Those closest to the resident, the CNAs, have the greatest authority for decision making. The core values of the facility are excellence in service, excellence in practice, excellence in leadership, and compassion. These four core values were redefined later as the eight pillars of service (see Table 15.1).

TABLE 15.1 Comparison of the Four Core Values and Eight Pillars of Service

FOUR CORE VALUES	EIGHT PILLARS OF SERVICE
1 Excellence in service	▪ Vision of excellence ▪ Respect dignity
2 Excellence in practice	▪ Self-determination (Choice) ▪ Employee empowerment
3 Excellence in leadership	▪ Flexibility ▪ Relationship
4 Compassion	▪ Compassion ▪ Integrity

Source: Ararat Nursing Home, (2010).

It has not always been this way. In the winter of 1994, life at the facility was very different. Crisis management was the dominant organizational behavior. Residents, families, and medical staff verbalized discontent regarding the care and various communication processes. Calling in sick (without being sick) was a common occurrence because a failure to have perfect attendance meant that the 12 vacation days were forfeited. Continuous piped-in music in combination with call-lights and loud conversations, created an uncaring atmosphere. The use of physical restraints was widespread. Risk management was a foreign term. Falls, misplaced belongings, weight loss, and dehydration were frequent. CNA documentation of resident care was incomplete and often inaccurate. For example, CNA charting was often done before the event occurred. CNA assignments were on rotation cycles so that residents and families did not know to whom questions could be addressed. "She is not my patient. I was not here yesterday" was a frequent response by CNAs. Because management was very dictatorial and controlling, morale was very low among the CNAs. Unprofessional behavior was demonstrated in poor grooming and by ignoring the needs of the other CNAs and the residents. There were many unresolved conflicts. There was no structured systematic orientation process.

During a CNA meeting in 1994, the new Director of Nursing (DON) made a statement that ushered in a new climate of organization. She said, "You are in a noble profession. Your work is noble. You are resident advocates. You are the most valuable players in this organization. We cannot do without you." The CNAs recognized these statements as genuine and knew that the existing system was not working and could not be repaired. It had to be replaced.

During the next weeks and months, the director and the CNAs designed a system that could systematically collect data, analyze the data, act upon the data, and evaluate the effectiveness of the interventions. It was named Performance Improvement Quality Improvement (PIQI). The focus of PIQI was on continuous improvement, proactive approaches, employee empowerment and recognition, professional growth, human resource excellence, and compassionate resident-centered care. The goal was to transform PIQI into a life style that would eventually replace the existing toxic culture. The steps taken in developing the quality performance program were as follows:

1. Establishment of standards
2. Monitoring the standards
3. Identification of areas of strength and weakness
4. Implementation of corrective actions
5. Evaluation of corrective action
6. Periodic re-evaluation

Some of the principles used in developing the program were: 1) quality can always get better, 2) quality is everybody's business, 3) some of the best plans will come from the most unexpected sources, and 4) departmental territoriality is the biggest obstacle to a quality program. You must know why and when something goes wrong and think beyond cutting costs. Little by little, cultural change became evident, and three distinct programs for CNAs were initiated. The changes observed in the facility are summarized as follows:

- A structured orientation program was implemented based on individualized needs.
- The CNA team, empowered and acknowledged, started demonstrating professional behavior, accountability, and empathy.
- Time clocks became obsolete.
- Paid Time Off promoted near-perfect attendance.
- Problems became "issues."
- Departments meant "services."
- Bosses were transformed into coaches, mentors, and role models.
- Family and resident satisfaction rates sky-rocketed.
- The turnover rate declined.
- CNAs rose to the position of "ambassadors."
- Recruitment ceased.
- Resident falls, weight loss, pressure ulcers, and lost belongings became rarities.

- Physical restraints became obsolete.
- Telephone calls were handled with finesse.

"There is a sense of serenity in this place," remarked a first time visitor. "Do your CNAs carry pagers?" Our CNAs did not carry pagers. They carried poise, tact, and empathy. By 1997, incomplete and inaccurate CNA documentation was considered ancient history. Group consensus became the norm. Fresh ideas and new dreams created a professional vitality. Unsightly appearances were converted into well-groomed CNAs. Attractive pastel colored outfits adorned the facility. CNA names were engraved on the Wall of Fame. Pins of Excellence caught the attention of the bystanders. The worst enemies—complacency, apathy, and mediocrity—vanished. A sense of excellence permeated throughout the organization. A culture of trust was being nurtured.

The transformation of the Ararat Nursing Facility from one of dictatorial management to one of shared management took place within the Caring for the Caregiver program. The senior management made a commitment to role model nurturing relationships with all the staff. All staff members were to be treated with dignity and respect. No employee would be criticized publicly, and positive behaviors would be commended. Mistakes would be considered to be an opportunity for teaching. Empowerment is the core of this program. The freedom to be a vital part of the decision-making process is the most valued privilege of the entire staff. A major component of this program is cross training and career ladder progression for all services. Environmental, dietary, and laundry staff are provided with 100% scholarships to obtain CNA certifications. CNAs are promoted to RNA (Restorative Nursing Assistant) positions. RNAs are encouraged to attend Licensed Vocational Nursing programs, and licensed vocational nurses (LVNs) are given the opportunity to attend Registered Nursing programs. At all service levels, employees are encouraged to attend seminars, workshops, and conferences with all expenses paid.

The PIQI-CNA program has the purpose of providing professional growth for the CNAs so that they in turn would be empowered to provide compassionate resident-centered care. The program has three distinct entities: CNA Career Ladder, CNA Primary Care, and CNA Recognition.

CNA CAREER LADDER

The career ladder has six levels and responsibilities and pay increases from one level to another. The levels are identified in Table 15.2.

TABLE 15.2 CNA Career Ladder

JOB LEVEL	JOB TITLE	RESPONSIBILITIES
CNA I	Entry Level Novice	Provides basic care
CNA II	Alternate Team Leader	Assumes some leadership responsibility
CNA III	Team Leader	Mentors the CNAs of her team and is responsible for flexible scheduling and management of her team
CNA IV	Certified RNA	Is responsible for restorative activities such as therapeutic dining, strengthening exercises, and ambulation
CNA V	Senior Team Leader	Functions as a resource person throughout the facility
CNA VI	Facility-Wide Staffing Coordinator	Is a member of nursing administration and works closely with the entire CNA team

Source: Ararat Nursing Home, (2010). CNA, certified nursing assistant; RNA, restorative nursing assistant.

Access to progression in the career ladder is by application, and CNAs are eligible to begin the process within 9–12 months of employment. The applicant undergoes peer review and if determined to be eligible for promotion, the application is forwarded to the DON for approval.

In addition to meeting regulatory requirements and a lengthy in-house orientation that provides 1:1 training, there are in-service education sessions for CNAs. These sessions concentrate on value-focused management, guest relations, therapeutic humor, conflict resolution, behavioral management programs for residents with dementia, quality improvement activities, team building, and sensitivity training. Competency-based in-service education is continuous through the facility in addition to weekly sessions on critical thinking, maintaining positive relationships, and implementing evidence-based criteria for patient care.

The expectations for each level are well defined. Pathways to leadership are in place. In order to motivate the CNA to move to an area of greater leadership, the team leader asks: (1) What are your goals? (2) Where would you like to be, and (3) How can I help you get there? Qualified CNAs may direct their advancement activities by entering an LVN or registered nurse (RN) educational program at any time. To encourage their efforts, partial or full scholarship tuition is provided.

CNA Primary Care Program

Every CNA is assigned to a group of residents. The intent of primary care is continuity of care, knowledge of the resident's proficiencies in daily living, bonding with the residents and their families, and promoting CNA self-worth. The CNA, within the scope of the job description, has the authority to make as many decisions as may be applicable. For example, CNAs schedule shower time, room transfers, shopping with residents, doctor office visits, dining off campus with residents, and communicating appropriate information with the families.

The CNA actively participates in the IDT Care Conferences by giving verbal reports about the residents in the group. It is customary for the nursing management staff to seek the opinions of the CNAs about residents in the group. The CNAs conduct clinical rounds with the DON. Because they have learned about the needs of the residents from the resident focused care program, CNAs have implemented programs such as resident hand washing, fall prevention, therapeutic dining, doll therapy, nonpharmacological pain interventions, a hydration program, restraint reduction techniques, a hospitality protocol for weight gain, and hug therapy. Each resident is "adopted" by a staff member who writes the life story of the resident and identifies life style issues. This information becomes part of the care plan.

CNAs do their own flexible scheduling. Last minute changes are acceptable as long as coverage is arranged. CNAs plan their own vacations as well. Because of their shared sense of mission, they do not plan any time off around annual survey time. An example of the autonomy the CNAs are given in scheduling is given in the following account:

> Recently, one of the CNAs lost her 1-year-old nephew in a tragic drowning accident. The CNA Team Leader called the grieving teammate at home and expressed her heartfelt sympathy on behalf of the team. Without consulting the DON Services, she said: "We do not want you to worry about your schedule. Take some time off. We have already arranged CNA coverage for your days off." When the DON learned about the incident, she posted the following memorandum: "Once again you have proved that corporate excellence begins with individual excellence. I commend you for utilizing your CNA authority. Your unwavering dedicated service is heartwarming. Truly, you are a never-ending source of encouragement to me. I should not be surprised. After all, you are our CNAs. I will always salute you."

CNA Recognition Program

The primary focus of the CNA recognition program is to unleash the potential of every single CNA and to recognize the smallest acts of positive behavior. The program is designed so that the recognition can be made in public. One form of recognition is to have the name placed on the Wall of Fame as employee of the month. Not everyone can achieve this, but the Pin of Excellence is often achieved. The Pin of Excellence is publicly bestowed by the DON on all those CNAs who have made a difference in the quality of life of a resident. Some examples of differences are weight gain by a malnourished resident, improvement in ambulation, or a praiseworthy remark by a family member in a difficult situation. The Pin of Excellence is also given to those who have achieved mini-goals such as adopting a resident and writing the life story of the resident in any form such as a scrapbook, album, creative memories, art work, a booklet or a case study, an effective IDT report, serving on a committee, completing a QI activity, or calling a team conference for an identified need of a resident or teammate. Every month, a coworker is recommended to the DON for acknowledgment. The person acknowledged is usually a CNA. Within 24 hours after the recommendation, an official memo is circulated praising the CNA for the specified reason.

In addition to recognition for outstanding service, other personnel policies enhance the work environment. Once a year, the CNAs evaluate the DON, the management staff, and the overall organizational performance. In addition, the CNAs evaluate their own performance every year in terms of goals accomplished and receive a merit raise for their professional performance. Each year, a member of the management team spends a whole day with a CNA learning to provide care for the residents. The CNAs see it as an honor to supervise and to teach their own supervisors. CNAs are allowed to take time off for educational leave and for any unavoidable emergency. After three years of employment, CNAs become eligible for the retirement plan. Five-year, 10-year, and 15-year anniversaries are celebrated in a pompous manner. At the gala banquet, the Executive Director depicts the accomplishments of the honoree with praiseworthy remarks. As a tribute to their commitment to quality care and professional behavior, scenic window sites at the facility are named after CNAs.

CONTINUOUS QUALITY IMPROVEMENT

The facility had been collecting and analyzing data for use in evaluating the quality of programs for a number of years. The data indicated a need for new systems to be developed to enhance the quality of service. These included:

- Redesigning a communication system so that all of the physicians would be informed about PIQI data, especially information about

antibiotic usage, susceptibility reports, and accessibility and availability of physician services.
- Formulating concrete criteria with specific thresholds and treatment plans for all of the residents who had the diagnosis of anemia, diabetes, and osteoporosis.
- Redesigning the award-winning (2000) pain management system to make documentation more manageable.

These system designs enhanced collaboration and effective communication and simplified charting into a manageable tool. In addition, higher standards of care were implemented for the resident.

BUILDING POSITIVE RELATIONSHIPS WITH FAMILIES

In addition to providing programs for all employees that foster dignity and respect, a program was developed to make family members of residents feel welcome and respected. When a resident is admitted to the facility, he or she is welcomed with a basket of silk flowers and a welcome card from the CNA caregiver. The Executive Director meets with the family around a table, explains some procedures, and listens to their fears and guilt feelings. This time with the family is considered to be a "teaching awareness moment." Families are encouraged to participate in future care conferences and to communicate with the CNA anytime the need arises. Families are instructed about issues affecting the oldest of the old population such as depression, anemia, osteoporosis, diabetes, flu/pneumococcal vaccination, polypharmacy, and stroke prevention. The admission paperwork was revised to include simple information for the purpose of educating families and raising consciousness for wellness such as a statement "Depression is not a part of normal aging."

On the day of admission, family members are the guests of the home for lunch. Members of all the services (activities coordinator, dietary services, environmental services, laundry services, social services, and the business department) individually meet with the family, thus assuring a smooth adjustment process for all concerned. The morning following the admission of the resident, the family is called to inform them how the new resident slept at night. Training sessions are conducted for all staff members to teach them how to be proactive in addressing family concerns, questions, and issues.

When the families of the residents were encouraged to organize a family council, they declined stating that is unnecessary because "Communication with and by the facility staff is always open and great." Communication with the family has been further increased by the development of a resident adoption program. Every employee, including the senior management and all ancillary services, is encouraged to adopt a resident of his/her choice and write the life story of the adoptee. For a full life story, the family has to be contacted for photographs and historical information about the resident. The families are gratified by the interest of the employee and provide pictures of the resident's past and family members. Information about the past experiences of the resident becomes available through verbal and written messages from the family. This active involvement has built lasting positive relationships not only with families but also with the residents. Appropriate information becomes a part of the permanent record of the resident's individualized care plan. After the death of a resident, the life storybook is given to the family.

VALIDATION OF TAYLOR'S RECOMMENDATIONS FOR A SALUTOGENIC PROGRAM IN THE RESIDENT-CENTERED CARE MODEL

Although the recommendations for the development of a treatment program based on salutogenic principles were identified by Taylor (1997) from his dissertation research with spinal cord–injured patients, it was found that his recommendations have been in practice at the Ararat Nursing Facility for a number of years. Based upon organizational assessment and the need for improvement, these practices were organized into the Resident-Centered Care Model in 2003. Ways in which the nursing facility carries out Taylor's recommendations identified in Chapter 2 are discussed as follows:

Recommendation 1

Use the salutogenic model. When a resident is admitted to the nursing facility, the emphasis of the program is to assist the resident to live a life as similar to that he or she was able to live at home as it is possible. The focus of the rehabilitation program is to teach the person to live safely with any disability that is present. This is accomplished in the IDT Care Conference that is held for every resident on admission and every 3 months. The resident is an active participant of the Care Conference. It is about the residents, their needs, their concerns, their problems, their values, their identities, and their families. It is a partnership between the resident, the family of the resident, and the Ararat Nursing Facility staff. A representative from every service participates in the IDT Care Conference along with the resident and a family member.

Staff members include the primary CNA, the primary nurse, the primary activity coordinator, the primary RNA, the Director of Clinical Services, and surprisingly, Administration. The Executive Director chairs the IDT Care Conference, which is an interlocking team. Every team member relates to every other member by listening, communicating, and assisting each other to help the resident experience quality care and quality life.

Recommendation 2

Use a systems approach. Residents also attend the Resident Council Meetings that are coordinated by one of the residents. This open environment of trust enhances communication with the entire IDT. Residents may make suggestions about changes they would like to see in the program. For example, they may make requests for a different menu, a new outing location, or meaningful activities such as planting flowers, taking care of birds, and so on. Minutes of the Resident Council Meetings are submitted to the Executive Director for immediate action. Often, the council chairperson acknowledges the extraordinary performance of a particular staff member or a service that has been appreciated. The Executive Director communicates these suggestions to the ITD team. In this way, the parts of the system are integrated into the whole system and a mechanism is provided for interpersonal interactions.

Recommendation 3

Focus on problem prevention. A proactive approach is the essence of the IDT approach. For example, to prevent falls related to dizziness, residents are taught to sit at the bedside and to count to 20 before getting up early in the morning. Likewise, caregivers are educated in conflict resolution and sensitivity training. As an example of conflict resolution, a resident with dementia who insisted on going home to cook for the family had her wishes satisfied by providing her with kitchen utensils and ingredients to prepare some food.

Recommendation 4

Assume that the behavior of the patient is a normal consequence of the illness event. Aging is a ripening process. We do not place pathogenic interpretations on the normal responses to aging such as denial, feelings of loss, anger, and grief. Once a relationship of trust is established, residents are encouraged to verbalize their feelings. One such resident, who was experiencing severe catatonic status upon admission, was provided with mega doses of gentle touch, therapeutic presence, coloring books, and materials. Little by little she came to accept her caregiver as her family. We located her estranged daughter in another state. The daughter was contacted to find out if she could visit her mother. We said that we would provide the means for transportation. After some silence, the daughter sent a Christmas card with a picture of her children to the Executive Director to be given to her mother. The IDT presented the Christmas card to the resident at a special occasion. For the first time, we witnessed a smile on the resident's apathetic face. The staff members were tearful. The card was later placed at the resident's bedside. We are still waiting for the daughter's arrival. It will be a day of great celebration. Today, this resident volunteers in the dining room by distributing napkins and fresh water.

Recommendation 5

Use a care manager to coordinate all services. The IDT functions as a case manager. It is rare for our residents to be placed in another setting, but if it happens, the team convenes to mutually identify the best placement for the resident.

Recommendation 6

Be sure that the patient is an active participant in planning for all health interventions. The day the resident arrives at our Home, the resident is greeted by the caregivers and given a basketful of flowers. The resident is introduced to his or her roommate and to the roommate's family. Lifestyle questions are asked to identify the resident's needs, concerns, or problems. We have a meaningful saying to all newcomers: "You have not come here to die. You have come to Ararat Nursing Home to live your sunset years, and live well." This is very comforting to the resident and his or her family. When medications are administered, the resident is informed about the purpose and benefits of the medications. The resident has the right to refuse any medication but will then be informed about the consequences. The resident is an active participant in the health process.

Recommendation 7

Aim to strengthen SSOC in the treatment process. Individual care plans can be made to resolve a resident's concern or a concern of a staff member about the resident. An example of such a care plan is presented in Chapter 16 illustrating the grounded theory of "Preserving Identity." Because the residents remain in the facility for long periods of time, it is possible to evaluate the effectiveness of the plan of care.

Recommendation 8

Identify level of SOC and strengthen it. We find out what the residents like to do and how we can support their beliefs and values to create a sense of coherence. To increase one resident's level of comprehensibility about her daily routine so that she could experience her environment as ordered, consistent, structured, and clear, we honored her desire to use the restroom right after the morning exercise as part of her bowel and bladder training became an integrated part of her individualized care plan.

Meaningfulness is seen when the staff and the family of a resident work together on problems experienced by the resident because they view all problems as worth investing energy in and as challenges they are willing to undertake. A resident, who was admitted because the daughter could not provide care for him at home in addition to the care for her mother who was dying, tried to leave the facility to visit his wife. An ankle transmitter was put on his leg so that the staff could keep track of him, and arrangements were made for him to go home on weekends. The daughter was very appreciative of the willingness of the staff to work with her to resolve this problem. Other examples of ways in which the staff helped the residents to find meaning in their lives were to provide ways in which the resident could be connected to important aspects of life at home. One resident was a violinist. Since his violin was an expensive one, it was left at home. When he expressed a wish to have his violin, the family was contacted and they were asked to bring it with them when they visited. In another case, a resident was expert in crocheting. When the staff found out about that, they provided her with yarn and needles. They praised her efforts, and her needlework is exhibited on a wall at the facility to this day.

An example of manageability is the effort of the staff to make the facility resources available to a resident so that he felt that his needs were met in a fair way. He liked to sleep until 11:00 a.m. and then be served a light breakfast. His care plan reads, "I will sleep until 11:00 a.m. I will then be served coffee and a cheese sandwich." Another example of the staff's willingness to make a special effort to help a resident accomplish the dream of his life was when they facilitated his becoming a citizen. A resident wished to become a U.S. citizen. Since he was not able to travel to the immigration office, the judge was invited to the Ararat facility to administer the oath. The event was photographed, and the picture is displayed in a prominent location.

Recommendation 9

Distribute power so that the patient is fully involved in all decisions. Liberalized diets are the norm. However, one resident's excessive weight was a great concern of the IDT. The resident was asked if she desired to lose some weight for more mobility. "Of course" she said. She decided that she would have small-portioned meals except when she visited her family off campus. The resident was fully involved in decision making concerning her weight reduction. Power was distributed so that all shared in the implementation of the plan.

Recommendation 10

Educate patient and staff to reinforce patient's self-care skills. The Ararat home is a learning organization. If we are not teaching then we are learning. Education is an ongoing process. Role modeling is one of the most effective ways of being change agents. Mentoring and coaching is the dominant teaching style. An example is validation therapy that is taught in a classroom setting with specific scenarios, but the actual elements are implemented at IDT meetings and during clinical rounds. Communication skills, building and maintaining positive relationships, conflict resolutions, and behavioral management are some of the ongoing training sessions.

Recommendation 11

Obtain feedback about the treatment program. Ongoing feedback on all aspects of every individual treatment program is evaluated at least every three months and as often as a need is identified. For example, Mrs. Y is a petite frail lady. She has only three teeth. She does not want her teeth extracted. The staff honors her wish but is open to changes in her wishes. However, her hat gets her undivided attention. She loves to wear it at all times except when in bed or taking showers. We cannot envision Mrs. Y without her hat; we make every effort to ensure that she has her hat at all times. The ongoing feedback of the treatment program covers the whole person and not fragments of her health care. Another resident had decided that her hair should never be trimmed or cut. Her wish was respected. One day, she reversed her decision because it would be easier to manage her hair. Her decision was implemented, and the care plan was revised.

Recommendation 12

Create a long-term relationship with the patient. In the total program at the Ararat Facility, there is an emphasis on creating long-term relationships—the commitment encompassing biological, psychosocial, and spiritual needs of the residents. For example, the staff goes shopping with residents and residents invite staff to attend significant family events, such as weddings. In one IDT meeting when the care of a middle-aged resident was discussed, the executive director said, "I guess I will have to visit her after I retire."

Recommendation 13

Integrate acute and rehabilitation phases of treatment. When residents are admitted with a need for rehabilitation training, the rehabilitation is done on an ongoing basis. The emphasis of the treatment program is on the resident's strength and potential to use his or her own resources when coping with life's challenges. When an acute condition occurs, a total rehabilitation plan is developed. When Mr. X's right leg was amputated because of diabetic complications, he was very anxious to use a prosthesis so that he could walk again. However, he could not afford the cost of the prosthesis. A mutually developed and mutually agreed upon treatment plan was implemented when we contacted outside sources to supply a prosthesis for him. Mr. X obtained his prosthetic right leg. The rehabilitation process was a great challenge. We were excited, but Mr. X was not. He could not tolerate the weight of the prosthesis. Then the rehabilitation had to be renegotiated on a quarterly basis. He chose not to walk, but to propel the wheelchair with his prosthesis on. He took on the task of picking up the daily newspaper and delivered it to the residents using his wheelchair. Examples such as this are communicated through inclusion in a bimonthly publication sent to supporters of the facility. The examples have also been used in reports for external review committees. These publications have been useful in a research study conducted at the Ararat facility.

Recommendation 14

Design the treatment program to maximize the patient's successful adaptation. When residents enter the Ararat Facility, many bring with them prescriptions for numerous medications. The IDT carefully evaluates each medication with the goal of reducing the resident's dependence on them. During the team conference, the resident is asked about how the medication helps and if it could be discontinued. When a decision is made that the medication is no longer needed, the physician is contacted to change the order.

Recommendation 15

Collect data to direct the treatment program and allow for research. The Ararat staff has observed that subtle changes do occur. These observations are recorded in IDT minutes and communicated to the appropriate caregivers for continuous monitoring. In addition, the Ararat staff has been very supportive of a grounded theory research about institutional practices and resident outcomes. The interviewers were given unlimited access to team meetings and resident activities to make observations, as well as access to records and published documents.

PROGRAM EFFECTIVENESS

In the eight years the Resident-Centered Care Program has been in operation, a number of milestones have occurred for the CNA staff:

- The turnover rate declined to 1.3%
- Accurate CNA documentation rose to 100%
- The Career Ladder was utilized by 70%
- The Wall of Fame consisted of 70% CNAs

Evidence of changes in patient outcomes was also significant:

- The facility became a restraint-free and pain-free environment
- Falls declined from 0.70 to 0.10 per bed
- The number of bedridden residents decreased to only one
- Little or no activity declined from 33% to 3%
- Hypnotic drug usage declined 25% to 5%
- Residents participating in daily restorative exercises increased to 93%

Satisfaction with the program was also significant:

- Family satisfaction rate rose to 98%
- The CNA satisfaction rate for the total organization performance rose to 95%
- The CNA satisfaction rate for management and the DON was 99%

The satisfaction ratings of the staff have importance for the overall operation of the nursing facility. It is estimated that it takes approximately $1,800 USD to train a CNA. Because the turnover rate declined to 1.3%, thousands of dollars have been saved. Building, nurturing, and maintaining relationships did not involve additional resources. The cost of the recognition programs including free meals, educational material, award, and certificates was less than $1,200 USD per year. A merit raise of 5% was built into the approved budget. The decline in falls that would have resulted in injuries and hospitalizations saved a minimum of $10,000, in the facility's estimation, for each prevented event. The decline in the use of expensive hypnotic and psychotropic medications had an estimated cost savings of $3,600 per month. A flat organizational structure with self-directed interlocking teams and team leaders eliminated middle management. This resulted in cost saving of thousands of dollars. Finally, the cost savings of the absence of liability lawsuits because of the high satisfaction rate of residents, families, and staff is significant.

FAMILY MAKING: A GROUNDED THEORY STUDY

A qualitative research study has been done by Winter and Artinian that describes the interaction among staff members (Winters, 2010). The purpose of this study was to describe the informal staff relationships that developed in a nursing home institution that has a resident care program based on the Artinian Intersystem Model. Staff members saw themselves as "family" and exhibited many of the characteristics of a family in their daily activities.

Classical grounded theory methodology developed by Glaser and Strauss (1967) and in the later writings of Glaser (1978, 1992, 2005) was utilized for this study. The researchers used open-ended interviewing to explore the background and motivation of these certified nursing assistants in order to determine their main concerns. The questions served as a guide for the interview process. This study was done strictly from the viewpoint of the CNA. Seven CNAs who work at the Ararat Nursing Home participated in this project on a voluntary basis. In-depth interviews were conducted with the subjects at the facility. Participant observation was also done in the common areas and in multidisciplinary conferences that were held every week at the facility. The interviews were recorded to provide clarity and detail to the data. Using constant comparative analysis, the data were simultaneously collected and analyzed to identify the core processes in the phenomenon under investigation in this study. The first author transcribed all of the interviews from the audiotapes. Line-by-line analysis of the written transcripts, along with frequent listening to the audiotapes, helped capture the powerful statements of the subjects that led to the development of the codes.

The findings of this study showed that the "family making" of the staff involved participatory leadership that started with the DON and involved all of the nursing staff. The theoretical code identified was functional reciprocity (Glaser, 2005), and it integrated five categories underlying the "work" of the family that emerged, which included the following: shared purpose, collectivity or seeing the family as part of something larger that itself, optimism that is grounded in reality, relativism which is living in the context of present circumstances, and finally, shared control with the family balancing internal control with trust in each other. This "family making" can be used to describe the informal family relationships that are developed in health care institutions in a multiplicity of settings.

VALIDATION OF THE RESEARCH FINDINGS

The benefits of the program as reported by the Executive Director and the research team in this chapter have been validated by an outside observer from the California Association of Health Facilities (CAHF), Jocelyn Montgomery, who described the program in two articles, "Is there anything more we can do for you? (April 6, 2007) and "Happy staff = happy residents" (April 20, 2007). These articles are available on the CAHF website.

CONCLUSION

It is possible to replicate the Resident-Centered Care Program. All that is needed is a genuine commitment by management to create a culture of trust in which staff experience high morale, security, and a sense of pride and creativity. Even though it was risky for senior management to create a partnership by distributing their power to the team, the outcomes were beneficial when self-directed interlocking teams and a respectful work place were created. Change has been managed in such a creative manner that cooperation and collaboration among residents, families, facility teams, and the medical staff has emerged. In a culture of trust, it is very fulfilling to unleash the potential of staff, to recognize positive behaviors, and to reward professional growth. It is a core value of the facility to give dignity and respect to the residents so that their identities will be preserved. It is equally important to provide this dignity and respect for the staff.

A number of evaluation forms have been developed by the Ararat Home committees for assessment of the patient at admission. Forms for evaluation of self and the program and staff and instruments to measure satisfaction of residents and families, physicians, and staff are used periodically. In addition to these forms, a number of published assessment forms are used. Information about these instruments can be obtained by contacting Executive Director Margo Babikian at her email address: margob@ararathome.org.

INTRODUCTION TO ONLINE CARE PLAN

A group care plan has been written by Artinian based on interviews with CNAs at the Ararat Nursing Home as part of a research study done by Victoria Winter and Barbara Artinian. The major research finding was that there is group consensus about how care should be given. Therefore, this care plan has been prepared as a generic group care plan illustrating how the nursing assistants approach the care of residents. The full text of the group care plan is available in the online adjunct manual.

REFERENCES

Artinian, B. M. (1997). Overview of the Intersystem Model. In B. M. Artinian & M. Conger (Eds.), *The Intersystem Model: Integrating theory and practice* (pp. 1–17). Thousand Oaks, CA: Sage Publications.
Glaser, B. (1978). *Theoretical sensitivity*. Mill Valley, CA: Sociology Press.
Glaser, B. (1992). *Basics of grounded theory analysis: Emergence versus forcing*. Mill Valley, CA: Sociology Press.
Glaser, B. (2005). *Grounded theory perspective III: Theoretical coding*. Mill Valley, CA: Sociology Press.
Glaser, B., & Strauss, A. (1967). *The discovery of grounded theory*. Chicago, IL: Aldine.
Montgomery, J. (2007, April 6). Is there anything more we can do for you: Part 1 of a two-part visit to Ararat Nursing Home. *CAHF News*. Retrieved from http://calculturechange.com/CultureChangeinCalifornia/Resources/Articles/Anything.aspx
Montgomery, J. (2007, April 20). Excellence in workforce practices: Part 2 of a two-part visit to Ararat Nursing Home. *CAHF News*. Retrieved from http://calculturechange.com/CultureChangeinCalifornia/Resources/Articles/Excellence.aspx

Taylor, D. (1997). *The implications of sense of coherence for the early treatment of people who have had a traumatic spinal cord injury.* Doctoral dissertation, University of Wollongong, Wollongong, Australia.

Winter, V. (2010, October). *Family Making: A grounded theory study.* Paper presented at the Joint Southern California Sigma Theta Tau International Chapters' Conference—Nursing Odyssey 2010, San Diego, CA.

16

Integrating Theory and Practice Using the Artinian Intersystem Model

Barbara M. Artinian

The Artinian Intersystem Model (AIM) was developed by integrating and extending a number of theories especially those of Chin (1969), Kuhn (1974), Antonovsky (1987), Knickrehm (1994), Blumer (1969), Stallwood and Stoll (1975), and Hill (1949). These theories were used to describe the interactional process that takes place when patient/client and nurse/health provider come together to form a mutual plan of care. The model can be used by the novice practitioner as well as by the advanced practice nurse or other experienced health care provider because the complexity of the model derives from the knowledge base of the user, not from the structure of the model as stated in Chapter 1. However, when additional theories are used to inform practice, the practitioner operates from a much wider knowledge base and the approaches to understanding the concern of the client are multiplied. The purpose of this chapter is to demonstrate how theories developed using grounded theory (GT) methodology (Glaser, 1978, 1998, 2001, 2005) can be used to enhance the effectiveness of the use of the model.

Walker and Avant (1995) describe a theory as "an internally consistent group of relational statements that present a systematic view about a phenomenon and that is useful for description, explanation, prediction, and/or control" (p. 26). Although theory developed from any type of research can be used to increase nursing knowledge and enhance practice, theories developed using GT are especially appropriate for use in the AIM because both GT research and the model have a similar orientation. In GT research, the researcher attempts to identify the main concern of the subjects and the patterns of behavior they use to resolve their main concern. In the AIM, the practitioner attempts to identify the main concern of either the client or the nurse and uses the process of the model to resolve the concern.

Ervin (2002) argues that middle range theories are more appropriate than abstract theories to use as a basis for developing interventions in the practice area. The middle range theories developed using the GT method are very useful because they provide insight into the patient concerns since they have been generated from actual experiences of client groups. Therefore, they are relevant to similar client situations. Ervin (2002) also gives criteria for evaluating a theory for practice. One criterion is the validity of the theory. Glaser (2001) states that grounded theories have external validity because they "fit the situations from which the theory was generated and can be generalized to other situations" (p. 13).

The major strength of the GT method is its ability to move data from the descriptive level to the conceptual level. This allows understanding about the resolution of a problem in a patient situation because the behavior of many patients experiencing the same situation has already been analyzed to identify patterns of behavior. Substantive grounded theories integrated by a core category offer explanations of how people living through a variety of health-related life situations resolve their main concern. These theories have relevance for the subjects in the study and the academic community because they fit the situation under study having been derived from observations and interviews with the participants. Therefore, they can be easily applied to practice. These theories can also explain the influence of societal interactions on outcomes including nurse–patient interactions and critical junctures that affect the processes of adaptation. Habermas (1971) describes this type of information about social life as practical knowledge based on interpretive understanding. Because GT research focuses on the actual experiences of patients or caregivers, the studies that have been reported can be used to guide practice with particular aggregates of patients.

Burns and Grove (1997) stated, "The expected outcome of nursing research activities is to improve nursing practice. In order for research to have an impact on practice, the findings of studies must be utilized by practitioners" (p. 671). However, many nurses see research as an esoteric enterprise and do not know how to apply research theories in their practice. Burns and Grove (1997) have also stated, "The utilization of nursing research knowledge needs to produce measurable, quality patient outcomes, in a variety of clinical settings" (p. 671). Using the AIM, information is collected from the client who is experiencing the health concern. Information is analyzed to measure the level of situational sense of coherence and develop a mutual plan of care. After implementation of the plan of care, the patient is again scored on the same measures, thus providing an objective measure of the success of the plan. When the plan of care is based on insights from theories, there is a greater likelihood that it will be successful in resolving the concern of the patient. The final rescoring on SSOC provides evidence about the helpfulness of the plan for the patient. If the final score is low, it indicates that the strategies were not successful and it is necessary to gather new information to start the process again. It also indicates that other theories should be considered to understand the patient behavior. By being familiar with a variety of theories, the nurse brings a wider repertoire of possibilities for finding solutions to patient concerns.

Although any nurse can use the process of the AIM, not every nurse pursues a career in research and develops theory. Therefore, it is important for practitioners to understand how the research findings of other researchers can be applied to enhance clinical practice. The use of theories to guide practice is beneficial for both the client and for the development of nursing knowledge. Ervin (2002) commented that using theories in practice is an actual test of the theory. This is the premise of the intervention mode of GT. In the introduction to the Intervention Mode Part IV of the book, *Glaserian Grounded Theory in Nursing Research* (Artinian, Giske, & Cone, 2009), Artinian writes, "The purpose of the Intervention Mode is to test and modify an existing theory while improving clinical practice. When the relationships among the variables are adequately conceptualized, an intervention can be designed to improve practice and refine and extend the theory" (p. 319). Four intervention studies were presented in the Glaserian research book. In this chapter, the theories of three of those intervention studies have been used for case studies that illustrate the use of GT in clinical situations. These examples offer insight into how theories developed in GT research can be applied for both intervention studies and in practice with clients.

The case studies developed from grounded theories presented in this chapter provide excellent examples of how research and practice can be integrated. To make them more useful, each theory is described using a conceptual map that depicts the theory. Ervin (2002) states that the method of describing the relationships in a conceptual map makes the theory more understandable. In fact, Ervin (2002) suggests that a conceptual map of a theory should be made before attempting to use the theory in practice.

Because of the widespread acceptance of the GT method of research, many studies are available for use by the practitioner. What is needed is an understanding of how they can be used by the practitioner. In this chapter, we present six GT studies that were published in the companion volume to this book, *Glaserian Grounded Theory in Nursing Research: Trusting Emergence* (Artinian, Giske, & Cone, 2009). For each study, we present the abstract of the study, the conceptual map that was developed to illustrate the relationships among the variables, and a care plan based on patient situations presented in the interviews that were used as data for developing the theory. The purpose of this chapter is to demonstrate how the understandings of the patient situation developed in the analysis of the research data can be used to guide practice in specific situations.

CARE PLAN BASED ON PRESERVING IDENTITY THEORY[1]

The following care plan is based on interviews conducted by Victoria Winter and Barbara Artinian at the Ararat Nursing Facility in Mission Hills, California, and reported in the study "Preserving Identity in a Nursing Home Setting" in *Glaserian Grounded Theory: Trusting Emergence* (Artinian, Giske, & Cone, 2009). Identifying details have been changed to protect the privacy of the resident.

Abstract of Preserving Identity Theory

Aim

The purpose of the study was to identify organizational practices that are used by the Ararat Nursing Facility to achieve quality patient care.

Background

The decision to surrender an elderly family member to the care of others can be a time of crisis for a family. The choice of a facility that the family can trust and depend on to provide care for the loved one is a difficult one. A facility that focuses on quality of life and quality of care is the Ararat Nursing Facility. It has received numerous awards for excellence in nursing home care and has developed the innovative Resident-Centered Care Model that is based on the AIM.

Method

Classical GT methodology developed by Glaser and Strauss (1967) and in the later writings of Glaser (1978, 1992) was utilized for this study. The researchers used open-ended interviewing to explore the concerns of the nursing staff and their relationships with the residents. The seven certified nursing assistants who participated in the study were asked about the relationships they formed with selected patients and how they worked together to provide quality care for all the residents.

Findings

The core category "Preserving Identity" emerged from analysis of the interviews and it integrated all of the categories. In order to understand the danger

---

[1] Used with permission from Victoria Winter.

to a sense of identity that occurs when a person enters a nursing home, we turned to Role Theory to help in structuring the data. Strategies such as ceremonializing role change, making mutual decisions, reinforcing the identity of the resident, and paying attention to individual preferences were used

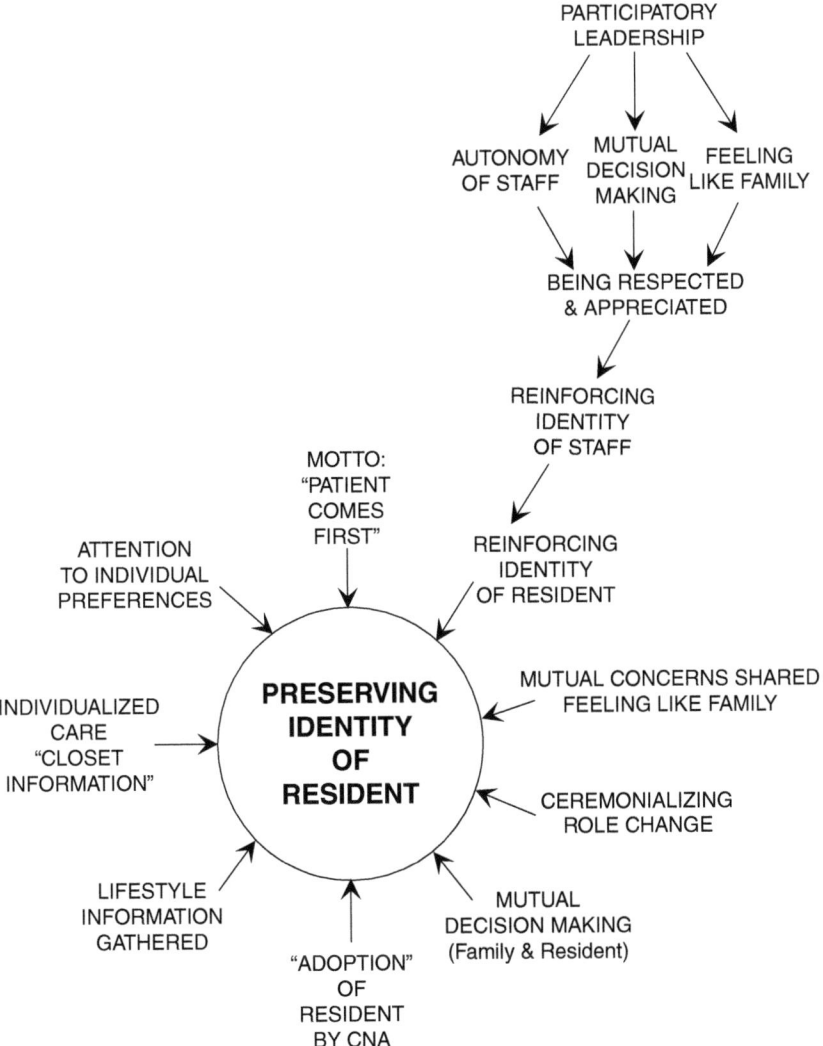

FIGURE 16.1 Conceptual map of Preserving Identity Theory.
Copyright © 2009 B. Artinian.

to preserve the identity of the resident in this role change. New nursing home residents must constantly negotiate their new role between themselves, the staff, and their family. Each individual tries to define the situation, choose a role that is advantageous or appealing, play that role, and persuade others to support it. Status and role represent conceptually the ideal patterns of behaviors that are to be expected in given situations. Nursing home residents must assume the status of a resident in a nursing home. To adjust to this new situation is to accept the fact that they are now patients.

Conclusion

Relatives involved with a family member experiencing a major role transition need to know the rights and obligations of the role and the behavior changes that the transition entails. For the residents at the Ararat Nursing Facility, their time in the nursing home becomes a rite of passage to a new role in life, where it matters to all who they are and how they can best live their final days. See Figure 16.1 for the conceptual map of this theory.

Introduction to Online Care Plan

A care plan was written addressing the problem of a resident who recently had entered a nursing home and who was having difficulty in accepting the resident role. The care plan illustrates the negotiation process used by the staff to maintain the resident's dignity and need for privacy and meet standards of safety. The full text of the care plan is available in the online adjunct manual.

CARE PLAN BASED ON PREPARATIVE WAITING THEORY[2]

The following care plan is based on interviews conducted by Tove Giske and reported in the research study "Patterns of balancing between hope and despair in the diagnostic phase on a gastroenterology ward" published in *Glaserian Grounded Theory: Trusting Emergence* (Artinian, Giske, & Cone, 2009). The name of the subject and certain aspects of demographic data have been changed to protect the privacy of the subjects.

---

[2] Used with permission from Tove Giske.

Abstract of Preparative Waiting Theory

Aim

The aim of this study is to present a GT "Preparative Waiting Theory" (PWT). This theory describes the experience of patients going through the diagnostic phase at a gastric ward and shows how the theoretical code of "balancing between hope and despair" integrates the theory. The intention is also to compare PWT with related research.

Background

Many studies report about the stressful diagnostic phase; however, none has presented a conceptual theory indicating how the concepts are sufficiently related to each other.

Method

The study used a classical GT design with data derived from 18 in-depth interviews with patients in a gastroenterology unit at a Norwegian University hospital. Interviews were conducted during 2002–2003.

Findings

Participants' main concern was found to be how they could prepare themselves for the diagnostic interview and life after diagnosis. The TC of balancing had four patterns: controlling pain, rational awaiting, denial, and accepting. These patterns of balancing demonstrated how participants used the categories of PWT: *seeking and giving information, interpreting clues, handling existential threats*, and *seeking respite* to resolve their main concern. Patterns were strategies, so one person could use more than one pattern.

Conclusion

The diagnostic phase was a difficult time for patients. PWT can assist nurses in assessing how patients prepare themselves differently for getting a diagnosis. All patients would find it helpful to be followed up by a designated contact person at the ward; however, patients who used the patterns of controlling pain and denial would benefit most from such support. See Figure 16.2 for the conceptual map of this theory.

Introduction to Online Care Plan

A care plan was written illustrating a patient took the initiative to get the information she needed to prepare for the final diagnostic meeting with the

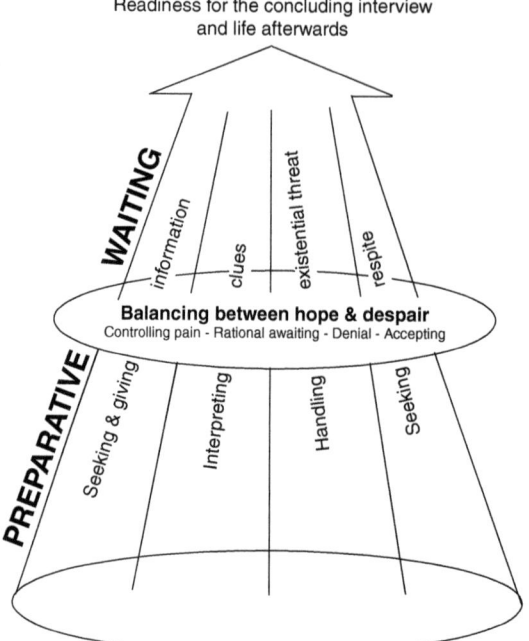

FIGURE 16.2 Conceptual map of Preparative Waiting Theory.
Copyright © 2009 T. Giske.

physician. She did this by negotiating with the nurse in charge of her care to receive information in a timely manner. The full text of the care plan is available in the online adjunct manual.

CARE PLAN BASED ON LETTING GO THEORY[3]

The following care plan is based on interviews conducted by Lynda Pash with hospice patients. The theory of "Letting Go" was developed from these interviews and was reported in the chapter "Letting go: the experience of dying from cancer in young middle age" in *Glaserian Grounded Theory: Trusting Emergence* (Artinian, Giske, & Cone, 2009). Identifying details have been changed to protect the privacy of the subject.

---

[3] Used with permission from Lynda Pash.

Abstract of Letting Go Theory

Aim

The purpose of this study was to examine the experiences of young middle-aged hospice cancer patients. The purpose was to learn from adults between the ages of 35 and 55 about the experience of dying "out of synchrony" or "out of time."

Background

Although there are studies of the dying experiences of pediatric and elderly patients, no studies were found targeting this age group.

Method

This was a qualitative study using GT methodology. Sixteen patients from three Southern California hospices were interviewed using an interview guide with broad, open-ended questions. The interviews were taped and transcribed. Content analysis was used to identify themes and categories, with constant comparative analysis occurring simultaneously with data collection.

Findings

A basic social process entitled "letting go" emerged. This theory describes an eight-stage developmental process by which study respondents let go of their lives. After *Awareness of Physical Changes and Failing Health*, respondents experienced *Loss of Control and Independence*. *Acceptance of Death* followed, leading to *Increased Closeness and a Desire for Openness*. Respondents made *Internal Preparations*. *Relinquishing Responsibilities* and *Finishing Things* were late stages. During *Looking Beyond*, the final stage, respondents withdrew from active participation in life. Though dying at a relatively young age, out of sync with normal expectations, the respondents were able to accomplish the tasks of old age. They seemed to condense many years of gradually *letting go* into a brief period of weeks or months.

Conclusion

Middle-aged cancer patients who are dying can reach the developmental goals of old age. See Figure 16.3 for the conceptual map of this theory.

Introduction to Online Care Plan

A care plan was written illustrating the way a hospice nurse was able to prepare the daughters for the death of their father. The nurse did this by providing

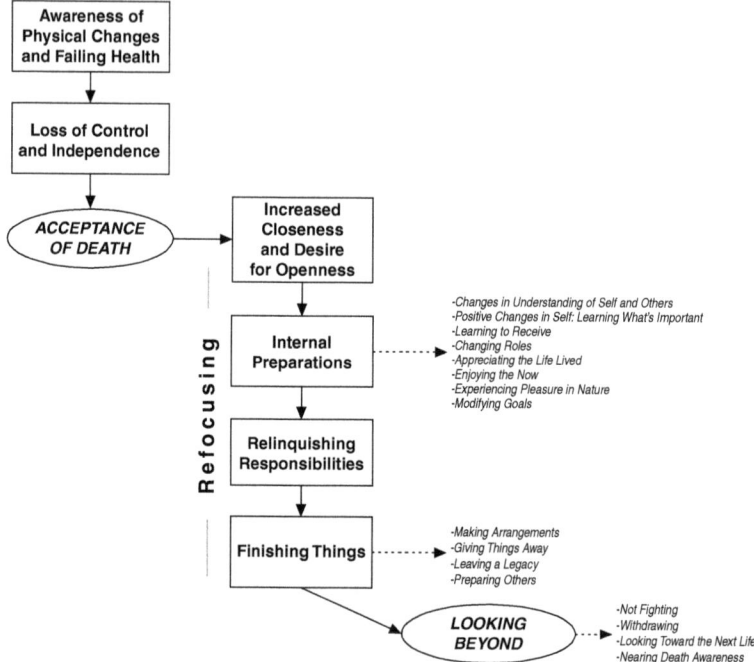

FIGURE 16.3 Conceptual map of Letting Go Theory.
Copyright © 2009 L. Pash.

comfort and knowledge about the dying process. The full text of the care plan is available in the online adjunct manual.

CARE PLAN BASED ON POSITIONING IN OPERATIONAL SPACE[4]

The following care plan is based on interviews conducted by Esther Hjälmhult with students in the public health nursing program in Norway. The theory of "Conquering Operational Space" was developed from these interviews and was reported in the chapter "Positioning in Operational Space" in *Glaserian Grounded Theory: Trusting Emergence* (Artinian, Giske, & Cone, 2009). Details have been changed to protect the privacy of the subjects.

---

[4] Used with permission from Esther Hjälmhult.

Abstract of Conquering Operational Space Theory

Aim

The purpose of this study was to develop understanding of how public health nursing students learn in clinical practice, identify the main concern for the students, and how they acted to resolve this main concern.

Background

How professionals perform their work directly affects individuals, but knowledge is lacking in understanding how learning is connected to clinical practice in public health nursing and in other professions.

Method

GT was used in gathering and analyzing data from 55 interviews and 108 weekly reports. The participants were 21 registered nurses who were public health nursing students.

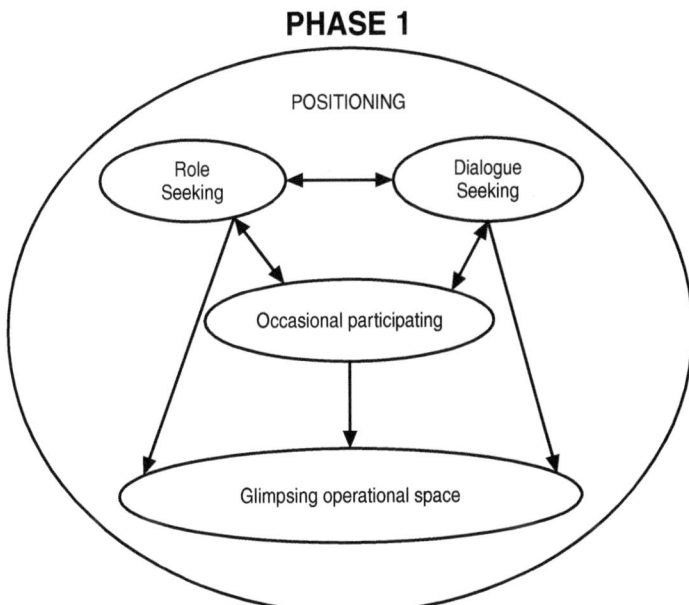

FIGURE 16.4 Conceptual map of Positioning in Conquering Operational Space Theory.
Copyright © 2009 E. Hjälmhult.

Findings

The GT of "conquering operational space" explains how the students work to resolve their main concern. A social process with three identified phases, *positioning, involving,* and *integrating,* was generated from analyzing the data. The subcategories and dimensions of these phases are related to the student role, relations with a supervisor, student activity, and the consequences of each phase. Public health nursing students had to work toward gaining independence, often working against "the system" and managing tension by taking a risk. Many of them lost, changed, and expanded their professional identity during practical placements.

Conclusion

Public health nursing students' learning processes in clinical training is complex and dynamic and the theory of "conquering operational space" can assist supervisors in further developing their role in relation to guiding students in practice. Relationships are one key to opening or closing access to situations of learning and directly affect the students' achievement of mastering operational space. See Figure 16.4 for the conceptual map of this theory.

Introduction to Online Care Plan

A care plan was written illustrating the organization of behaviors of a public health nursing student and her nurse supervisor when the student was afraid that her knowledge base was inadequate to work with a patient. The full text of the care plan is available in the online adjunct manual.

CARE PLAN BASED ON CAREGIVING BEHAVIORS OF INTRAPARTUM NURSES STUDY[5]

The following care plan is based on interviews conducted by Maureen Friesen and reported in the research study "Caregiving Behaviors of Intrapartum Nurses" published in *Glaserian Grounded Theory: Trusting Emergence* (Artinian, Giske, & Cone, 2009). The names of the subjects and certain aspects of demographic data have been changed to protect the privacy of the participants.

---

[5] Used with permission from Maureen Friesen.

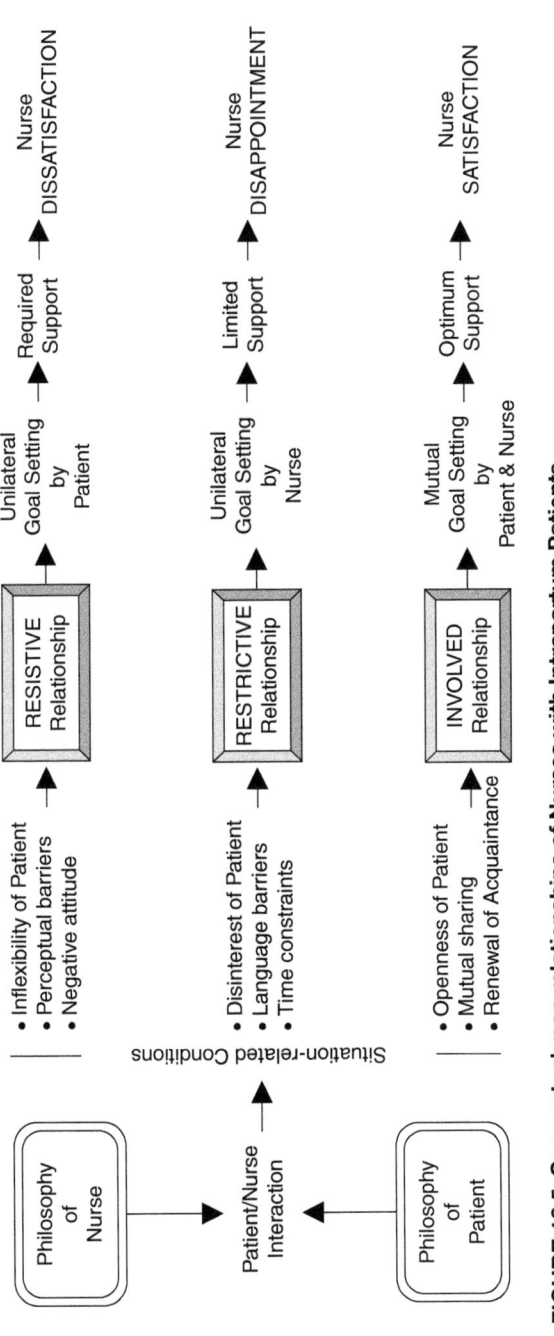

FIGURE 16.5 Conceptual map relationships of Nurses with Intrapartum Patients.
Copyright © 2009 M. Friesen.

Abstract of Caregiving Behaviors Descriptive Study

Aim

The purpose of the study was to better understand how intrapartum nurses perceived their caregiver behaviors during the labor process.

Background

Information was desired to understand the relationship between intrapartum nurses and their patients in a tertiary care medical center.

Method

An exploratory descriptive design was used. Data were analyzed using the constant comparative approach of the GT method (Glaser, 1978). Interviews were conducted with the nurses either at the hospital or in their homes. The participants were 12 intrapartum nurses between the ages of 31 and 60 with 11–25 years of obstetrical experience. They were recruited from a nonprofit, private, tertiary-level referral hospital in the Southwest, which had an average of 4,000 deliveries per year.

Findings

It was found that variations in care resulted from the type of nurse–patient relationship that developed in the caregiving encounter. Three distinct types of relationships emerged: (1) *resistive relationships*, (2) *restrictive relationships*, and (3) *involved relationships*.

Conclusion

In order for a satisfying nurse–patient relationship to be established, several factors need to be considered. First, the patient needs to be the nurse's focus, not the task. Second, there needs to be time for relationship development, and third, there must be a rapport between the nurse and patient so that mutual plans for caregiving can be developed. See Figure 16.5 for the conceptual map of this theory.

Introduction to Online Care Plan

A care plan was written illustrating the failure of the negotiating process. When the value systems of the patient and nurse are in conflict, no mutual plan of care could be made. The full text of the care plan is available in the online adjunct manual.

CARE PLAN BASED ON RECONNECTING THEORY[6]

The following care plan is based on interviews conducted by Pamela Cone and reported in the research study "Mutuality: Reconnecting to Overcome Homelessness" published in *Glaserian Grounded Theory in Nursing Research: Trusting Emergence* (Artinian, Giske, & Cone, 2009). The names of the subjects and certain aspects of demographic data have been changed to protect the privacy of the participants.

Abstract of Reconnecting Theory

Aim

The aim of this study was to explore the experience of formerly homeless mothers to discover the process whereby they overcame their homelessness. The aim of this study is to present a GT "Reconnecting Theory" (RT) of homeless mothers.

Background

Homelessness is a worldwide phenomenon that continues to increase every year. The most rapidly growing segment of the homeless population is single mothers with at least two small children. Many studies report the conditions of homelessness, but few have looked at getting out of homelessness from the perspective of those experiencing it. Understanding how these overcame homelessness can inform the practice of those who serve the homeless.

Method

The study used a classical GT design with data derived from 18 in-depth interviews with homeless mothers and 12 first-hand reports in the literature. Interviews were conducted during 2003–2006. Constant comparative analysis began with the first interview and continued identification of the main concern and the selecting of the categories through the saturation of categories and theoretical sampling.

Findings

Participants told their stories of becoming homeless, surviving homelessness, and overcoming homelessness. The main concern of the participants was found to be getting off the streets into stable housing for the sake of their children. The process they used to accomplish this resolved this concern and

---

[6] Used with permission from Pamela H. Cone.

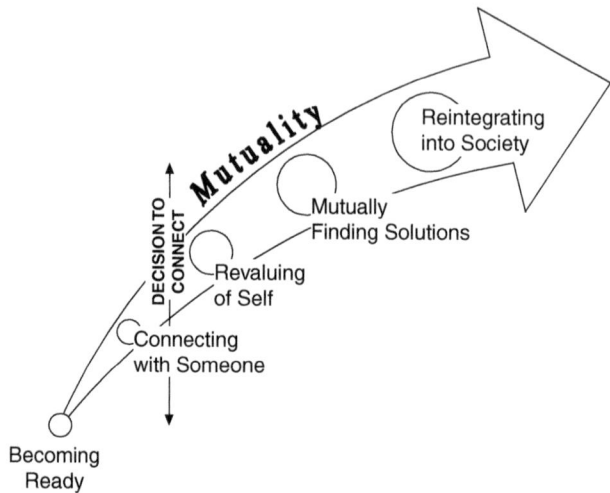

FIGURE 16.6 Conceptual map of Reconnecting Theory.
Copyright © 2009 P. H. Cone.

moved these women toward integration into mainstream society. The steps of the process were "Connecting with Someone," "Revaluing of Self," "Finding Solutions," and "Reintegrating into Society." Developing a mutual connection with one genuinely caring person was the key to reconnecting with society and overcoming homelessness.

Conclusion

The process of reconnecting enabled homeless mothers to come to a decision point and begin the mutual process of making choices, revaluing self, strategizing solutions to problems, and getting into a home and reinvesting into society. This one-on-one process is simple in execution but profound impact. Through the use of the principles of RT, caring people can bring about transformational change in the lives of homeless mothers as they mutually negotiate their plan of care. See Figure 16.6 for the conceptual map of this theory.

Introduction to Online Care Plan

A care plan was written illustrating how Serena, the mother of a teenage girl, and a nurse mutually negotiated the process of reconnecting to overcome homelessness through the revaluing of self. The full text of the care plan is available in the online adjunct manual.

REFERENCES

Antonovsky, A. (1987). *Unraveling the mysteries of health: How people manage stress and stay well*. San Francisco, CA: Jossey-Bass.

Artinian, B. M., Giske, T., & Cone, P. H. (2009). *Glaserian grounded theory: Trusting emergence*. New York, NY: Springer Publishing.

Blumer, H. (1969). *Symbolic interactionism*. Englewood Cliffs, NJ: Prentice Hall.

Burns, N., & Grove, S. (1997). *The practice of nursing research: Conduct, critique, & utilization* (3rd ed.). Philadelphia, PA: W.B. Saunders Company.

Chin, R. (1969). The utility of system models and developmental models for practitioners. In W. Bennis, K., Benne, & R. Chin, *The planning of change* (pp. 297–312). New York, NY: Holt, Rinehart & Winston, Inc.

Ervin, N. E. (2002). *Advanced community health nursing practice: Population-focused care*. Upper Saddle River, NJ: Prentice-Hall.

Glaser, B. B., & Strauss, A. L. (1967). *The discovery of grounded theory: Strategies for qualitative research*. Hawthorne, NY: Aldine de Gruyter.

Glaser, B. G. (1978). *Theoretical sensitivity*. Mill Valley, CA: Sociology Press.

Glaser, B. G. (1992). *Basics of grounded theory analysis*. Mill Valley, CA: Sociology Press.

Glaser, B. G. (1998). *Doing grounded theory: Issues and discussions*. Mill Valley, CA: Sociology Press.

Glaser, B. G. (2001). *The grounded theory perspective: Conceptualization contrasted with description*. Mill Valley, CA: Sociology Press.

Glaser, B. G. (2005). *The grounded theory perspective III: Theoretical coding*. Mill Valley, CA: Sociology Press.

Habermas, J. (1971). *Knowledge and human interest*. Boston, MA: Beacon Press.

Hill, R. (1949). *Families under stress*. New York, NY: Harper & Row.

Knickrehm, B. (1994, August). *The origins of inequality: A theoretical synthesis*. Paper presented at the 1994 American Sociological Association Meeting, Los Angeles, CA.

Kuhn, A. (1974). *The logic of social systems: A unified deductive, system-based approach to social science*. San Francisco, CA: Jossey-Bass.

Stallwood, J., & Stoll, R. (1975). Spiritual dimensions of nursing practice, Part C. In I. Beland & J. Passos (Eds.), *Clinical nursing* (3rd ed., pp. 1086–1098). New York, NY: Macmillan.

Walker, L. O., & Avant, K. C. (1994). *Strategies for theory construction in nursing* (3rd ed.). Upper Saddle River, NJ: Prentice Hall.

Appendix A: AIM Block Care Plan Template for Undergraduate Students

DEVELOPMENTAL ENVIRONMENT[1]

COLLECTION OF INTRASYSTEM DATA TO IDENTIFY MAIN CONCERN		
Describe Focus of Interaction		
Assess Organizational Memory		
Assess Patient Subsystems Biological Subsystem		
Psychosocial Subsystem		
Spiritual Subsystem		

[1] See Figure 1.8
Copyright © 2011 B. Artinian, PhD. From *The Artinian Intersystem Model: Integrating Theory and Practice for Professional Nursing*, 2nd ed. New York, NY: Springer Publishing. May use with permission.

Tentative Identification of Main Concern of Patient or Nurse	
ASSESSMENT OF INTRASYSTEM FUNCTIONS RELATED TO MAIN CONCERN	
Intrasystem Data Collection About the Patient	**Intrasystem Analysis Data Collection About the Nurse**
Knowledge What does the patient know about the Main Concern?	Knowledge What do I know about the Main Concern?
Attitudes and Values What are the patient's attitudes and values about the Main Concern?	Attitudes and Values What are my attitudes and values about the Main Concern?
Behaviors What skills or resources does the patient have to deal with the Main Concern?	Behaviors What skills or resources do I have to deal with the Main Concern?
Validation of Main Concern of Patient or Nurse	

Copyright © 2011 B. Artinian, PhD. From *The Artinian Intersystem Model: Integrating Theory and Practice for Professional Nursing*, 2nd ed. New York, NY: Springer Publishing. May use with permission.

SITUATIONAL ENVIRONMENT

ANALYSIS OF INTRASYSTEM INFORMATION BY NURSE	
Identify Stressors of Patient	
Identify Coping Resources of Patient	
Score Patient on Situational Sense of Coherence (SSOC) (high = 3, medium = 2, or low = 1)	SCORE
Comprehensibility: In relation to what the patient needs to know about the Main Concern, how much is known?	
Meaningfulness: In relation to motivation, how much effort is the patient willing to put into resolving the Main Concern?	
Manageability: In relation to resources, what is available to manage this Main Concern?	

Copyright © 2011 B. Artinian, PhD. From *The Artinian Intersystem Model: Integrating Theory and Practice for Professional Nursing*, 2nd ed. New York, NY: Springer Publishing. May use with permission.

State Nursing Diagnosis/es	
Identify Goals to Increase SSOC	
Assess Ability of Patient and Nurse to Work Together to Resolve Main Concern	
INTERSYSTEM INTERACTION TO RESOLVE MAIN CONCERN	
Communicate Information	
Negotiate Values	
Develop Mutual Plan of Care	
Develop Joint Goals	
Develop Joint Objectives	
Develop Implementation Strategies	

Copyright © 2011 B. Artinian, PhD. From *The Artinian Intersystem Model: Integrating Theory and Practice for Professional Nursing*, 2nd ed. New York, NY: Springer Publishing. May use with permission.

Implement Strategies

EVALUATION OF THE RESOLUTION OF MAIN CONCERN

Re-score Patient on SSOC (high = 3, medium = 2, or low = 1)	SCORE	
Comprehensibility: In relation to what the patient needed to know about the Main Concern, how much was learned?		I did this: Because: It was/wasn't effective.
Meaningfulness: In relation to motivation, how much effort did the patient put into resolving the Main Concern?		I did this: Because: It was/wasn't effective.
Manageability: In relation to resources, what was available to manage the Main Concern?		I did this: Because: It was/wasn't effective.

Copyright © 2011 B. Artinian, PhD. From *The Artinian Intersystem Model: Integrating Theory and Practice for Professional Nursing*, 2nd ed. New York, NY: Springer Publishing. May use with permission.

Appendix B: AIM Community Health Care Plan Template

DEVELOPMENTAL ENVIRONMENT[1]

COLLECTION OF INTRASYSTEM DATA TO IDENTIFY MAIN CONCERN		
Describe Focus of Interaction		
Assess Community Memory		

Assess National Memory
    HP2020[2] Focus Area
    HP2020 Indicator
    HP2020 Objective		

[1] See Figure 1.8
[2] Healthy People 2020 – http://www.healthypeople.gov

Copyright © 2011 B. Artinian, PhD. From *The Artinian Intersystem Model: Integrating Theory and Practice for Professional Nursing*, 2nd ed. New York, NY: Springer Publishing. May use with permission.

Assess Community Subsystems

Physical/Biological Subsystem (Geography, Transportation, Health Agencies, Community Resources)

Psychosocial Subsystem (Cultural Networks, Social Resources)

Values/Spiritual Subsystem (Mission Statements, Beliefs and Values, Religious Groups)

Tentative Identification of Main Concern of Community

ASSESSMENT OF INTRASYSTEM FUNCTIONS RELATED TO MAIN CONCERN

Intrasystem Data Collection About the Community	Intrasystem Data Collection About the Nurse
Knowledge What does the community know about the Main Concern?	Knowledge What do I know about the Main Concern?
Attitudes and Values What are the community's attitudes and values about the Main Concern?	Attitudes and Values What are my attitudes and values about the Main Concern?
Behaviors What skills or resources does the community have to deal with the Main Concern?	Behaviors What skills or resources do I have to deal with the Main Concern?

Validation of Main Concern of Community or Public Health Nurse

Copyright © 2011 B. Artinian, PhD. From *The Artinian Intersystem Model: Integrating Theory and Practice for Professional Nursing*, 2nd ed. New York, NY: Springer Publishing. May use with permission.

SITUATIONAL ENVIRONMENT

ANALYSIS OF INTRASYSTEM INFORMATION

Identify Stressors in the Community	
Identify Coping Resources Available in the Community	
Score Community on Situational Sense of Coherence (SSOC) (high = 3, medium = 2, or low = 1)	SCORE
Comprehensibility: In relation to what the community needs to know about the Main Concern, how much is known?	
Meaningfulness: In relation to motivation, how much effort is the community willing to put into resolving the Main Concern?	
Manageability: In relation to resources, what is available to the community to manage the Main Concern?	

Copyright © 2011 B. Artinian, PhD. From *The Artinian Intersystem Model: Integrating Theory and Practice for Professional Nursing*, 2nd ed. New York, NY: Springer Publishing. May use with permission.

State Community Nursing Diagnosis (At Risk of _____, Among _____, Related to _____)	
Identify Goals to Increase SSOC	
Assess Ability of Community and Public Health Nurse to Work Together to Resolve Main Concern	
INTERSYSTEM INTERACTION TO RESOLVE MAIN CONCERN	
Communicate Information	
Negotiate Values	
Develop Mutual Plan of Care	
Develop Joint Goals	
Develop Joint Objectives	
Develop Implementation Strategies	
Implement Strategies	

Copyright © 2011 B. Artinian, PhD. From *The Artinian Intersystem Model: Integrating Theory and Practice for Professional Nursing*, 2nd ed. New York, NY: Springer Publishing. May use with permission.

EVALUATION OF THE RESOLUTION OF MAIN CONCERN
Interim evaluations of the community's progress may be needed.

Re-Score Community/Client on SSOC (high = 3, medium = 2, or low = 1)	SCORE	
Comprehensibility: In relation to what the community needed to know about the Main Concern, how much was learned?		I did this: Because: It was/wasn't effective (circle one).
Meaningfulness: In relation to motivation, how much effort did the community put into resolving the Main Concern?		I did this: Because: It was/wasn't effective (circle one).
Manageability: In relation to resources, what was available to the community to manage the Main Concern?		I did this: Because: It was/wasn't effective (circle one).

Copyright © 2011 B. Artinian, PhD. From *The Artinian Intersystem Model: Integrating Theory and Practice for Professional Nursing*, 2nd ed. New York, NY: Springer Publishing. May use with permission. Developed by K. S. West.

Appendix C: AIM Standard Care Plan Template

DEVELOPMENTAL ENVIRONMENT[1]	
COLLECTION OF INTRASYSTEM DATA TO IDENTIFY MAIN CONCERN	
Describe Focus of Interaction	
Access Organizational Memory	
Assess Patient/Client Subsystems	
Biological Subsystem	
Psychosocial Subsystem	
Spiritual Subsystem	
Tentative Identification of Main Concern of Patient or Provider	
ASSESSMENT OF INTRASYSTEM FUNCTIONS RELATED TO MAIN CONCERN	
Intrasystem Data Collection About Patient/Client Related to Main Concern	
Knowledge	
Values	
Behaviors	

[1] See Figure 1.8

Copyright © 2011 B. Artinian, PhD. From *The Artinian Intersystem Model: Integrating Theory and Practice for Professional Nursing*, 2nd ed. New York, NY: Springer Publishing. May use with permission.

Intrasystem Data Collection About Nurse/Provider Related to Main Concern	
Knowledge	
Values	
Behaviors	
Validation of Main Concern of Patient/Client or Nurse/Provider	

SITUATIONAL ENVIRONMENT

ANALYSIS OF INTRASYSTEM INFORMATION BY NURSE

Identify Stressors of Patient	
Identify Coping Resources of Patient	

Score Patient on Situational Sense of Coherence (SSOC)
(high = 3, medium = 2, or low = 1)

	SCORE	
Comprehensibility		
Meaningfulness		
Manageability		
State Nursing Diagnosis/es		
Identify Goals to Increase SSOC		
Assess Ability of Patient and Nurse to Work Together to Resolve Main Concern		

INTERSYSTEM INTERACTION TO RESOLVE MAIN CONCERN

Communicate Information	
Negotiate Values	

Develop Mutual Plan of Care

Develop Joint Goals	
Develop Joint Objectives	

Copyright © 2011 B. Artinian, PhD. From *The Artinian Intersystem Model: Integrating Theory and Practice for Professional Nursing*, 2nd ed. New York, NY: Springer Publishing. May use with permission.

Develop Implementation Strategies	
Implement Strategies	
EVALUATION OF THE RESOLUTION OF MAIN CONCERN	
Re-score Patient on SSOC (high = 3, medium = 2, or low = 1) SCORE	
Comprehensibility	
Meaningfulness	
Manageability	
Assess Effectiveness of Implementation Strategies	
Identify Strengths and Weaknesses of Implementation by Nurse	
Reassess Need for Further Interaction (select one of the following three options)	
Main Concern Is Not Resolved *Return to Intrasystem Data Collection and Care Plan Process.*	
Main Concern Is Resolved *Identification of New Main Concern.* *Start Over.*	
Main Concern Is Resolved *No Further Intervention.* *Storage of Information in Organizational Memory.*	

Copyright © 2011 B. Artinian, PhD. From *The Artinian Intersystem Model: Integrating Theory and Practice for Professional Nursing*, 2nd ed. New York, NY: Springer Publishing. May use with permission.

Appendix D: AIM Narrative Care Plan Template for Graduate Students

DEVELOPMENTAL ENVIRONMENT[1]

1. COLLECTION OF INTRASYSTEM DATA TO IDENTIFY MAIN CONCERN

- 1.1. Describe Focus of Interaction
- 1.2. Access Organizational Memory
- 1.3. Assess Patient/Client Subsystems
    - 1.3.1. Biological Subsystem
    - 1.3.2. Psychosocial Subsystem
    - 1.3.3. Spiritual Subsystem
- 1.4. Tentative Identification of Main Concern of Patient or Provider

2. ASSESSMENT OF INTRASYSTEM FUNCTIONS RELATED TO MAIN CONCERN

- 2.1. Intrasystem Data Collection About Patient/Client Related to Main Concern
    - 2.1.1. Knowledge
    - 2.1.2. Values
    - 2.1.3. Behaviors
- 2.2. Intrasystem Information About Nurse/Provider Related to Main Concern
    - 2.2.1. Knowledge
    - 2.2.2. Values
    - 2.2.3. Behaviors
- 2.3. Validation of Main Concern of Patient/Client or Nurse/Provider

---

[1] See Figure 1.8

Copyright © 2011 B. Artinian, PhD. From *The Artinian Intersystem Model: Integrating Theory and Practice for Professional Nursing*, 2nd ed. New York, NY: Springer Publishing. May use with permission.

SITUATIONAL ENVIRONMENT

3. ANALYSIS OF INTRASYSTEM INFORMATION BY NURSE

- 3.1. Identify Stressors of Patient
- 3.2. Identify Coping Resources of Patient
- 3.3. Score Patient on Situational Sense of Coherence (SSOC) (high = 3, medium = 2, or low = 1)
    - 3.3.1. Comprehensibility
    - 3.3.2. Meaningfulness
    - 3.3.3. Manageability
- 3.4. State Nursing Diagnosis/es
- 3.5. Identify Goals to Increase SSOC
- 3.6. Assess Ability of Patient and Nurse to Work Together to Resolve Main Concern

4. INTERSYSTEM INTERACTION TO RESOLVE MAIN CONCERN

- 4.1. Communicate Information
- 4.2. Negotiate Values
- 4.3. Develop Mutual Plan of Care
    - 4.3.1. Develop Joint Goals
    - 4.3.2. Develop Joint Objectives
    - 4.3.3. Develop Implementation Strategies
- 4.4. Implement Strategies

5. EVALUATION OF RESOLUTION OF MAIN CONCERN

- 5.1. Re-score Patient on SSOC (high = 3, medium = 2, or low = 1)
    - 5.1.1. Comprehensibility
    - 5.1.2. Meaningfulness
    - 5.1.3. Manageability
- 5.2. Assess Effectiveness of Implementation Strategies
    - 5.2.1. Identify Strengths and Weaknesses of Implementation by Nurse
- 5.3. Reassess Need for Further Interaction (*select one of the following three options*)
    - 5.3.1. Main Concern Is Not Resolved
        Return to Intrasystem Data Collection and Care Plan Process.
    - 5.3.2. Main Concern Is Resolved
        Identification of New Main Concern. Start Over.
    - 5.3.3. Main Concern Is Resolved
        No Further Intervention. Storage of Information in Organizational Memory.

Copyright © 2011 B. Artinian, PhD. From *The Artinian Intersystem Model: Integrating Theory and Practice for Professional Nursing*, 2nd ed. New York, NY: Springer Publishing. May use with permission.

Index

Note: Page references followed by "*f*" and "*t*" denote figures and tables, respectively.

ABC-X model of family stress, 33, 76–77
Acute illnesses, and SOC, 36, 38–39
Adeniran, R. K., 51
Advanced practice nursing
  in acute care setting, 98
  in ambulatory setting, 201–206
  in case management, 231
  in long term care, 237
AIM. *See* Artinian
    Intersystem Model
Anesthesiologist, 20, 23–25
Angle of recovery, 33, 78
Antonovsky, A., 10, 13, 14, 15, 16, 31, 33,
    34, 35, 40, 42, 47, 49, 60, 70, 77,
    79, 152, 173, 209, 257
  adolescence, and SOC
    development, 50
  adulthood, young
    and SOC development, 50, 72
Ararat Nursing Facility, 238, 260
Artinian Intersystem Model (AIM),
    3–30, 12*f*, 18*f*, 209, 220. *See also*
    Intersystem model
  development of, 6–11
  early phases, 3–6
  environment, 13–15
    developmental environment, 13–14,
      49–57
    situational environment, 15, 59–66
  Main Concern, 17

Assistive personnel (AP), 207, 211, 213
Atkins, S., 139
Avant, K. C., 257
Azusa Pacific University School of
    Nursing (APU-SON), 147–171
  adoption of AIM, 152–153
  approach to introducing models,
    163–164
  graduate nursing education at APU,
    159–160
  lesson plan for teaching the AIM,
    160–163
  philosophy of, 148–149
  undergraduate nursing education,
    153–159

Benner, Patricia, 64, 135, 137,
    139, 141, 167, 182, 183,
    216, 217
Bevis, E., 136, 137
Biological subsystem
  of community, 107*f*
  of family, 69–70, 70*t*
  of institutions, 83, 94
  of person, 13, 52–53
    assessment of, 54*t*
  of nation, 107*f*
  of state, 107*f*
Blumer, H., 13, 14, 64, 257
Boswell, C., 141

294   Index

Boyer, Ernest, 149–152
  centrality of language, 150
  climate for creative learning, 151–152
  climate that affirms the building of character for every student, 152
  curriculum with coherence, 151
  5 Priorities for Quality Schools, 149
  sense of community, 150
Budding RN (B-RN) program, 90–100. *See also* Citrus Valley Health Partners
Burundi, 173–175, 179

Cannon, S., 141
Caregiving behaviors of intrapartum nurses descriptive theory, abstract and conceptual map of, 65, 268–270
Case studies, 120–131, 186–195
  Bond, Margaret, 192–193
  Evangelista, Abigail, 125–126
  Hardianto, Antonius, 120–122
  Kirschner, Elena, 194–195
  Martinez, Vince, 188–191
  Ratliff, Darya, 127–128
  Song-Howe, Michelle, 122–124
  Stilley, Amy M., 186–187
Care plans, 7, 20, 56, 79
  Illustrating Resolution of Main Concern of Patient, Care Plan 1.1, 23–25
  Illustrating Resolution of Main Concern of Nurse, Care Plan 1.2, 25–30
  Illustrating Resolution of Main Concern of Institution, 93–100
  introductions to online care plans, 56, 79, 205, 255, 262
    Artinian, Barbara, 255
    Barkman, Mary, 56
    Brownell, Beverly, 79
    Cone, Pamela, 271

Erdmann-Nell, Christine, 205
Friesen, Maureen, 268
Giske, Tove, 262
Hjalmhult, Esther, 266
Pash, Lynda, 264
Winter, Victoria, 260
templates,
  AIM Block Care Plan, 275–279, & online
  AIM Care Plan, 287–288, & online
  AIM Care Plan Narrative Outline, 289–290, & online
  AIM Community Health Care Plan, 281–285, & online
Carter, E., 72, 73*t*
Certified nursing assistant (CNA) career ladder, 237, 239, 241
  primary care program, 242–243
  recognition program, 243–245
Change agent. *See* Nurse
  characteristics of, 60–61
  setting, 62–63
  interaction, 64
Children/childhood
  and SOC development, 49
  worldview of, 56
Chin, Robert
  Intersystem Model, 4, 5*f*
Chronic health conditions, 37*t*
Citrus Valley Health Partners, 92
Citrus Valley Health Partners, Mentorship, and Professional Development Program (CVHP MAP^{sm}), 93
Citrus Valley Medical Center (CVMC), 90, 92. *See also* Budding RN program
Clinical Analysis Record, 3–4, 7
Clinical learning, theories used in, 135–138
Clinical reasoning, 141–142
Closed-type families, 75
Cognitive learning theory, 136
Cognitive subsystem, 53

Communication, 60
  in management, 82, 82*f*
Community as client, 103–131
  case studies, 120–131
  definition of, 106
  public health nursing
    comparison with community health nursing, 104–106, 105*t*
    dimensions of, 104–109
    practice models, 109, 112
Community health care plan template, 281–285
Comprehensibility, 16, 32, 35, 96–97, 100, 103, 225. *See also* Sense of coherence (SOC)
Conquering operational space theory, abstract and conceptual map of, 267–268
Coping
  resources, identification of, 96. *See also* Generalized resistance resources (GRRs)
  strategies, definition of, 15
  successful, SOC and, 33–34
Cosmetic nursing practice, 203–205
Crisis, 36
  definition of, 33
Critical thinking, 137–138
Cultural brokering, 87–88
Cultural competence, definition of, 51
Cultural values
  organizational, 86–87
  personal, 85–86
Culture
  definition of, 50
  and delivery of care, 56
  and SOC development, 50–51

Davidhizar, R., 56
Delegation, definition of, 207–208
Delegation decision making, 207
  algorithm, 216*f*
  effective, learning, 208
  model for learning, 209
  Nursing Assessment Decision Grid (NADG), 211
    follow-up activities, 217
    outcome assessment, 216–217
    scoring strategies, 211–214
    teaching delegation skills, 214–216
Developmental environment, 13–14, 17, 49–51, 106, 109, 275, 281–282, 289
  definition of, 13–14
  institutions, 93–95
  assessment of, 82–87
Developmental tasks, family, 73–74
Disability
  and SOC, 38
  psychological consequences, 43–44
Divorced families, development cycle, 72, 73*t*
Doctor–nurse game, 86
Duvall, E., 71–72

Educational program development, 147, 149, 151, 153, 159, 164, 175. *See also* Azusa Pacific University; Citrus Valley Health Partners; Hope Africa University
Effective leader, 84
Environment, 13–15
  definition of, 13–14
  developmental, 13–14
  of health care setting, 63
  situational, 15
Ervin, Naomi, 257, 258, 259
Ethical concerns, intersystem interaction, 89–90
Ethical decisions, 89
Evidence-based practice (EBP), 135, 139–141

Facione, N., 138
Facione, P., 138

Family
- as client, 69–79
  - family developmental theory, 71–74
  - family stress theory, 76–79
  - SSOC theory of recovery, 77–79
- definition of, 69
- life cycle of divorce, 72, 73*t*
- orientation to life, 70
  - subsystems, 69–70, 70*t*
  - types, 74–75, 75*t*

Family developmental theory, 71–74
Family making theory, abstract and conceptual map of, 69, 253–254
Family stress theory, 76–79
Friesen, Maureen, 65, 268, 269*f*
Futility, principle of, 89

Gadow, S., 86
Gagne, R., 136, 137
Gender, workforce, 83
Generalized resistance resources (GRRs), 33, 40, 70, 72
Giger, J., 56
Glaser, Barney, 258, 260
Glaserian Grounded Theory, 257, 258. *See also* Grounded theory studies
- intervention mode, 259

Gordon, M., 182
Grounded theory (GT), 257, 258, 259
- Cone, Pamela, 153, 160, 271
- Friesen, Maureen, 65, 268
- Giske, Tove, 262
- Hjalmhult, Esther, 266
- Pash, Lynda, 264
- Vuckovich, Paula, 19–20
- Winter, Victoria, 69, 253, 260

Group culture, 86

Health, 15–16
Health care, and SOC, 36–39, 37*t*
Health policies, 83
Health promotion
- across community, 112–117
- at local level, 117
- in multilevel comprehensive integrated program, 113–117

Heart Failure Outreach Patient Program (HFOPP), 219, 231
- power distribution, 226–229
- salutogenic model, using, 221
- situational sense of coherence (SSOC), strengthening, 224–225
- SOC level, identifying and strengthening, 225–226
- specific interventions of, 220

Hierarchy of Intrasystems, 107*f*
Hill, R., 71, 76, 78
- ABC-X Model, 33
- SSOC Theory of Recovery, 36*f*, 78*f*

Hope Africa University (HAU), 173
- Bachelors of Science Nursing (BSN) program, 175–179
- Masters of Science in Nursing (MSN) program, 177–179
- required courses, 177*t*
- course outline based on Intersystem Model (1987) for "Readings in Nursing Theory, Practice, and Research," 178*t*
- philosophy of, 176

Howell, T., 86
Human body, subsystems, 52
Human relationships, workers, 84

Illness
- experience, SSOC in understanding, 34–35, 36–39, 37*f*
- meaning of, 64

Individual boundaries, 74
Individual learning styles, 214–215
Inequality of power, 60, 61
Infancy, and SOC development, 49
Information, communication of, 97–98
In-service education, 90
- worksheet for, 91–92*t*

Institutional leadership theory, 81–82

Institution as client, 81–101
　AIM, application of, 90–93
　care plan, 93
Interaction
　characteristics, 64
　failure of, 65
　intersystem. *See* Intersystem interaction
Interactive nursing. *See* Mutuality
Interpersonal relationships, 4
Interpersonal subsystem
　boundaries, 74
Intersystem interaction, 3, 13, 15, 81
　cultural brokering, 87
　ethical concerns, 89–90
　families, 78–79
　government, 118–119*t*
　institutions, 87–90, 97–100
　　negotiation, 87–89
　polarity management, 88, 88*f*
Intersystem Model (1997), 10*f*, 16–17.
　　See also Artinian Intersystem
　　Model (AIM)
　characteristics of, 4, 5*f*
　development of, 6–11
　Hope Africa University, 173, 176,
　　177, 178
　nursing process in
　　implementing, 11*f*
　transition to AIM, 11–13
Intervention programs, development
　to increase SOC, 42–47
Intrasystem analysis, 15, 16–17, 65
Intrasystem(s)
　data collection
　　about client, 94–95
　　about provider, 95
　functions (knowledge, values,
　　behaviors)
　　of families, 79
　　of institutions, 94–95
　　of persons, 38
　　of public health clients, 114–115*t*
　hierarchy of, 107*f*

information, analysis, 96
　overview, 16–17
Involvement, context of, 59–66. *See also*
　Situational environment

Jezewski, M., 87
Johnson, B., 88

Kantor, D., and Lehr, W.
　family types, 74–75, 75*t*
Knickrehm, B., 61
Knowledgeable client, 38*f*, 39
Knowledgeable nurse, 38*f*, 39
Kuhn, Alfred, 6–7, 16, 52, 79, 81,
　152, 162

Leadership, 81–82, 83–84
　person-centered, 84
　task-oriented, 84
Learning
　theories, 135
　typology, 136–137
Leininger, M., 50
Letting go theory, abstract and
　conceptual map of, 264–266
Life-threatening illness, and SOC, 38

Main concern, 13, 15, 17, 20, 23–30, 60,
　66, 78–79, 94–95, 97–100, 109,
　112, 116, 117, 120, 122, 125, 127,
　143, 151, 155, 158, 201, 209, 257,
　263, 271, 279, 285, 287
　identification of, 55,
　negotiated Plan of Care, 153
　resolution of
　　client and provider's ability to
　　　work together, 97
　　evaluation of, 100. *See also* SSOC,
　　　rescoring of; SSOC, scoring of
　　nurse–patient interaction, 64–65
Malloch, K., 82, 84
Manageability, 16, 32, 35, 97, 100,
　103, 225. *See also* SOC

Management, structure, 82, 82f
Manthey, M., 211
Matheney, R., 3
McCarthy, B., 214, 215
McCarthy, D., 214, 215
McCown, Darlene, 173
McCubbin, H., 71, 77, 78
McCubbin, M., 71, 77, 78
McGoldrick, M., 72, 73t
Meaningfulness, 16, 32, 35, 97, 100, 103, 225. *See also* SOC
Miller, B., 71–72
Model as map, 18f, 164
Murray, K., 139
Mutuality in clinical practice, 64, 181–197
  interactive nursing, 181–183
  teaching methodology, 183–196

Nation, as client. *See* Community as client
Negotiated order, 62–63, 62f
  and social order, 63
Negotiation context, 62
Neumann, T., 211
Newborn Hearing Screening Program (NHSP), 116
  intersystem interactions in, 118–119t
Northern Arizona University, 181
Nurse
  characteristics, 60–61
  knowledgeable, 38f, 39
Nurse–patient relationship, 65
Nurse–patient interaction
  to resolve main concern, 64–65
Nursing action, 16–17, 19–20
Nursing assessment decision grid (NADG), use of, 209, 210t, 211
Nursing problem, definition of, 4
Nursing Process Systems Model 9f

Open-type families, 76
Organizational culture, 85–87
  levels of, 85
Orlando, I. J., 181–182, 196, 197

Parsons, L., 207, 208, 214, 216
Pathogenic model of treatment, characteristics of, 40–41
Person, 8, 8f, 13
  subsystems of, 13, 51–54, 54t
Personal cultural values, 85–86
Person-centered leadership, 84
Philosophies of graduate student nurses, 164–170
  Hull, Mary, 169–170
  Templeton, Sarah, 165–166
Plans of care. *See* Care plans
Polarity management, 88–89, 88f
Porter-O'Grady, T., 82, 84
Positioning in conquering operational space, Phase 1, abstract and conceptual map of, 266–268
Power, 60, 61
  distribution, 44–45, 226–227, 229
Preparative waiting theory (PWT), abstract and conceptual map of, 262–264
Preserving identity theory, abstract and conceptual map of, 260–262
Priorities for Quality Schools, 149–152
Problem prevention, 43, 222–223
Process, interaction, 62
Programs using AIM, 90–93, 237
  Ararat Nursing Facility, 237, 238, 241, 246
    Resident-Centered Care Model, 237, 246–252
  Citrus Valley Medical Center
    Budding RN, 92, 93
    Mentoring & Professional Development (MAP) Program, 93
  Saddleback Memorial Medical Center, 219
    Heart Failure Outreach Patient Program, 219
Provider, intrasystem data collection about, 95

Psychosocial subsystem
of community, 107f
of family, 69–70, 70t
of institutions, 83, 94
of person, 13, 52–53
assessment of, 54t
of nation, 107f
of state, 107f
Public health nursing. *See also*
Community as client
and community health nursing,
comparison, 104–106, 105t
dimensions of, 104–109

Reconnecting theory, abstract and
conceptual map of, 270–272
Reiss, David, 69
Resident-centered care program,
in long-term facility, 237
Family making: A Grounded Theory
Study, abstract of, 253–254
Taylor's recommendations, validation
of, 246–252
Resolution of Main Concern. *See* Main
Concern
Rodgers, R., 74
Saddleback Memorial Medical
Center, 219
Salutogenic model, 41, 43, 46, 221,
246–252. *See also* Taylor, David
Sense of coherence (SOC), 3, 15,
31–34, 59, 70, 77, 81, 150,
152, 160, 162
components of, 32
definition of, 31
development of, 49–57
cultural context, 50–51
intervention programs, 40
recommendations for programs, 42.
See also Taylor, David
strengthening, 44, 224–225
successful coping, relationship to,
33–34

Situational environment, 15, 17, 59–66
change agent characteristics, 60–61
client characteristics, 59–60
definition of, 59
institutions, 96–97
assessment of, 85–87
interaction characteristics, 64
nurse–patient interaction to resolve
Main Concern, 64–65
setting characteristics, 62–63
Situational Sense of Coherence (SSOC),
3, 10, 16, 17, 31–47, 59, 81,
96–97, 143, 150, 209,
224–225, 248–249, 283–284.
See also Sense of
coherence (SOC)
construct, description of, 35
evaluation of
rescoring of, 34
scoring of, 34
family, 70
in chronic health conditions, 36–39, 37t
theory of recovery, 36, 36f, 77–79, 78f
development of, 39–40
SOC. *See* Sense of Coherence
Social interactions, inequality in, 60–61
Social order, and negotiated order, 63
Social self, 53
Social value, of client
and interaction, 60
Spiritual subsystem
of community, 107f
of family, 70, 70t
of institutions, 85, 94
of person, 13, 52–53
assessment of, 54t
of nation, 107f
of state, 107f
SSOC. *See* Situational Sense of
Coherence
State as client. *See* Community as client
Stein, L. L., 86
Strauss, Anselm, 59, 62

Stress, management of, 15–16
Stressors
    identification of, 96
    interaction in family, 69–70
    management, and SOC, 33
    organization, 86–88
Stress theory, family, 76–79
Structural context, institutional, 62
Stallwood, J., 8, 9, 13
Stoll, R., 8, 9, 13
Subsystems, 8, 8*f*, 9*f*, 13, 14, 51–54, 69–70, 70*t*, 74, 78–79, 83–85, 94, 143, 151, 154*t*, 155, 201, 209, 211, 275, 281
    biological, 8, 13, 52–53, 54*t*, 69–70, 70*t*, 83, 94, 154*t*, 211
    psychosocial, 8, 13, 53, 54*t*, 70, 70*t*, 83–85, 94, 99, 107*f*, 154*t*, 211
    spiritual, 8, 13, 53–54, 54*t*, 70, 70*t*, 85, 94, 107*t*, 154*t*, 211
Symbolic interaction theory, 14, 60, 64
Systems theory, 14, 31

Tanner, C., 135, 141
Task-oriented leadership, 84
T-Double ABC-X model of adaptation, 77
Taylor, David, 34, 35, 40, 41, 42–43, 44, 45, 46, 220–234, 246–252
    Recommendations for a Salutogenic Program, 42–46, 220–234, 246–252

Teaching-learning environment, 214
    individual learning styles, 214–215
Tension
    in families, 76
    management of, 33
Theory of recovery, SSOC, 36, 36*f*, 77–79, 78*f*
    development of, 39–40
Therapist-Family Intersystem Model, 5*t*, 6
Trieschmann, R. B., 40, 42, 43, 44
Treatment, 45, 46
    pathogenic model of, 40
    salutogenic model of, 41
    ongoing feedback of, 250

Values. *See* Intrasystem Functions

Walker, L. O., 257
Watson, J., 136, 137
Watts, D. T., 86
White, J., 74
Workers, empowerment of, 83
Workplace, 63
Worksheet for in-service education, use of AIM, 91–92*t*
Worldview, 14, 49, 55, 56, 93
Wrubel, J., 64, 167, 182, 183

Young adulthood, and SOC development, 50

www.ingramcontent.com/pod-product-compliance
Ingram Content Group UK Ltd.
Pitfield, Milton Keynes, MK11 3LW, UK
UKHW021833140426
5217IPUK00021B/1417